The
Hands-on Guide
to the Foundation
Programme

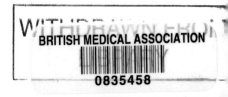

The Hands-on Guide to the Foundation Programme

Fifth Edition

ANNA DONALD
BA (Sydney), BM, BCh (Oxon), MPP (Harvard)
Late of Bazian Ltd, London, UK

MICHAEL STEIN
MB ChB, BSc (Hons) (UCT), DPhil (Oxon)
Chief Medical Officer, Map of Medicine, London, UK
and Medical Advisor, Hearst Business Media
Hearst Corporation, New York, NY, USA

CIARAN SCOTT HILL
BSc (Hons), MSc (Clin. Neuro.), MBBS, MCSP, MRCS, MRCP, DMCC, DOHNS
Neurosurgery Registrar, The Royal London Hospital
Honorary Senior Lecturer, in Neuroscience, University College London,
and Prehospital Care Physician, London Air Ambulance, London, UK

SELINA J CHAVDA
MBBS, BSc (Hons), MRCP
NIHR Academic Clinical Fellow in Haemato-Oncology
The Royal Marsden NHS Foundation Trust and the Institute of Cancer
Research, London, UK

WILEY Blackwell

Library of Congress Cataloging-in-Publication Data

Donald, Anna, author.
  The hands-on guide to the Foundation Programme / Anna Donald, Michael Stein, Ciaran Scott Hill,
Selina Chavda. – Fifth edition.
    1 online resource.

    Preceded by The hands-on guide for junior doctors / Anna Donald, Michael Stein, Ciaran Scott Hill. 4th ed. 2011.
  Includes bibliographical references and index.
    Description based on print version record and CIP data provided by publisher; resource not viewed.
    ISBN 978-1-118-76744-3 (Adobe PDF) – ISBN 978-1-118-76745-0 (ePub) – ISBN 978-1-118-76746-7 (pbk.)
I. Stein, Michael, 1963 May 25– , author. II. Hill, Ciaran, author. III. Chavda, Selina, author. IV. Title.
    [DNLM: 1. Foundation Programme (Great Britain. National Health Service) 2. Medical Staff,
Hospital–organization & administration–Great Britain–Handbooks. 3. Clinical Competence–Great
Britain–Handbooks. 4. Internship and Residency–organization & administration–Great Britain–Handbooks.
5. Medicine–Great Britain–Handbooks. WX 203]
    RA972
    616–dc23
                                                2014028668

A catalogue record for this book is available from the British Library.

Wiley also publishes its books in a variety of electronic formats. Some content that appears in print may not be available in electronic books.

Cover image: Hand MRI © kemie /iStockphoto; Heartbeat © Rinelle /iStockphoto; Pills and capsules © FotografiaBasica / iStockphoto; ECG © enot-poloskun /iStockphoto; Filled vials and syringe © Liuhsihsiang /iStockphoto

Set in 7.5/9pt Gill Sans by SPi Publisher Services, Pondicherry, India
Printed in Great Britain by TJ International Ltd, Padstow, Cornwall

1   2014

Dedication

The wonderful Anna Donald died during the preparation of the fourth edition of *Hands-on Guide for Junior Doctors*. For those who never had the privilege of meeting Anna, here is a little bit about an extraordinary friend and colleague (also see her obituary in the *BMJ* – 4 February 2009 – by Richard Smith and Sir Muir Gray).

Anna had a brilliant and inquisitive mind, receiving degrees from not one but three top-flight universities:

■ University of Sydney: Bachelor of Arts, majoring in history and preclinical medicine
■ University of Oxford: Bachelor of Medicine and Surgery degree (Rhodes Scholar)
■ Harvard University: Master's degree in Public Policy

Anna worked as a doctor and lecturer in epidemiology and public policy at University College London and was founding editor of the British Medical Journal's *Clinical Evidence*, the journal of evidence-based health care and evidence-based health policy. Anna's professional passion was the delivery of high-quality health care for everyone. Indeed, in 1998, as a pioneer in evidence-based health care, Anna founded Bazian, one of the first companies in the world to provide specialist evidence-based consulting and analysis to support the delivery of health care.

In 2007, Anna learned that her breast cancer, first diagnosed in 2003, had metastasized. Anna remained incredibly positive and said this: 'When you discover you have metastatic cancer you think you've picked a black ball in the lottery. But I've discovered it's a luminescent ball. I'm becoming the person I want to be. I'm not putting it off until I retire'.

Anna died 2 years later on 1 February 2009 having become the person she wanted to be. And she was always a person that everyone who met her, loved.

For more about Anna Donald, see her entry in Wikipedia.

Contents

13   Practical procedures   163

14   Radiology   191

15   Approach to the surgical patient   198

Introduction

I expect to pass through this world but once. Any good, therefore, that I can do or any kindness I can show, let me do it now. Let me not defer or neglect it for I shall not pass this way again.

Etienne de Grellet (1773–1855)

Your first years as a doctor are guaranteed to contain some of the most memorable experiences of your life. Free at last from rote learning and endless exams, your first job is intensely practical. The trouble is that the theoretical training in medical school does not usually prepare you for the physical and emotional rigours of hundreds of tasks being thrust upon you around the clock. Similarly, medical textbooks rarely deal with the practical know-how which makes all the difference between clumsy and elegant doctoring.

This book is based on the collective experience of junior doctors who remember only too well the highs and lows of their first few years. It contains information not readily available in standard texts that will help you to feel competent and confident despite sleepless nights and low blood sugars. It assumes minimal practical know-how.

Whatever you do, keep your head up and keep smiling. Hospitals are funny places. Lots of people love their first job; we hope you are one of them. Take care and good luck!

Anna Donald
Michael Stein
Ciaran Scott Hill
Selina J Chavda

How to use this book

This book is designed as a user-friendly manual. We recommend skimming through it when you first buy it and then referring to relevant sections for particular problems that you come across.

This book provides standard algorithms for diagnosis and management of clinical problems that worked for us and our colleagues, in different settings throughout Britain. Please don't follow our instructions slavishly. We realize that every firm has its own way of doing things and that there may be more appropriate algorithms for specialist wards or unusual situations. Like a recipe book, feel free to scrawl in the margins to make it more usable for you. We have included some blank pages at the back for extra notes.

We want to emphasize that this book is not the *Oxford Textbook of Medicine*, so please don't expect to find the 337 causes of tropical swollen legs here!

To keep the book compact and maximally relevant to what you need, we have not attempted to replicate the *British National Formulary* (BNF). Whilst we do suggest drugs where relevant, we realized from our own experience that the safest and most efficient way to prescribe drugs is to use the *BNF* in conjunction with your hospital's drug formulary.

Finally, if you discover a better way of doing something, please let us know. If we can use your suggestion, you will be acknowledged in the next edition of the book.

Acknowledgements

This book is dedicated to Uncle Ivan Harris and to Bruce, Janet and Tom Donald for the support and love that made writing this book possible.

Fifty per cent of the authors' royalties for this book are donated to the University of Cape Town Medical School.

Abbreviations

We include a long list of abbreviations to aid reading medical notes and for reference throughout this book.

μg	micrograms
A&E	accident and emergency
ABC	airway, breathing, circulation
ABG	arterial blood gases
ac	*ante cibum* (before food)
ACE	angiotensin-converting enzyme
ACTH	adrenocorticotrophic hormone
AED	automated external defibrillator
AF	atrial fibrillation
AFB	acid-fast bacillus
AIDS	acquired immunodeficiency syndrome
ALS	Advanced Life Support
ANA	antinuclear antigen
APTT	activated partial thromboplastin time
ARCP	Annual Review of Competence Progression
AS	aortic stenosis
AV	atrioventricular
AVCs	additional voluntary contributions
AXR	abdominal X-ray (plain)
BBB	bundle branch block
bd	*bis die* (twice per day)
bHCG	beta-human chorionic gonadotrophin
BMA	British Medical Association
BMJ	*British Medical Journal*
BNF	*British National Formulary*
BP	blood pressure
bpm	beats/minute
Ca	carcinoma
Ca	calcium
CCF	congestive cardiac failure
CK	creatinine kinase
CNS	central nervous system
COPD	Chronic Obstructive Pulmonary Disease
CPR	cardiopulmonary resuscitation
CRP	C-reactive protein
CSF	cerebrospinal fluid
CT	computed tomography
CV	curriculum vitae
CVA	cerebrovascular accident
CVP	central venous pressure
CVS	cardiovascular system
CXR	chest X-ray
DC	direct current
DIC	disseminated intravascular coagulation
DKA	diabetic ketoacidosis
dl	decilitre(s)
DM	diabetes mellitus
DOB	date of birth
DVT	deep venous thrombosis
ECG	electrocardiogram
ECHO	echocardiography
EM	electron microscope
ENT	ear, nose and throat
EPC	early pregnancy clinic
ESR	erythrocyte sedimentation rate
FBC	full blood count
FDP	fibrin degradation product
FEV_1	forced expiratory volume in first second
FFP	fresh frozen plasma
FOB	faecal occult blood
FVC	forced vital capacity
FY1	Foundation Year 1
FY2	Foundation Year 2
g	gram(s)
G&S	group and save
G6PD	glucose-6-phosphate dehydrogenase
GCS	Glasgow Coma Scale
GGT	gamma-glutamyl transferase
GI (GIT)	gastrointestinal
GMC	General Medical Council
GP	general practitioner
GTN	glyceryl trinitrate
GUM	Genitourinary Medicine
HB	heart block
Hb	haemoglobin
Hep	hepatitis

HepSal	heparinized saline	MST	morphine sulphate tablets
HHS	hyperosmolar hyperglycaemic state	MSU	midstream urine
		N&V	nausea and vomiting
HIV	human immunodeficiency virus	Na	sodium
HOCM	hypertrophic obstructive cardiomyopathy	NB	*nota bene* (note well)
		NBM	nil by mouth
IBD	inflammatory bowel disease	*NEJM*	*New England Journal of Medicine*
IBS	irritable bowel syndrome		
ICP	intracranial pressure	NGT	nasogastric tube
ID	identification	*nocte*	in the evening
Ig	immunoglobulin	NR	normal range
IHD	ischaemic heart disease	NSAIDs	non-steroidal anti-inflammatory drugs
IM	intramuscular		
INR	international normalized ratio (prothrombin ratio)	obs	observations
		OCP	oral contraceptive pill
ITU	intensive therapy unit	OD	overdose
iu (IU)	international unit	od	once a day
IV	intravenous	$PaCO_2$	partial pressure of CO_2 in arterial blood
IVU	intravenous urography		
JVP	jugular venous pressure	Pap	Papanicolaou
K^+	potassium	PaO_2	partial pressure of O_2 in arterial blood
KCl	potassium chloride		
kg	kilograms	PAYE	pay as you earn
kPa	kilopascals	PCR	polymerase chain reaction
L	left	PE	pulmonary embolism
l	litres	PEFR	peak expiratory flow rate
LBBB	left bundle branch block	PID	pelvic inflammatory disease
LDH	lactate dehydrogenase	PM	*post mortem*
LFT	liver function test	PMH	past medical history
LMP	last menstrual period	PO	*per orum* (by mouth)
LMWH	low molecular weight heparin	PPD	purified protein derivative
LP	lumbar puncture	PR	*per rectum*
LV	left ventricle	PRN	*pro re nata* (as required)
LVF	left ventricular failure	PSA	prostate specific antigen
LVH	left ventricular hypertrophy	PTH	parathyroid hormone
mane	in the morning	PV	*per vaginum*
MC&S	microscopy, culture and sensitivity	qds	*quarte in die somemdum* (to be taken four times a day)
MCV	mean cell volume		
MDU	Medical Defence Union	R	right
Mg	magnesium	RBBB	right bundle branch block
mg	milligrams	RIF	right iliac fossa
MI	myocardial infarction	RV	right ventricle
ml	millilitres	RVH	right ventricular hypertrophy
mmHg	millimetres of mercury		
MPS	Medical Protection Society	SAH	subarachnoid haemorrhage
MRI	magnetic resonance imaging	SBE	subacute bacterial endocarditis
MRSA	methicillin-resistant *Staphylococcus aureus*		
		SC (sub cut)	subcutaneous
MS	multiple sclerosis	SHO	Senior House Officer

SIADH	syndrome of inappropriate ADH secretion	TOP	termination of pregnancy
SJTs	situational judgement tests	TPN	total parenteral nutrition
SL	sublingual	TSH	thyroid stimulating hormone
SLE	systemic lupus erythematosus	TTA	to take away
SOB	shortness of breath	TTO	to take out
SpR	specialist registrar	TU	tuberculin units
SSRV	structured small round virus	u (U)	units
stat	*statim* (immediately)	U&E	urea and electrolytes
STD/STI	sexually transmitted disease/infection	US	ultrasound
		UTI	urinary tract infection
SVCO	superior vena cava obstruction	VDRL	venereal diseases research laboratory
SVT	supraventricular tachycardia		
T	temperature	VF	ventricular fibrillation
$T_{1/2}$	biological half life	VMA (also	
T3	triiodothyronine	HMMA)	vanillyl-mandelic acid
T4	thyroxine (tetraiodothyronine)	VQ scan	ventilation perfusion scan
TB	tuberculosis	VT	ventricular tachycardia
tds	*ter die somemdum* (to be taken three times a day)	WBC	white blood cell
		WCC	white cell count
TFTs	thyroid function tests	WPW	Wolff–Parkinson–White syndrome
TIA	transient ischaemic attack		
tid	*ter in die* (three times a day)	ZN	Ziehl–Nielsen stain

Chapter 1
STARTING UP

The first day of a junior doctor's working life is often filled with fear and trepidation. However, there really is no reason to be scared. Day 1 is usually filled with induction, meetings with your seniors and supervisors and tours of the hospital. Before you know it, the dreaded first day is over. Day 2 begins and then you are on the wards finally as a real doctor. That is when the real excitement begins.

Panic?

Never panic. One of the main things that terrifies junior doctors is that they will be expected to act beyond their level of competency and to run a cardiac arrest on their own when they don't even know where the patient is, let alone where the arrest trolley is.

At the start, the wards and the hospital can be unfamiliar, daunting places. The whole situation is enough to cause excessive sweating and palpitations, something that regularly occurs to junior doctors.

The most important thing to remember is that you are never alone. There is always someone that will be able to help you. Your seniors will not expect you to know much on your first day and will help you develop during your time with them. Everyone will show you what to do, and soon it will become second nature to you.

People to help you

You are surrounded by people who can help you. All you need to do is to ask them. They include:

1 Nurses who often know a great deal about what needs to be done for each patient. Many are very experienced and have been doing their jobs for years. Their advice can often be invaluable. They often also know individual patients very well. They generally have fewer patients on their lists than the doctors and may have spent considerable time with both the individual patient and their relatives. Every time they take a patient's observations or administer drugs they are exposed to the subtle signs of disease. This gives them a great 'intuition' for when patients are developing a problem. If you are unsure about the current issues or plan with a patient then their nurse will hopefully be able to help.

2 Patients who want to be treated kindly and properly and with as little pain as possible. Developing an open and honest approach with patients will make your life infinitely easier. If there is an issue you do not know the answer to or cannot fix immediately it is usually best to acknowledge this. A partnership with patients empowers them and also reduces the stress that comes from pretending to be an omniscient doctor.

3 Other doctors who love to demonstrate their skill at just about everything. Most people are secretly happy to be asked by a junior doctor for help; it makes them feel useful and gives them a chance to shine. If you ask for help you will almost certainly get it. There is no shame in it, and you will be helping others by developing a culture of honesty and cooperation. If you are unfortunate enough to

The Hands-on Guide to the Foundation Programme, Fifth Edition. Anna Donald, Michael Stein,
Ciaran Scott Hill and Selina J Chavda.
© 2015 John Wiley & Sons, Ltd. Published 2015 by John Wiley & Sons, Ltd.

initially meet with some degree of apparent resistance or negativity do not take it personally. Some doctors (usually the busy ones) won't always be overjoyed by having another thing added to their list; however, this does not mean that you should not have asked or that they are critical of you. Try not to take any emotional outbursts personally.

4 Other members of the multidisciplinary team. These allied healthcare professionals can be really helpful in providing you with useful information about your patient.

- Problems arise when junior doctors do NOT ask for help. This can be a disaster. If you feel panic rising in your throat, *please* just ask for help. This is counter-intuitive for self-reliant medics, but it saves lives (yours and the patient's).
- Make sure you attend orientation day for junior doctors if the hospital has one. It is useful for finding out what the hospital can do for you. They can be painful and bureaucratic but are often sources of important information. Most hospitals now have a mandatory shadowing week when you start your FY1. Use this to your advantage to get acquainted with the hospital.
- If possible contact your predecessors before their last day on the job. They can give you invaluable information about what to expect (the idea for this book originally came from a request for help from a new junior doctor). In particular, ask them for any nuggets of information, for example, what your new consultants do and do not like, how to access the computer systems, if there are any specific specialist investigations you may be required to request and how to do so.
- Most people find that they are physically exhausted during their first week of work. Such fatigue passes as you get used to the hospital and new routines. Plan to be kind to yourself during this time and try to avoid planning too many late nights. Hospital life is always much easier when you are well rested.

Three basic tips

1 Take the initiative in hospitals. If things are not working, do something about it. If there is a problem, try to think of a solution for it, and contact the person in charge. You may need more firepower, and this can come from your senior sister on the ward, your consultant or even the general ward managers. Junior doctors can achieve amazing changes when they make the effort to do so.

2 Similarly, take initiative in managing patients. Try to know why each patient came to hospital and what their current problem is. This may sound insultingly basic but it is not unusual to see a patient on a ward round when no one has this information to hand. Again, nurses are usually quite good at knowing what a patient's current problems are. Present seniors with a plan for your patients rather than just asking them what to do. You will learn how to manage problems much more quickly if you think about them yourself first. Don't be afraid to look beyond what is asked of you. If you feel that a patient has a problem that your team is not interested in then don't just ignore it, take the initiative. The fact that a senior doctor has not addressed a problem does not necessarily mean that it is okay to ignore it. Thinking strategically actually makes work more fun and prepares you for more responsibility.

3 Prioritize your work. When tasks are being fired at you from all directions, priority setting is really important. Try to learn early on which things are very urgent and which can wait. Despite the hype, in between moments of chaos, there is quite a lot of downtime in your junior doctor year (unless you are very unlucky or disorganized!). Keeping a list of written jobs is essential, especially when you are really busy. If it's not written down clearly, you will at some point forget it no matter how important you know it is.

Other useful start-up information

Dress

It is worth bearing in mind that patients often dress up to the nines to 'visit the doctor'. I once watched an elderly woman with deteriorating eyesight, high-heeled shoes and lop-sided make-up hobble over the hospital lawn to visit the diabetes clinic. Having always dressed casually, I dressed my best from then on.

■ Changing from student to doctor mode can put grave dents into your early pay cheques. If nothing else, buy good-quality shoes which will look good and will stay comfortable after a hard day on the wards.

You may get stained with all sorts of unmentionable substances as a junior doctor. Stain removers from supermarkets and household stores can fix most things. Soaking garments in cold water and lots of soap followed by a normal machine wash removes blood stains.

■ Whilst wearing theatre scrubs ('blues') on the wards can be all the rage, doing so is a theoretical infection risk and frowned on by some hospitals. If you have to wear them outside theatre, remember to change regularly and return them to the hospital laundry to be washed! Wearing them outside hospital grounds is definitely not acceptable.

A general rule of thumb is to dress modestly and smartly. Avoid flashy jewellery as this poses an infection risk, and open toe shoes should be avoided. High heels can be cumbersome and in some specialities rather inappropriate, for example, intensive care unit (ICU).

Equipment

Always carry the following things:

1 Pen (more than one). Black is the only acceptable colour unless you are a pharmacist.

2 Notebook/personal digital assistant/piece of paper.

3 Stethoscope.

4 Pen torch to assess pupillary reflexes and for looking in mouths.

5 Pager/bleep.

6 Cash for food/drink/newspaper.

7 Ophthalmoscope (if not readily accessible on wards).

8 You should also have access to a neurology kit (tendon hammer, orange sticks, neuropins, tuning fork and Snellen's eye chart; remember that neurotips and orange sticks should be disposed of in a sharps bin after use on a patient and should never be reused).

9 Contact details of your seniors and colleagues:

● You may wish to carry everything in a traveller's pouch or a small shoulder bag.

● Things often get misplaced so you should label anything you cannot afford to lose with your name, either by engraving or hospital wrist bands.

● Junior doctors definitely need access to ophthalmoscopes. Ward ophthalmoscopes have an amazing tendency to walk and to run out of batteries. Therefore, buy your own portable ophthalmoscope, and examine people's eyes at every opportunity. They are expensive but definitely worth every penny. It is a great skill to have but takes time to acquire. Pocket veterinary ophthalmoscopes are sometimes the most portable, cheap and reliable, and little known to medics – as they are advertised for vets.

● Ask your ward pharmacist for a couple of aliquots of tropicamide (0.5%) to carry in your top pocket. One to two drops greatly facilitate ophthalmic examination. It takes a few minutes to work. Warn the patient that they may have blurred vision and sensitivity to light for a few hours; record the procedure in the notes and tell the nurse. Having failed to do the latter, you are liable to be fast bleeped by a nurse who thinks the patient is coning. It is sensible to dilate both eyes, not only to avoid mistaken neurology but also to allow you to view and compare the fundi. Never use tropicamide in patients with a history of glaucoma, eye surgery or who need neurological monitoring. You should also avoid alternatives like cyclopentolate as these can take weeks for the eye to return to normal.

● Consider carrying a ring binder or folder (see Chapter 2) containing important team info, a handful of blood forms, radiology requests, blank drug charts and history, discharge summary and to take out (TTO) sheets (if your hospital still uses them). Such a binder allows you to do a lot of the paperwork on ward rounds, before it gets forgotten.

First-day paperwork

The first day is mainly paperwork. Each trust may have slightly different requirements and will send you documentation before you start of exactly what you will need to bring.

Try to fill out as much of the documentation as possible prior to your meeting with payroll and HR. Making copies in advance will save you long queues at the photocopier.

Here is a checklist of essential documents to bring:

■ GMC registration certificate
■ Passport and/or driver's licence with its counterpart
■ Medical indemnity certificate (e.g. Medical Defence Union or Medical Protection Society)
■ Bank details – last bank statement:

- Utility bill
- CRB certificate

■ Induction pack and contract from the trust
■ Occupational health report (and data card if you have one with a list of your immunizations and blood results)

Geography

■ Get a map of the hospital from reception to help you learn where everything is.
■ Specifically, find out the location of blood gas machines, canteen, casualty, ITU, wards that you are working on, radiology department, doctors' mess, drink machines, endoscopy, labs for crucial bloods, nuclear medicine and on-call rooms if available.

Ward rounds

Think of yourself as the ward round producer (much of it *is* performance). Give yourself at least 20 minutes' preparation time to have everything ready. For each patient, be prepared to supply at the drop of a hat the following details:

1 Patient ID (name, age, date of admission, occupation, presenting complaint)

2 Changes in condition and management since last round (with dates of change)

3 Results (any investigations carried out recently from blood tests to imaging reports)

4 Assessment (physical, social, psychological)

5 Plan for inpatient management (future investigations, ops, drugs, reviews by specialist teams)

6 Plan for discharge (see Discharging patients)

It is helpful to print off a list of patients to give to consultants and the senior registrar, which includes the preceding points. Before the ward round, check with the ward clerk, nurse in charge or online system that no patients have moved overnight.

Encounters with patients on the ward round

■ Unless the patient asks for relatives to remain present, it is generally a good idea to ask them to leave the room whilst the team examines the patient. People will often give more information if their relatives are absent.
■ Ask your registrar which investigations to have available. If your hospital uses an electronic reporting system such as PACS (picture archiving and communications system) then you may wish to access the important scans before the ward round so that your seniors can look at them without too much disruption. Alternatively, print out the reports and have them to hand.
■ Each consultant will have their own pet details that he or she wants to know about each patient. Find out what these are from your predecessor and supply them tirelessly at ward rounds. These could range from occupation to ESR to whether or not the patient has ever travelled to the tropics.
■ Never say that you have done something you haven't, and never make up a result to please anyone. It is bound to backfire. If you realize you have given a piece of information that is wrong, admit it sooner rather than later. It is much better to admit ignorance than to make up something incorrect that could affect patient safety.
■ Do not argue with colleagues (or anyone else) in front of patients – it is unprofessional.
■ Get a clear idea of the management plan for each patient. Make definite 'action points' and if your consultant cannot be pressed into being clear, then ask your registrar. This is

particularly important when making decisions regarding ceilings of care.

■ If you work with a partner, such as a fellow junior doctor, make sure that jobs arising from the round are clearly allocated. Meet up later for a 'paper round' to check important results, prioritize jobs and make sure that everyone is clear about what remains outstanding.

● As the junior doctor, you are expected to know everything about the patient, both medically and socially. Developing a rapport with other members of the multidisciplinary team is therefore vital.

Social rounds

You need to let the social team know how your patient is going to cope (or not) on discharge:

1 Ask yourself: how is this patient going to manage physically, socially and mentally? Specifically, draw up a list of 'activities of daily living'. Find out if there are any activities that the patient is having difficulty with especially in elderly patients. These are essential to ensure a patient is discharged safely and to assess if they may need more care in the community.

2 Have relevant patient details ready (see the succeeding points). Most are available from the medical notes and the front-page admissions sheet. Otherwise, try the nurses, nursing notes, patient, relatives and general practitioner (GP).

3 If you are required to give a history, try to include the following points:

● Patient ID
● Prognosis: short and long term
● GP and admitting rights to local hospitals (usually in the admission sheet at the front of the notes and dependent on home address)
● Type of residence and limitations (e.g. stairs)
● Home support and previous reliance on social services such as packages of care, telecare and pendant alarms
● Financial status
● Issues regarding capacity if there are any
● Special problems which need to be addressed (physical, social, mental, legal)

4 Go to the meeting with specific questions you want to be answered. Make sure you come away with 'action points' – not just vague gestures from various team members about your patient's care (this goes for all ward rounds).

5 Translate medical jargon into normal English for social rounds, as some members of the social team may not be fully fluent in medical acronyms.

6 Familiarize yourself with key people from local rehabilitation services, residential homes, nursing homes and alcohol support services. Effective liaison can prevent or at least curtail hospital admission.

Night rounds

As a junior doctor your experience of night shifts may be limited. However, it is important to do a quick night round before you leave for home. If you are covering overnight this can mean the difference between a relatively happy night and a sleepless nightmare. Even if you are not on overnight you still have a responsibility to leave your patients well tended to for the evening shift. This will reduce the stress of the night cover (which will one day be you) and protect your patients from being neglected whilst you are away. If you do nothing else, make sure you have checked off the following before going to bed:

1 Analgesia

2 Fluids

3 Infusions

4 Sedation if needed

5 Ask each team nurse on the night shift if he or she has problems that need sorting out before the morning:

● If possible start your night round *after* the night nurses' start of shift and drug rounds have been completed. This is when they identify problems that you need to deal with before going to bed.

● If you are the covering doctor then tell night staff to bleep you if they are concerned about a patient. Paradoxically, this combined with reassurance and information about worrisome patients cuts down bleeps.

• Inform every team nurse of what to do if a sick patient's condition changes. Sometimes you can set limits for relevant signs (e.g. pulse, CVP, T, BP) beyond which you want a doctor to be called. Write these in the notes. Many hospitals have 'early warning systems' that do this job for you and tell nurses when they should contact a doctor or nurse specialist.

• If bleeped for an apparently trivial matter overnight, try your best not to sound irritated. Be ready to go to the ward, even if only to provide reassurance. Again, paradoxically, this reduces bleeps. If nurses are confident that you will turn up if requested, they will not bleep you ahead of time. If you do have a problem with a large number of bleeps that seem inappropriate or unnecessary it is best to speak to the nurse in charge rather than getting upset or angry.

• Fewer and fewer hospitals provide on-call rooms for junior doctors. If there is one and if it is a long way from the wards, there may be somewhere that you can sleep on the ward. Ask the sister or charge nurse. Be very careful though as some trusts have taken disciplinary action against doctors sleeping in side rooms at night.

Discharging patients

Clearing hospital beds is an invaluable skill that will earn you lots of brownie points from virtually everyone. To clear beds effectively:

1 Make plans for people's discharge on the day they arrive. Ask yourself the following points:

• When will they be likely to leave?
• What will get in the way of this person going home or being transferred?
• What can be followed up in clinic?

2 If possible, write discharge summaries at least 24 hours in advance (Chapter 3, Discharge summaries (TTO/to take away [TTA])) and send the TTO (drug prescriptions) to the pharmacists early in the day to avoid delays.

Work environment

Evidence suggests that upgrading your environment upgrades your work – and you. There are ways you can make your particular corner of the hospital a great place to work, even if the rest of the hospital has miles of yellow peeling paint and dripping pipes:

■ Consider buying a music player. Label it clearly and lock it away. It can do wonders for long winter weekends and nights on call.

■ Put postcards/pictures/photos up in your work area provided it is not accessible by patients. If you don't have a bulletin board, order one from hospital supplies. Some managers frown at this, but if it is in an area to which patients do not have access, like the doctor's room, then it should be fine.

■ Most hospitals provide a computer in the doctor's room. Make sure you get as much Internet access as local policy allows. Carry an encrypted trust approved portable USB hard drive. It will allow you to carry your work with you. Ensure that you maintain patient confidentiality at all times by anonymizing patient information. A password is not enough, and the drive must be encrypted.

■ Bring decent coffee, tea or cocoa supplies to work. A single-cup cafetière, some packs of coffee at the back of the ward fridge and a jar of your favourite spread can upgrade your existence no end. The expense of this can be shared with your colleagues.

Bibliography

Most junior doctors read little other than fiction during their job. You probably don't need to buy anything you don't already have. A few recommended texts and online resources are as follows:

■ *Pocket Prescriber:* Nicholson T., Gunarathne A., Singer D. (2013) Hodder Arnold, London. A brilliant and truly portable little text, useful for checking those common drugs on a ward round.

■ *Acute Medicine:* Sprigings D., Chambers J. (2007) Wiley Blackwell, Oxford. A comprehensive guide to emergencies.

■ *Pocket Examiner*: Hill C.S. (2009) Wiley Blackwell, London. A pocket-text of clinical examinations.

■ *Oxford Handbook of Clinical Medicine*: Hope R.A. (Editor), Longmore J.M., Wilkinson I., Davidson E., Foulkes A., Mafi A. (2010) Oxford University Press, Oxford. A great pocket reference text for medical conditions.

■ *Surgical Talk*: Goldberg A., Stansby G. (2011) Imperial College Press, London. Commonly asked topics for those awkward theatre moments.

■ *The ECG Made Easy* (and sequel, *The ECG in Practice*): Hampton J. (2013) Churchill Livingstone, Edinburgh. An approachable guide to the mysteries of the ECG.

■ *Clinical Medicine*: Kumar P., Clark M. (2012) Saunders, London. Love it or hate it, it probably answers most of the medical questions you could ever ask. The pocket version is an excellent reference guide and fits into most shoulder bags.

■ *Rapid Medicine*: Sam A.H. et al. (2010) and *Rapid Surgery*, Baker C. et al. (2010) Wiley Blackwell, Oxford. Both are memory joggers for core facts.

■ *Junior Doctors' Handbook*: Published annually by the BMA and free to members. An excellent summary of your rights and useful information for your early years as a doctor.

■ *Map of Medicine*: A set of 300 flow charts covering the community and specialist aspects of the 300 'top' conditions. An excellent and interactive quick reference. It is free to NHS professionals in England and Wales; you need an Athens password for the professional version (www.mapofmedicine.com). The read-only version is available through NHS Choices. Recommended texts for the medical specialties (SHO-level texts) include:

■ *Lecture Notes: Respiratory Medicine*: Bourke S., Burns G. (2011) Wiley Blackwell, Oxford. Beautiful explanations of the pathophysiology and principles of management of respiratory disease. A very good primer for a chest unit job.

■ *The Little Black Book of Neurology*: Zaidat O., Lerner A. (2008) Saunders, New York. A concise but very detailed guide to clinical neurology.

■ *Essential Haematology*: Hoffbrand A., Pettit J., Moss P. (updated every reprint; the most recent edition, 2011) Wiley Blackwell, Oxford. A superb book!

■ *Essential Endocrinology and Diabetes*: Holt R., Hanley N. (2012) Wiley Blackwell, Oxford. Another very useful primer for an endocrine job.

We haven't found any particularly good small books for rheumatology or nephrology, so we recommend using the appropriate chapter in any medical textbook such as Kumar and Clark. If you want a really detailed text, then the Oxford Handbooks for both rheumatology and nephrology and hypertension are excellent and small enough to take on the ward with you.

For fun and rapid insight into the world you are entering, try the classic *House of God* by Sham S. (1978).

Chapter 2
GETTING ORGANIZED
OR 'THE FOLDER'

Keeping track of patients and their details is extremely important as a doctor. This can quickly become an arduous task if you are not organized. Filling in forms after work is a waste of precious evenings and should be avoided at all costs if possible. Fortunately, you can greatly reduce the time you spend chasing paper, patients and results with the core weapon in a junior doctor's arsenal: a folder.

Personal folder and the lists

A well-organized ring binder or slot-in folder can save days of time. Unlike a Filofax or tablet/iPad, a folder doubles up as a clipboard, providing a decent writing surface at the bedside and an immediate supply of forms during ward rounds, so that you can do all the paperwork during rounds. As well as saving time, a folder means you are less likely to forget things because you can do many tasks as soon as they are requested. Although they look great and are very useful as a reference source, tablets and iPads unfortunately don't synchronize (yet) with hospital electronic medical record systems. There are also multiple issues with patient confidentiality that still exist with personal computer devices.

How to make a personal folder

You need one A4 ring-binder folder and multiple brightly coloured dividers. Sheets of pre-punched transparent plastic pockets for each section are also very useful. Fill the folder with all the different forms you use regularly during the day, stacking each type of form behind different dividers. Label the dividers. You can keep spare blank forms (e.g. blood forms) in the plastic pockets. Useful contents include spare continuation/history sheets, blood forms (biochemistry, haematology, microbiology/virology and group and save/cross match), radiology and nuclear medicine request cards, ECHO and cardiology request forms, endoscopy request forms, drug charts, discharge forms (if these are still paper in your hospital) and commonly used telephone numbers:

1 You can almost always find a hole puncher at the ward clerk's desk to use.

2 Consider keeping common drug regimens in the front of the folder for easy reference. These might include heparin dosing, insulin sliding scales, glyceryl trinitrate and morphine infusions and gentamicin dosing. Common antibiotic regimens and doses specific to your hospital are also really helpful.

3 Hospitals have their own days for doing specialty procedures (such as isotope scans and endoscopy). Colleagues and relevant departments will know when these are. Find out from your colleagues what you need to bring for team activities such as radiology conferences, academic events and mortality/morbidity meetings. Find out if there is a pro forma that you can use for these events, and if so make sure you have plenty of copies.

4 Phone numbers are essential. Making a list early saves a lot of time. You can shrink the list and stick it on the front of your ward folder

The Hands-on Guide to the Foundation Programme, Fifth Edition. Anna Donald, Michael Stein, Ciaran Scott Hill and Selina J Chavda.
© 2015 John Wiley & Sons, Ltd. Published 2015 by John Wiley & Sons, Ltd.

for easy reference. Another option is to include it in a small font on the bottom of your patient list so it is reprinted each day. Get out-of-hours contact numbers as well. It is important to have senior colleagues' bleeps, the critical care outreach team's numbers and medical/surgical registrar's numbers close to hand. From experience, it is easier to find names if the list is strictly alphabetical. Copy or modify Figure 2.1 if you like.

5 Your folder should also contain relevant patient information such as up-to-date blood test results or scan results.

In addition to the sundry paperwork in the preceding text, you will also need to generate three lists daily. Spreadsheets are usually better than word processors for organizing lists, as they have all kinds of sorting functions. The necessary lists are as follows:

1 The patient list (i.e. the master list), which should be updated at least daily

2 The job list

3 Results sheet

Many doctors combine the three but it can often be useful to have a paper copy of each,

Name	Extension	Name	Extension
Accident and emergency		Occupational therapy	
Anaesthetist on-call bleep		Outpatient clinics	
Bed manager		Pain team	
Biochemistry		Pharmacy – general	
Blood transfusion		Pharmacy – drug information	
Cardiology on-call bleep		Physiotherapy	
Coronary care unit		Porters	
Discharge coordinator		Psychiatry team	
Doctors' mess		Radiology – CT scanning	
Electrophysiology unit		Radiology – general	
Echocardiogram		Radiology – portable films	
Endoscopy		Radiology – MRI	
Ophthalmology clinic		Radiology – secretaries	
Food – local takeaway		Registrar bleeps (your dept.)	
Haematology		Rota coordinator	
Histology		Secretaries (your dept.)	
Intensive care unit		SHO bleeps (your dept.)	
IT department		Surrounding hosp. quick dial	
Matron		Stroke reg bleep	
Medical records		Theatre list coordinator	
Medical staffing		Thrombolysis nurse bleep	
Microbiology		Ward extensions	

Figure 2.1 Essential telephone numbers.

particularly if you are sharing out jobs with colleagues.

Keeping track of patients (List 1)

This is a hassle. People have devised many complex strategies for ensuring that they have up-to-date details for each patient. However you do it, you need information to hand so that you can answer questions on ward rounds; discuss patients over the phone with general practitioners, nurses and colleagues; write in the notes and do the discharge summary; and request and find results of investigations. The minimum information for this includes:

■ Patient name, hospital number and date of birth
■ Reason for admission and major details from PMH
■ Main problems now
■ Mainstay of management (e.g. drugs, surgery)
■ Recent results
■ Social history and their activities of daily living in brief

One way of keeping track of such information is to stick patient labels onto history sheets, leaving a space between each to fill in patient details. Put a line through patients who have been discharged. The labels contain patient IDs. A sheet like this can be made up as patients are admitted in casualty and stored at the front of a personal folder.

An alternative is to keep a summary sheet on each patient with the preceding details, and if any changes develop in the management, the sheet can be updated. This can be kept in your file or in the front of the medical notes.

List of things to do (List 2)

The simplest ways to keep track of many tasks are as follows:

1 Keep a daily list on the back of a card that you can update regularly.

2 Keep a small diary to note down requests for days and weeks ahead (this can be done electronically if you have access to a shared file):

● Write down all requests as soon as you receive them, on your list next to each patient. There is no job too big or important that it cannot be forgotten in the heat of a busy shift if you haven't written it down.

● It is useful to sit down after each ward round with your colleagues and run through each patient to make sure you know what is needed for each of them.

● Try subdividing tasks in terms of *where* they have to be done. This enables you to choreograph your movements around the hospital rather than endlessly dashing from one ward to another and going to the same place in the hospital repeatedly. For example:

X-ray	Give in forms from ward round
	Ask Dr A about Mr B's CT request barium enema for Mr C
Ward 6A	IV line for Mrs D
	Talk to Mr E for colonoscopy
Ward 7B	Vitamin K for Ms F
	Sign verbal for paracetamol

● Use a checkbox system so you know what things have been done. One system is to tick the box once the task is initiated (i.e. form handed in, referral made, blood test taken) and then convert it into a cross when the result of that is back (an alternative is to colour half a square then complete it).

Results sheet (List 3)

Most hospital systems are able to print off all results from blood or urine tests for the day for a particular consultant, department or ward. Print off one at the beginning of the day and carry it about for the occasion when your registrar asks about the patient's eosinophil count. If the computers fail (as they often will) or you work in a security conscious hospital you may not be able to do this, so just record the results (e.g. from phone calls, lab computers) onto blank labels and you can just peel them off to stick them into patient notes without having to laboriously copy them out. You may still need to record the important results into a table in the notes to chart progress. As a starting point, it is recommended to make sure that you note haemoglobin, mean cell volume, white count with predominant differential, creatinine, urea, sodium, potassium and C-reactive protein. Certain firms will require different results, for example, a liver job will obviously require liver function tests and clotting on most patients. Those patients on warfarin should always have international normalized ratio (prothrombin ratio) noted. Don't forget to check the date on which the blood was sent for each of the patients and check the trends. Writing results in notes is important for patients staying longer than a few days or who have stepped down from intensive care, but you don't need to do it for every single patient.

Data protection and confidentiality

Beware of leaving your folder or any list or USB memory stick lying about. Always carry it in your pocket or in a shoulder satchel. If needing to use your hands to examine a patient or to perform a procedure, make sure you put your folder/list where you won't forget it and where a casual bystander will not be able to just glance at it. Pick up any such lists that your seniors or colleagues are apt to leave about, and dispose of them accordingly. After you are done with the lists for the day it is good practice to dispose of them in a confidential waste bin. Some doctors like to keep their lists for a few days before disposing of them. NEVER take your lists home with you or out of the hospital. NEVER leave them in a public place, as this is considered a breach of patient confidentiality. You may wish to have your teams name and bleep number automatically noted on the top of all lists, so that you have ownership over each list. In a day and age where technology is rapidly advancing, it is important to make sure that whatever form of information technology you use (tablet, iPad, laptop, etc.) is not only password protected but encrypted and the trust you work at is happy for you to use that form of technology. This is particularly relevant for portable storage devices like USBs. So far, the cases of breached confidentially with hacked emails are infrequent, but with some email providers having quite liberal security policies, it is probably wisest to stick to using your trust email or ideally NHS mail for all patient-related correspondence. The importance of avoiding any posting related to patient information on social media does not, I hope, require highlighting. I would offer caution to any doctor using social media that there are many people out there who would like to see a young doctor publicly attacked/humiliated. It is somewhat like the 'Miranda rights', '*anything you say or do may be used against you*'.

Chapter 3
PAPERWORK AND ELECTRONIC MEDICAL RECORDS

Lots of junior doctors do not realize the importance of accurate note keeping, and at the time, it may seem irritating. However, if the worst were to happen and an adverse event occurred, accurate medical paperwork can make a huge difference if a lawsuit was brought against the hospital. As doctors communicate with many people through forms and notes, it is important that they contain clear, accurate information. The most important part of paperwork is writing clear, legible patient notes. One of the most important parts of using an EMR is accurately typing information. When you start at your new hospital, ask your predecessors to show you any short-cuts for EMRs or if there are any favourite lists they use for blood requests. Ask them to show you how to do these on your own version of EMR.

The following chapter mainly refers to paper records, but most of it is also applicable to EMRs.

Although most medical records are still written, particularly notes made on ward rounds and reviews, it is becoming increasingly common for hospitals to move towards 'paperless' systems. Some trusts now require all emergency admissions and clerking to be recorded on EMR.

As an aside, given the ubiquity of computers, it is worth making sure your typing skills are up to scratch. If you haven't already developed a fast typing style, it is worth spending a few evenings learning to touch type. This can dramatically improve your productivity and is a skill that will remain useful throughout your career. You can find good teaching programmes in most computer stores or online.

Patient notes

Doctors are expected to write in patients' notes at least once every 72 hours. However, it is good practice to write something daily and waiting 2 days to fill in notes is unlikely to endear you to the powers that be. More importantly, you may well forget what you have said to your patients on that particular day. It is much more sensible to write in the notes as you go along, or, if there are two of you, for someone to scribe whilst you are with the patient on your ward round:

1 Always sign notes with your signature and print your surname clearly with your level and bleep number. Some hospitals provide stamps for this purpose. If you make a mistake and cross anything out, also put your initials or sign your name by this as well.

2 It is useful to ask two things when writing patient notes:

- Do the notes give enough information to treat the patient when I'm not available?
- Will I be legally covered if these notes were ever before a court?

3 For daily notes, there are various standardized ways but the most popular is SOAP (see the succeeding text).

4 The most crucial aspect of any entry in the patient's notes is the plan. If you know when a scan or test is going to be done, it is helpful to document this in the notes, so the next person who sees them will have this information

The Hands-on Guide to the Foundation Programme, Fifth Edition. Anna Donald, Michael Stein, Ciaran Scott Hill and Selina J Chavda.
© 2015 John Wiley & Sons, Ltd. Published 2015 by John Wiley & Sons, Ltd.

available to them. With shift systems in place and plenty of handovers, it is often difficult for someone reading the notes to tell what is already in motion. For decisions that may have to be made in your absence, it is essential to document clearly a decision tree, for example, 'If systolic BP drops below 100 mmHg, stop GTN infusion'.

5 If you're not sure about how to document a patient's condition, flick back through previous notes and see how others approached it.

6 It is imperative to include the time and date in the margin of notes. Also, if you are documenting a ward round, you should always note the surname and designation of the person leading the round at the top of your entry.

SOAP

Subjective data (e.g. history and examination)

Objective data (e.g. blood results, imaging)

Assessment (e.g. active and inactive problems)

Plan for future

---

7 If you are called to see a patient, briefly document (even if the call was trivial):

- That you saw the patient
- The time and date
- Your plan of action (even if you just want to continue with the current treatment plan)

8 It is foolhardy to write anything in the notes that you would not want the patient or relatives to read; they have legal access to the notes. When writing in notes, it is best to remain objective at all times, and simply document discussions as they happen without putting an emotional slant on things. This is particularly helpful when documenting discussions with patients about 'do not attempt resuscitation' orders or advanced care planning. Often it can be helpful to put what patients or their relatives have said in quotation marks in the notes, if you feel this will benefit the documentation.

9 It is perfectly admissible to write 'no change' if nothing has happened to the patient but be careful that there hasn't been an important

change you have missed. Writing 'Patient well, continue' doesn't look good if they've actually been spiking temperatures or have deteriorating renal function! If you are worried that you don't know what changes to make, it is always better to ask your seniors earlier in the day rather than later. Some consultants or registrars do 'board rounds' or 'paper rounds' where they discuss patients verbally. Ask them what changes they want to make in each patient's plan at that time, so you can press on organizing the jobs in a timely manner.

10 Don't forget to document the social or psychological aspects (e.g. whether the patient is cheerful, sad or fed up).

Incident forms

When called to see a patient who has had an adverse incident (e.g. fell out of bed):

1 See the patient as soon as possible. Nurses are legally liable unless they make sure you see the patient. Never be short with a nurse who is making a reasonable request even if you are very busy. It is their job to call you with their concerns.

2 Ask the patient what happened. Get a history from the nurse or any witnesses. After a quick 'airway, breathing and circulation (ABC)' emergency assessment, check the following:

- Routine observations, after observation with: temp, BP, pulse, O_2 saturations and respiratory rate.
- Consciousness level and pupils to ensure they are reacting (see Appendix, Glasgow Coma Scale, GCS). It is always alarming to find unequal pupils, but before panicking take time to check the notes to see if it was pre-existing. Also take such findings in the broader context. If the patient is otherwise entirely well and has a GCS of 15 they will not be dying of an intracranial herniation regardless of their pupils.
- A brief neurological examination, including cranial nerves. Checking the patient's plantars is also a must.
- Skin for bruising, bleeding, cuts and fractures. If you think there may be a fracture but assessment is difficult due to patient age or

responsiveness it is generally better to err on the side of caution and get imaging.

● Bone tenderness and shape for fractures. Frail patients can sustain fractures with remarkably little fuss. Especially look for hip, wrist, humeral and scaphoid fractures. Examine the skull carefully if the patient hit their head for lacerations, haematomas or open wounds that may need gluing or suturing. Consult with your senior if there is sign of serious injury or drowsiness – the patient may well need a CT head scan (see Chapter 14, Skull X-rays; CT head – some emergency indications).

3 Sign an 'incident form' or 'Datix form' (the nurses will give you one). Filling it in is self-explanatory. In some hospitals, the nurses will do this online, in which case you don't need to worry unless there is particular information or concerns you want to pass on.

4 Also write in the patient's notes. Include the following:

● Your name and designation.

● Time and date.

● Brief history of accident, witnesses or nurses history of the incident.

● Examination findings. Often doctors document their assessment as an ABC approach in the notes. Make sure you document your examination findings clearly, so if the patient clinically deteriorates, this can be seen easily.

● A plan including a note that you must be contacted if the patient's vital signs deteriorate or there is concern.

● That the nurses have filled in an incident form.

5 Ask the nurses to continue doing neurological observations at regular intervals. This includes calculating the patient's GCS, usual observations, pupil reaction and limb movement. Specify how often you need them done. Try and be reasonable so as not to overburden the nurses with unreasonable requests. However, if you are worried and feel that a certain frequency is required then you must be firm about this. You are responsible for making sure the patient does not come to harm.

6 Think about how the incident occurred. Consider referral to other teams as necessary, for example, a hospital falls team. Depending on the history, the patient may need an electrocardiogram (ECG), lying and standing BP to exclude postural hypotension, echocardiography or a 24-hour tape to look for arrhythmias (see common calls).

7 Consider carrying a couple of incident forms in your personal folder or at least knowing where to find them. It can save time in the middle of the night.

Blood forms and requesting blood tests

■ Again, many of these forms are now electronic.

■ Ask the lab which details on blood cards are essential. Often there are spaces on the card for information that isn't needed.

■ Write your bleep and ward number clearly on blood cards so the labs can contact you if necessary.

■ Good times to fill in forms are during the ward round, when writing in patients' notes or when you are checking each patient's blood results. Having forms ready saves time.

■ Where possible, anticipate patients' blood needs and write forms in bulk. Conditions for which it is sometimes possible to fill in serial forms include those shown in Table 3.1.

■ Try having a separate plastic bag or paper clamp for each day of the week in the doctors' office. You can write serial forms at the start of the week. Many hospitals now have phlebotomy folders that can be used for this very purpose.

■ If you don't have a phlebotomist, don't despair. Taking bloods in the morning enables you to sort out patients' problems before the ward round. Make sure you take round a trolley like the phlebotomists do. This has remarkable effects on one's efficacy. Make sure you label each patient's bottles as you take the bloods. This avoids mix-ups and confusion between different patients. Having your blood forms written in advance also saves vast amounts of time.

Table 3.1 Conditions for which it may be possible to fill out serial forms.

Acute coronary syndromes	
On admission	
Days 1–3	Lipids (only worth doing within 12 hours of infarct, unreliable post-MI for 3 months)
	Serial troponins
	Serial ECGs
Warfarin initiation	Check the INR at least
	Every day for 1 week
	Every week for 3 weeks
	Every month for 3 months
	Every 8 weeks after that
Renal failure	
Daily	Urea, creatinine and electrolytes
TPN	
Daily	Creatinine and electrolytes
Monday, Wednesday, Friday	LFT, calcium, phosphate, alkaline phosphatase
Weekly	Magnesium, zinc, FBC, urea
IV fluids	Daily urea, creatinine and electrolytes
Post-op bloods	
Next day	Urea, creatinine, electrolytes and FBC

Discharge summaries (TTO/TTA)

The discharge summary or 'TTO'/'TTA' (to take out or away) is a sheet or electronic form that junior doctors write for patients to take to their general practitioner (GPs). It enables GPs to continue with outpatient care. The TTO is also the prescription form that the nurses use to order drugs for patients to take home with them. The vast majority of units now have electronic TTAs that incorporate the medications with space for a free-hand discharge letter, and so you may not have to do both. Paper TTOs are commonly still used on day surgery units or for those having elective day cases, where they are generally used for prescribing medication and summarizing the result of the procedure:

1 Get the GP's name and address from the patient, the front page of the notes or the EMR.

2 Complete the TTO before the patient leaves! Include the following:

- Patient details (name, DOB, hospital number)
- Name of consultant
- Diagnosis
- Important results (positive and negative) including blood test results, ECG changes or scan results
- Treatments given during admission
- If the patient saw any specialist teams during their inpatient stay
- Whether they were seen by the allied healthcare professionals, for example, dieticians, physiotherapists, occupational therapists, social workers, etc., and if any changes have been made to their social setup in the community
- Treatment on discharge
- Follow-up arrangements, for example, outpatient appointments with the consultant (dates and times are useful), or any follow-up procedures or scans

- What the patient has been told
- Your name and bleep number

3 Patients are often delayed in hospital because TTAs have not been written. Write them as soon as possible so that drugs can be fetched from the pharmacy and ideally 24 hours in advance. Patients will love you for this as it avoids them sitting around all day waiting for their medications to arrive from pharmacy. Nurses and the bed manager will love you as you have now freed up a bed for them that they desperately need. Some hospitals in fact now have a pre-11 a.m. discharge policy and require all discharge summaries to be written 24 hours prior to the patient leaving to ensure a smooth discharge process. Remember that this is work you are going to have to do anyway and not only is doing this in advance a marker of being a 'good' efficient doctor who is popular with seniors and nurses but it also means that there will be less patients on the ward for you to have to manage as they will be ready for discharge. It will similarly cut down the inevitable bleeps that will start coming from nurses as soon as the decision to discharge is made (when you will still be on the ward round and unable to help). However, DO NOT sign off TTAs until the day the patient is leaving. It goes without saying that prepared TTAs will need a final check for any recent changes.

4 If you have a paper system, you can carry a bunch of TTOs on ward rounds so that you can write them on the spot when the decision is made to send someone home. If you are on an electronic system and a decision is made to send a patient home on the ward round, do a quick mental check to make sure that there are no outstanding issues you are unsure about like follow-up time or anticoagulant plans.

5 Phone the GP on discharge if the patient:

- Self-discharges
- Is in an unstable condition
- Has complex home circumstances/care needs
- Is elderly/terminally ill
- Dies
- Needs an early visit or a repeat blood test done locally soon after discharge

Handovers

Before you go home or away for the weekend you will need to 'hand over' your patients to the doctor who replaces you. A formal handover is really helpful for your colleagues taking over. I would recommend that you avoid a handover like 'There's a Mrs Smith on Ward 4 to be seen. See you in the morning' – your colleagues will not thank you and Mrs Smith may never get the review that she needs. At best you will then have to do it yourself tomorrow, at worst the patient may come to harm. Obviously how much detail you tell your successor depends on whether or not they are familiar with the patients – bear in mind that they may not know them at all. In these changing times of the European Working Time Directive, handover is becoming ever more frequent and important. Sometimes handover is done verbally, but some hospitals have an electronic system that requires you to fill out a form that the weekend or night doctors on call use. You need to make sure your successors know the following:

1 Who your patients are, which ward they are on and why they are in hospital.

2 A brief summary of the management of each patient (e.g. awaiting surgery tomorrow, NBM, needs continuous morphine infusion for pain relief but stable). Also state specifically what jobs they need to do and why. If asking someone to check some bloods, tell them what to look for and what to do if there is an abnormality, for example, please check Mrs X's bloods, specifically her creatinine. If it has continued to rise please adjust her IV fluid supplementation.

3 Likely complications or difficulties and how you have been dealing with these to date, as well as what to do should they arise.

4 Anyone (doctor/nurse/relatives) who may be contacted if problems arise.

5 What the patient's ceilings of care are if they deteriorate, that is, resuscitation status or if they are for intensive therapy unit- or ward-based care.

6 It is good practice to ask for a 'hand back' in the morning or after the weekend to find out what has happened in your absence.

Referral letters

If you need to refer a patient to another team, you can phone the registrar to make a verbal referral and leave relevant details in the patient's notes. Alternatively, you can write the consultant a letter. You may also be required to write email referrals. If you write a letter, include the following:

1 Address the letter to the consultant of the other team.

2 Name of your consultant, yourself and your bleep number.

3 Name of patient, age, sex, DOB, hospital ID and current location (e.g. ward/home).

4 Name of patient's GP.

5 Specific question(s) your team needs to be answered and the reasons for referral.

6 Relevant clinical history and examination findings.

7 Recent investigations (including negatives).

8 When you need his or her advice by (write this in a humble way!).

Try to anticipate which investigations the other team might need and include them in your referral letter. For example, surgeons almost always need a recent full blood count (FBC), clotting, group and save and maybe an ECG and chest X-ray if they are considering theatre. Gastroenterologists, or any specialist doing a biopsy, will want an international normalized ratio (INR (prothrombin ratio)) and platelet count if investigating liver complaints.

Self-discharge

However it may feel, hospitals are not prisons. Unless patients seem likely to incur life-threatening harm to themselves or lack capacity to make decisions regarding discharge, you cannot restrain them from leaving hospital – even when it is patently a bad idea for them to do so.

If your patient decides to leave against your advice, try the following:

■ Explain to them why they should stay and the risks they are taking by leaving.

■ Try to find out why they want to leave, and see if there are any issues you can help them resolve.

■ Inform your senior and the sister in charge of the ward.

■ Have the patient sign a self-discharge note. This is usually available from the ward clerk. If necessary, you can write one yourself. You need to have a second witness to sign the note. Ensure the patient's name, DOB, hospital number and the name of the hospital you work in are on the form, and then file this in the patient's medical notes.

> I, (*Jo Bloggs*) of (insert address of patient here), wish to discharge myself/take my child on (insert date here) against medical advice and accept full responsibility for my actions. Witnessed by Dr (*your surname, today's date*) and (*colleague's name, today's date*)
> (Jo Bloggs' signature)
> (Your name and signature)
> (Second witness name and signature)

■ Rarely, you may consider using the Mental Health Act to section a patient and restrain them from leaving. Always seek senior advice before doing this (Appendix, Mental Health Act). Usually, there will be a member of the mental health team you can contact for advice or ask them to review the patient in question.

■ Make a brief note of what happened in the patient's notes.

■ Inform the patient's GP that the patient has self-discharged.

Sick notes

You may be asked to write a sick note for patients to verify that they have been unable to work. There are two types of sick notes you can write:

1 If the patient is *not* trying to claim state benefit, they may request a handwritten note on hospital-headed paper. The easiest way to address it is 'To Whom It May Concern' along the top, followed by something like 'Mrs A has been an inpatient at the X Hospital from 24–30 April and will be unable to return to work until 7 May'. Sign and date it, and block print your name and position under your signature as well as the name of the patient's consultant. In this kind of letter, you should *not* disclose the diagnosis. It is worth writing the letter and getting the patient to check they are happy with it.

2 If the patient *is* trying to claim state benefit after leaving hospital, they can self-certify for the first 5 days of absence from work due to ill health. They can obtain the SC2 form from their employer. Similarly, for the self- or unemployed, an SC1 form can be obtained from the department of work and pensions. This means that you shouldn't have to write one for a patient unless they will clearly need an extended period of absence in which case you can normally find forms on the ward that require a signature. I would always check that the patient is happy for you to write any medical details on such a form before issuing it. Most doctors will give a maximum of 2 weeks' worth of sick leave to patients and then ask them to see their GP to renew the sick note or review the need for it.

Chapter 4
ACCIDENT AND EMERGENCY

With contributions from Dr Kimberly Ashton

Working in accident and emergency (A&E) is likely to be the rotation in which you learn the most and have the greatest opportunity to put your skills into practice. You will almost certainly feel unprepared and out of your depth when you start. This chapter aims to provide some advice on surviving and thriving in A&E as well as guidance on coping with the more common medical and surgical conditions that you will treat.

General advice

Whilst there is an enormous variety of pathology to be encountered in A&E, you will soon realize that you see the same handful of conditions repeatedly most of the time.

A&E operates on a shift system. There will always be a consultant in charge for the day. Depending on whether you are working in a hospital that takes emergency medicine trainees, there may also be registrars or ACCS trainees.

As a junior doctor, you will be expected to see patients and initiate appropriate investigations and treatment, before referring to the appropriate specialty, or considering sending them home. If you have any problems, there should be someone in your own department to ask for advice, but if this is not the case, then you should phone someone senior from an appropriate specialty. Generally, if you plan on sending a patient home, you should discuss with someone senior before doing so to check that there is nothing you have missed. This is particularly important at the beginning of the rotation, when you may not have much experience of how things work.

Structure of A&E

A&Es have a majors and a minors or 'injuries' department. When a patient arrives, a relatively senior nurse or doctor will triage the person to the section they think suitable.

The minors department will see patients with a variety of problems. People may have fractures, cuts or other minor injuries. If you feel a patient has been inappropriately triaged as 'minor', you should arrange to have them transferred to majors as they will receive more urgent and thorough attention. You should make clear with your colleagues at this point whether you will see them, or whether someone else will, to avoid patients 'falling through the cracks'.

Majors will have a section called 'resus' (short for resuscitation) where the most unwell patients go. This area can get quite full of people from different departments and can occasionally become noisy and chaotic. If you have started seeing a patient, you should make sure that you know who everyone is and what their role in the situation is. It may be that someone more senior than you takes over, but until this happens, try to maintain an overview of the situation to avoid confusion and inefficiency. Again, if it turns out that a patient is more unwell than first thought, they

The Hands-on Guide to the Foundation Programme, Fifth Edition. Anna Donald, Michael Stein, Ciaran Scott Hill and Selina J Chavda.
© 2015 John Wiley & Sons, Ltd. Published 2015 by John Wiley & Sons, Ltd.

can be moved from majors or minors to the resus area:

■ Do not be afraid to ask nurses for advice. They have generally seen it all before and they know the regular patients. Senior nurses or advanced nurse practitioners can be a goldmine of information and are often particularly skilled at managing minor injuries.

■ You can waste a lot of time looking for equipment. Ensure that you know where important items are kept, including where IV fluids and giving sets are stored as you may need to put these up yourself.

■ There is likely to be a shortage of metal trolleys, so make sure you clear up after yourself to leave them free for others. It makes life much easier if you have a reasonable space for working from rather than depositing everything on a nearby chair or bin lid.

■ A small yellow sharps bin is ideal if you can find one. If not, dispose of your sharps as you go. It may take time, but it's the safest way to avoid a needlestick injury.

■ If you are on-take for a specialty and are seeing patients in A&E, tape two or three sheets of paper to an available desk. Use these to note down accepted patients, so as not to lose track of expected (and received) patients. These sheets can also be used to document tentative and confirmed diagnoses, the results of initial tests and the ward to which the patient is sent from casualty. You can then remove and use this information for handover or post-take rounds. Sticking patient labels on the list is a good way to get all the relevant details for your patient in one place legible. Remember to dispose of this in the confidential waste bin at the end of handover.

■ Dehydration is a real problem if you work without a break in A&E (or anywhere else for that matter). Drink as much fluid as you can! Otherwise, always take a bottle of water onto the 'shop floor' with you. Keep it in a nonclinical area, and label it clearly with your name.

■ Take meal breaks ruthlessly. Hold the fort for your colleagues and have them do the same for you. No one works efficiently with

hypoglycaemia. You should find out when you come on shift whether the person on the shift before has taken their break. If not, encourage them to organize a suitable time, and then plan to take yours when the next person is due to arrive. Most A&E departments allow you the equivalent of 30 minutes break per 6 hours of work, either in one go or as two split breaks. Make sure you take them! Rest, recuperate, eat, and if you can then try and mental switch off from work for a few minutes.

Admitting and allocating patients

1 If you are working in A&E on-take for a specialty, ask medical and nursing colleagues about the local routine for admitting and allocating patients during take. If anyone in particular needs to be informed, such as the bed manager, make sure you make a note of how to contact them. Remember that referral from the emergency team is generally a one-way street. Once you have agreed to see a patient, you have 'accepted them' and are then responsible for their care. If it turns out that they should have been referred to a different specialty, you cannot then ask the emergency team to do this – you will have to make that further referral.

2 When a general practitioner (GP) telephones you to admit a patient:

● Be polite. Remember that the GP almost certainly has more experience than you, and it is not respectful to take the attitude that you know more than they do because they are referring to you.

● Have paper and pen ready.

● Listen first. This will provide less frustration for both parties.

● Take down the name, age, problem (in as much detail as is feasible), hospital number, GP name and number and when to expect the patient's arrival.

● Phone A&E or the ward with the patient's details, and if necessary, inform the site manager.

• Let your senior know that the patient is coming in and what their main complaint is.

3 If you accept a patient from a GP, then you are obliged to review them, even if it is obvious that they need to be transferred to another specialty. Try, therefore, to obtain as much information as you can during the referral and triage if you can to the right speciality, or you will end up seeing the patient, however, inappropriately.

4 In many hospitals nearly all patients will be shipped to an 'Acute or Medical Assessment Unit' from where they will be either discharged home or, if their stay is likely to be more than a few days, to a more long-term ward elsewhere in the hospital. If a patient is admitted directly to a normal ward, investigations and the instigation of treatment can take much longer than if they are seen in A&E. If you think someone is likely to be very unwell, try to insist that you can at least review them in A&E first. This makes obtaining tests such as portable CXRs much easier.

Keeping track of patients

■ Try keeping a sheet of paper with patient stickers down one side with results of baseline tests and diagnosis next to each sticker. This is invaluable for handing over to colleagues and ensuring nothing important is missed. It is easy to get overwhelmed when you have seen three or four patients and are waiting for multiple tests to come back before referring to the appropriate specialty or discharging. It is vital to keep a record of what has and has not been done.

If you are missing results, be conscientious in checking them before going home. It is better to spot an unexpected abnormal result late and when you are looking forward to leaving rather than when you return the next day and something tragic has happened. Alternatively, make sure you have handed over to someone else to check. If at all possible, it is better to check it yourself as you will know the story better and be in a better position to deal

efficiently with the results. If you have handed over results to someone else to review, you should document who you spoke to, what you asked them to check and the plan of action. Remember that taking responsibility is absolutely central to being a good doctor, and if you do not follow up investigations and results, it is unlikely that anyone else will. It is your diligence in such a situation that will determine the type of doctor you become.

■ If you urgently need a result out of hours, you may need to phone the laboratory technician on call. This can be particularly important for tests like lumbar punctures, where the samples can otherwise sit unnoticed on the microbiology desk until the next morning. Likewise, there is usually a duty biochemist or haematologist on call.

Medicine

On admission, complete for each medical patient:

1 A focused history and examination

2 Baseline tests:

• Bloods: FBC, U&E, glucose, ESR and CRP (consider clotting screen and LFT)
• Urine: MSU and dipstick
• ECG
• Radiology: CXR

3 IV access

4 IV fluid

5 Drug charts

Patients refusing treatment

The vast majority of patients have capacity to refuse treatment. This is the default position and capacity is normally assumed unless something suggests otherwise. Routine capacity tests are not necessary simply because a patient disagrees with your recommendation. You can section someone who refuses to be treated (see Appendix, Mental Health Act) if you think they do not have capacity to refuse treatment. You can then treat them according to their best interests. This should be used as an absolute last resort. Sectioning someone is a complex process and may have serious consequences for them and is likely to require specialist help from the psychiatry team. This is in contrast to a simple capacity assessment that any doctor should be able to perform. Sectioning a patient is not something that a patient should ever be threatened with.

Medical and surgical assessment units

Over the past 10 years, these units have become integrated into hospitals, chiefly not only to take the pressure off A&E and meet the 4-hour target but also to begin the initial assessment and management of patients within the first 24 hours of admission. If your hospital has these units, it is likely you will see many of your medical or surgical patients here rather than in A&E. All the same principles in A&E apply to these units with the added benefit of having the entire team available and the majority of the patients in one place.

Fast-track patients

Some patients (usually with time-critical conditions although many others are beginning to fall under this banner) will be triaged directly into pathways for rapid assessment, investigation and treatment. Common pathways include acute coronary syndrome, acute stroke, GI bleeding and trauma:

■ Be familiar with the local policy as these pathways are designed to lighten bureaucracy, reduce errors and generally make things easier for you.
■ These pathways will be audited, so be aware of the critical factors in these pathways (e.g. thrombolysis times, grading of severity).
■ Also, remember that these pathways also apply to inpatients, not just to new patients coming in.

Chapter 5
BECOMING A BETTER DOCTOR

With contributions from Dr Rahul Mukherjee

Postgraduate medical training in the United Kingdom has undergone significant reforms in the last decade. Newly qualified doctors embark on a 2-year Foundation Programme to develop core generic skills and take responsibility for patient care. Trainees may then complete specialty training before gaining entrance onto the specialist register or the general practitioner (GP) register. The duration of this additional specialty training varies from 3 to 8 years depending on specialty. During this period, trainees can do a number of things to develop their clinical skills, increase their knowledge and become a better doctor.

Foundation Programmes (United Kingdom)

Foundation Programmes are compulsory for all UK graduating doctors. The programme is intended to streamline training so as to ensure that all junior doctors develop a set of core transferable skills and to reduce the bottleneck when entering the registrar grade. Foundation Programmes are divided into 2 years (FY1 and FY2) that are now usually paired within the same training deanery.

FY1 trainees are comparable to the pre-registration house officers in the older system and are frequently still called that. Placements are of variable length between 3 and 6 months, but most programmes have six placements of 4 months each across a 2-year programme. Typically trainees spend a minimum of 4 months in surgery and medicine. During FY2, many programmes contain a general practice placement recognizing the importance of primary care in healthcare delivery in the United Kingdom. During the first year, if not already allocated during your job selection, you will have an opportunity to put forwards your preferences for placements in FY2. Ultimately you should choose your placements based on your interests as well as any gaps you may have in your experience. It will be useful when applying for specialist training posts if you can demonstrate a clear path from your initial foundation jobs to the specialty you wish to pursue. For example, a GP trainee may want initial experience in general medicine and surgery before undertaking specialized rotations in paediatrics and obstetrics/gynaecology. Although it is emphasized that the foundation jobs you undertake will not influence selection to specialist training, most trainees who are successful in securing specialist training posts have demonstrated significant commitment to their specialty through audit experience, logbook of procedures and attendance at relevant courses. Having gained some experience in the specialty you want to go into during foundation training certainly helps but is not mandatory.

It may be worth noting that a core commitment of the NHS is to try to accommodate flexible training. This includes the foundation years. Trainees may elect to complete their training less than full time at the outset and the arrangements for this vary between trusts.

The Hands-on Guide to the Foundation Programme, Fifth Edition. Anna Donald, Michael Stein, Ciaran Scott Hill and Selina J Chavda.

Some trusts offer a slot-sharing arrangement, for example, where two trainees share one full time post and the pro rata out of hours. It is possible to take time out of the Foundation Programme (e.g. due to maternity leave), but this may lead to a delay in the completion date of your programme. In these circumstances, it is advisable to speak to your Foundation Programme training director and educational supervisor at the earliest opportunity to ensure that appropriate procedures are in place and arrangements made for your return to training.

Academic Foundation Programmes

In addition to the clinical Foundation Programmes, there are a number of academic programmes (around 400 in the United Kingdom) where trainees have protected time to develop their research, teaching or leadership skills. These are prestigious posts and form part of the Integrated Academic Training Pathway to help develop the next generation of academic clinicians and research leaders. All academic trainees must complete the same clinical competencies as standard clinical trainees but get less 'clinical' time to do so. This means that you have to be highly motivated and organized to fulfil your academic and clinical aspirations.

During your academic Foundation Programme, you will have a period of 'protected research time'. The protected research time can be delivered in a number of ways. Most jobs provide a dedicated 4-month block with no clinical duties, but others offer a day release every week or even weekly blocks of research separated by longer periods of clinical work. Some trainees choose to spend this time in a laboratory developing their knowledge of basic science whilst others complete a clinical project. This protected time gives an invaluable opportunity to produce work that can be presented at national and international conferences as well as published in peer-reviewed journals. Completing an academic Foundation Programme also demonstrates your commitment to a particular specialty and gives a distinct advantage when applying

for the next stage in the Integrated Academic Training Pathway – the Academic Clinical Fellowship phase.

Assessments

Your meetings with your educational supervisor should be focused on the progress of your training. This will largely be based on your assessments. Although a rapidly changing area, the assessment tools currently in use include the following:

1 Multi-source feedback (peer assessment tool) and team assessment behaviour (TAB)

You should pick a range of assessors from amongst your peers, consultants and other healthcare professionals (including physiotherapists, pharmacists, nursing staff and healthcare assistants) and ask them to complete specific questionnaires about your clinical skills and conduct on the wards. You also complete a self-assessment and the results are collected and presented to you in your meetings with the educational supervisor. This exercise is aimed at finding out your strengths and weaknesses. It can be very demoralizing to discover your weaknesses (or what other people *think* are your weaknesses) but you should not shy away from selecting more critical assessors. Although compulsory for progression, these assessments are not currently used in any competitive sense so you should choose assessors who are likely to give you an honest appraisal. The most critical assessments are often the ones that help you learn the most about yourself and how you are perceived by different members of the multi-disciplinary team. It can also be very useful to gain feedback from patients, and some specialty programmes are beginning to incorporate 'patient surveys' into the assessment process.

2 Mini-clinical evaluation exercise (CEX)

You will have to find several clinical scenarios to be assessed on. These are extremely varied and can be found in the curriculum of your Foundation Programme on your ePortfolio. The assessor is usually a senior registrar, consultant or GP. It can be difficult to arrange an occasion where a real clinical scenario, assessor and you coincide. You may be able to go to a clinic and be observed whilst taking a history or doing a clinical examination. The post-take ward round can also be a good place to conduct a brief clinical exam in front of your consultant. It is usually best to complete the assessment on ePortfolio as soon as you have done it, but often sending your consultant a reminder via an ePortfolio link at a later time, with a brief summary of the clinical scenario, is needed.

3 Direct observation of procedural skills (DOPS)

You will have to find a variety of clinical opportunities to demonstrate your prowess. The procedural skills do not need to be complex; they can be fairly routine and straightforward (e.g. venepuncture, taking an ECG) and will happen at least once a day on every ward. As such, there will be no shortage of occasions to be assessed. That said, if you have a mind to go into a particular specialty (e.g. anaesthetics) an interview panel will probably be more impressed if you pull out examples of several central line insertions you have done than if you can only prove your ability to take blood. The trick again is to find the assessor first and then offer to perform the task that the assessor was going to do. It can often be difficult to find the opportunities to perform certain procedures (e.g. chest drain insertion, central line insertion, abdominal paracentesis). Some hospitals have pleural intervention units where a respiratory physician with a special interest may perform lists where they insert chest drains under ultrasound guidance. It may be worth getting in touch with these consultants and expressing your interest to observe one of their lists and perhaps get an opportunity to do one yourself under supervision. If your hospital has an interventional radiology unit, they may have lists when they perform procedures under ultrasound guidance. Cardiology units will routinely perform diagnostic angiography via femoral/radial arterial line insertion.

4 Case-based discussion (CBD)

This is the more traditional format where you pick cases you have seen to discuss with your consultant or other senior medical team member. History-taking, examination, differential diagnosis, investigation, management, record-keeping and ethical aspects are areas you will have to cover. If you see surgical pre-admissions or patients on an acute take, then these are easy opportunities to complete the task. If you rotate through accident and emergency, this also offers many opportunities for near complete clinical encounters.

There are minimum numbers of assessments you will need to do, but do not be limited by them. The more assessments you have, the more you will learn and the more you will have in your logbook as evidence of adequate training. Surgical logbooks are not essential at foundation level of training, but if you are an aspiring surgeon it is useful to keep a log that you can show at interview to the panel.

In addition to these 'minimum' prescribed assessments, you are expected to be a lifelong learner and a 'reflective practitioner'. The latter means taking time to think about events that you have been involved in (both positive and negative) and searching for the underlying lessons they can teach you.

Reflective pieces in practice should be done at least once a month and uploaded to your ePortfolio. In some foundation schools, they are a mandatory requirement to pass the year and are easier to do monthly rather than have a huge number at the end of the year prior to your Annual Review of Competence Progression (ARCP).

Situational judgement tests

In order to improve recruitment practices in the United Kingdom, many programmes including the Foundation Programme are using situational judgement tests (SJTs) to assess job relevant behaviours and select the best candidates for any given post. SJTs consist of a series of hypothetical scenarios that you may encounter as a junior doctor. Questions are either 'ranking questions' where candidates rank five responses to a clinical scenario or 'multiple-choice questions' where candidates may choose the three most appropriate actions. These aim to test the candidates' professionalism, communication, teamworking and coping with pressure.

There are still many unanswered questions about the discriminatory power of SJTs and whether they represent a robust and reliable method for selecting trainees to UK training programmes. Many specialty training programmes however, including core medical training, are piloting the use of SJTs to assess recruitment into programmes. There are now a number of books and online resources dedicated to preparing candidates taking SJTs for postgraduate medical training.

Moving on from the Foundation Programme

Selection into specialist training can differ markedly depending on your specialty choice. In addition, it is liable to change rapidly over the coming years. There are currently two main groups of specialties – those that have a period of core training (general surgery/core medicine/psychiatry/acute care common stem) followed by further competitive selection into subspecialties and those that are 'run-through' and do not have a stage of further selection. The latter includes specialties such as general practice, histopathology, neurosurgery, ophthalmology, microbiology, paediatrics, radiology, obstetrics and gynaecology and public health. For more information on the selection process, see http://www.medicalcareers.nhs.uk/.

In terms of postgraduate exams, it is currently possible to enter for the first part of the MRCS (surgical membership) exam as soon as you are granted a medical certificate; the final part can then be completed whenever the candidate is ready. For MRCP (medical membership) you need at least 12 months experience (i.e. complete FY1) to enter the first part. Once this is completed you can again sit for the final two parts whenever you are ready. In the past, it was not encouraged for trainees to take postgraduate exams during foundation training. However, it is now compulsory for core medical trainees to complete all parts of the MRCP in order to fulfil requirements for their ARCP sign-off and be able to take up

ST3 posts. It is therefore advisable to complete the MRCP as soon as you are able to. For the other specialties (anaesthetics, pathology, psychiatry, radiology emergency medicine, etc.), it is not usually possible to sit any exams until on a training programme. There are lots of diplomas that can be completed if you are itching to work on your postgraduate CV; the *British Medical Journal (BMJ)* careers section has good articles on most of them.

Around a third of Foundation Programme graduates do not immediately progress to specialty training in the United Kingdom. Some choose to work and travel abroad in order to gain new work and life experiences. Australia is particularly popular as no entry exams are currently required, working hours are flexible and trainees report gaining more hands-on experience and enhancing their skills. Some trainees seek more clinical experience doing 'trust grade' posts in the United Kingdom – these posts can sometimes provide an advantage if the trainee chooses to apply for that specialty in the future or failed to secure a training post at the first attempt. Other valuable learning experiences include the National Medical Director's Clinical Fellow Scheme where junior doctors can be seconded to organizations such as the Department of Health, the NICE or the Royal College of Physicians and develop skills in leadership, management and health policy. It is also possible for Foundation Programme graduates to pursue higher degrees (e.g. MD or PhD) or research experience before committing to specialty training.

Information technology

It is becoming impossible to practice medicine without a basic level of technical knowledge. Most people will be familiar with using computers for word processing, email and web surfing, but there is a lot more out there:

■ Junior doctors move around a lot, and with the plummeting cost of computers, laptops are much more practical. Decent laptops or an iPad has become cheaper in price and having an iPad handy might allow you to work on a case report or read the latest issue of the *BMJ* during a quiet on-call period. Be sure to get permission if connecting your computer to hospital equipment (e.g. printers, network points). There are numerous smaller alternative devices now available, and many of the more business-oriented mobile phones have word-processing capability.

■ Electronic tablets and smartphones such as the iPhone/iPad and alternative Android devices are becoming ever more popular with medical professionals. Each can be loaded with a lot of medical software including formularies, patient list software, medical calculators and textbooks. Many of these are free and some trusts are now also using trust-specific apps for easy access to guidelines, such as antibiotic prescribing. Most medical software (especially formularies) are designed for North American doctors, so they may not always be relevant.

■ All UK hospitals now have networked computer systems for accessing patient details, blood results and ordering tests.

■ The use of mobile phones in hospitals is a controversial area. The best advice is to follow local hospital policy (and not the behaviour of your consultant!). At the very least, it will make it less likely for patients and relatives to follow suit and start answering calls during ward rounds!

■ Digital photos or videos are best taken formally. The written consent of the patient should be explicit about what the images can be used for, and a copy of it should be filed with the patient's notes. Remember that you are responsible for the images. The medical photography department can help for more difficult photos (e.g. fundi) or get better pictures of clinical signs for case reports. Taking images without patient consent, even if anonymized and strictly for educational purposes, is rarely supported.

The Internet

Using the Internet in the NHS is fraught with precautions and limitations. All hospitals will have local policy about the level of Internet access and what is allowed. Be aware of these. A few pointers:

■ Be careful with confidential or potentially sensitive information in emails, particularly if you try to forward emails from work to home email addresses (the opposite way round is generally much easier).

■ Keep discussions of clinical cases anonymous even in closed teaching sessions like grand rounds.

■ The hospital intranet will often have archives of local policy, the local formulary and contact details of various people.

■ Keep hospital email and personal email distinct. Most hospitals are giving doctors' their own email account. You can get a universal NHS one at www.nhs.net; this is highly recommended as it is likely that you will be working within the NHS for a long time and can be used to get patient information from different trusts in the form of secure email. In addition, many people like www.doctors.net. uk although it is not recommended by the NHS for transference of patient data.

Online medical databases

NHS Evidence is a good starting point for clinical information. This includes useful resources like clinical pathways represented in the Map of Medicine (NHS-approved clinical flow charts) and Clinical Knowledge Summaries (formally Prodigy), a summary of evidence-based information provided for the National Institute for Health and Care Excellence. Take a little time to familiarize yourself with this NHS service — it is improving all the time!

Other websites rich in online content are:

■ The *British National Formulary* at www.bnf. org can save you time if you cannot find the ward's *BNF*. Your hospital should have a subscription to it.

■ PubMed at www.ncbi.nlm.nih.gov/PubMed.

■ The General Medical Council (GMC) at www.gmc-uk.org.

■ *British Medical Journal* at www.bmj.com

■ The *New England Journal of Medicine* at www.nejm.org.

■ The British Thoracic Society at www.britthoracic.org.uk has very detailed guidelines on the diagnosis, investigation and management of respiratory disease.

■ eMedicine at www.emedicine.com is a useful quick reference on common and rare diseases. It is directed towards US doctors, though. A comparable UK service is offered by www.gpnotebook.co.uk

Keeping up with the literature

The information and technology explosion is real. There are several ways to keep up to date with stacks of international journals with minimal fuss; we wish we had known about these when we were students!

■ Adopt a 'problem-based' approach to reading. This means reading whatever you need to answer real questions rather than blindly scanning journals with minimal retention and maximum boredom (see Evidence-based medicine). You will remember much more of what you read if your patient depends upon it, and you'll probably also find it more interesting. The age-old advice of reading up on clinical conditions you see still holds true. Good review articles are often excellent, up-to-date sources of information on a particular clinical topic.

■ Good-quality systematic reviews, especially those using meta-analysis, are the most efficient studies to read [1] because they combine the results of many individual studies, adding statistical power and giving you an efficient overview of the topic. Much of the write-up in these studies flows around methodology and may be difficult to read unless you are specifically appraising the literature. However, if you can convince yourself relatively quickly that this is adequate, then the conclusions are often very useful and clinically relevant.

■ Learn to critically appraise what you read so that you can evaluate studies yourself rather than relying on the authors' conclusions. It is true that most published studies, even in leading medical journals, do not have reliable results because the study methodology was not rigorous enough. Critical appraisal is a simple process that enables you to be much

more discriminating in what you read (see Evidence-based medicine).

■ If you are a member of the BMA, you will automatically receive a copy of the *BMJ* every week. There is a 'research news' section of the *BMJ* which contains summaries of the latest clinical studies in other general medical journals. This can be a useful way of keeping up to date on research developments.

Evidence-based medicine

Evidence-based medicine is a central tenet of being a good doctor. Basically, evidence-based medicine involves using research findings to give clinicians much more statistical power in interpreting everyday clinical data rather than relying on anecdotal evidence. Not only do people who practice evidence-based medicine find that they become more aware – and critical – of research findings, but they quickly become adept at solving difficult problems and find that they can engage better in medical debates. Evidence-based medicine can be practiced by teams or by individuals.

Evidence-based medicine involves carrying out three key steps:

1 Ask a clear question about the problem you are trying to solve (e.g. should I anticoagulate an elderly woman with asymptomatic atrial fibrillation?).

2 Search the literature for good-quality evidence using a structured, hierarchical search that gives you the most statistically powerful research first. Search first for systematic reviews, second for randomized controlled trials and lastly for other types of studies.

3 Critically appraise the evidence you have found to see whether or not its findings are reliable and relevant to your situation. To do this you need a list of questions, which help you to assess the methodology of the research. There are various books and courses to boost these skills. The evidence then should be combined with your clinical knowledge and practically applied to the patient in question, taking into account their wishes.

If in doubt, look it up and discuss with your seniors or ideally at a formal journal club.

Clinical governance and paraclinical work

In addition to all the work directly involving patients, you should strongly consider getting involved in the other aspects of medicine. Not only is it a worthwhile learning experience, but also it is good on your CV and occasionally enjoyable! The amount of paperwork and the organizational obstacles can be very daunting but your seniors should be supportive.

Clinical governance is increasingly important for all doctors. As a minimum, you should know what it means and how to go about the process of audit.

Clinical governance is defined by the system through which NHS organizations are accountable for continuously improving the quality of their services and safeguarding high standards of care by creating an environment in which clinical excellence will flourish. It is traditionally classified in terms of the seven 'pillars':

1 Clinical effectiveness and research

2 Audit

3 Risk management

4 Education and training

5 Patient and public involvement

6 Using information and information technology

7 Staffing and staff management

Clinical audit

Clinical audit is simply the measurement of clinical practice against a specific standard and its effectiveness with the aim of improving it. It is useful to get involved in clinical audit as you will learn about management, common pitfalls and the difficulties in implementing change in a large organization. You can easily get involved in an existing audit by speaking to the relevant consultant or your hospital audit department. Alternatively, you can start a new one. Retrospective audits are generally easier to conduct than prospective

ones unless your daily work overlaps with audit. You can start by looking at local or national guidelines that the service you work in should ideally meet. Then you need to decide how to measure whether the guidelines are being followed or the standards achieved. Here are some 'tips':

■ Design a form with all the data parameters you want to collect.

■ Use the clinical coding department to your advantage. Here you can get a list of clinical codes that fit the scope of your audit. From there, you can get hold of a list of patients.

■ Don't try to track down all the notes yourself. Your clinical audit department is far more efficient at getting them. The ward clerk or the secretary for your department/consultant should also be able to request patient notes.

■ Spreadsheet programmes are very good at sorting out the data once you have collected it.

■ Find an occasion to present it. Invite everyone involved. Monthly local audit meetings are a good way to present your data to a wide range of healthcare professionals including consultants.

■ Do not forget to think up solutions to any deficits you discover and make these recommendations as part of your presentation.

■ If you are working in the same hospital for more than a few months, consider repeating your audit once your recommended changes have been implemented. An audit cycle is not truly complete until it has been repeated at least once. In this way, you can see if your changes have effected a change for the better.

The audit cycle involves the following steps:

Step 1: Identify an issue or problem.

Step 2: Set criteria and establish a 'gold standard'.

Step 3: Observe practice and collect data.

Step 4: Compare performance with criteria and standards (data interpretation).

Step 5: Make recommendations to implement change.

Step 6: Re-audit to establish effectiveness of change and 'close' the loop. If the process is repeated again, it becomes an audit 'spiral'.

Quality improvement projects

The GMC expects all doctors to take part in systems of quality assurance and quality improvement, and this forms part of the appraisal and revalidation process. Quality improvement projects aim to improve patient experience and outcomes using systematic change methods and through changing provider behaviour. Quality improvement projects use a plan-do-study-act cycle and aim to make a difference in a relatively short space of time rather than the traditional audit model.

Successful quality improvement projects need to have specific, measurable, achievable, relevant and time-bound (SMART) goals. An example could be to improve weekend handover by introducing a patient pro forma with specific and relevant clinical information. There are a number of journals and conferences that encourage innovation and creative thinking to improve healthcare. You could consider submitting your completed project for publication in one of these journals (e.g. *BMJ Quality and Safety*) or present work at relevant conferences.

Case reports

There is an element of luck in writing a case report, since you need an interesting case to write about. However, a good case need not be a rare one; common cases can be just as good, especially if there were pitfalls in the diagnosis or management of the patient:

■ You will likely need pictures or videos of any diagnostic imaging, so make sure you get consent from the patient and involve the photographic unit.
■ The *BMJ* or the *Journal of the Royal Society of Medicine* has good formats to follow.
■ Good case reports are short and succinct. Journals are rarely interested in any superfluous details.
■ Your case report does not need to follow strictly the chronology of events in the patient. By holding back on the result of a key investigation until the end of the case report, you can create necessary drama!

A popular choice amongst trainees is to submit a case report article or clinical image (as a picture quiz) for *BMJ* Endgames. This is a weekly section published in the *BMJ* intended to help junior doctors prepare for their postgraduate examinations and professional development.

Courses

Education is more than just working on the wards, attending grand rounds and reading books. There is a wide array of courses one can take on; these are regularly advertised in the *BMJ* careers classified sections and fall into several broad groups:

■ Examination courses are aimed at doctors sitting postgraduate exams and try to condense everything you need to know in a short period of time (5 days or a weekend). They are often overbooked, so apply early. Despite what you may hear, it is not necessary to attend these courses to pass an exam. They are largely based around boosting confidence.
■ Skills training courses are extremely varied from the more clinical ones like the Resuscitation Council's advanced life support (ALS) courses to less clinical ones like courses teaching interview technique. Resuscitation Council courses are invaluable and should be top on the list of courses you do. It is now a requirement that ALS is completed by the end of FY2 in most foundation schools. ATLS is a popular choice amongst the more trauma/surgery minded. Check which courses are compulsory or organized by the deanery before using up your own time and money. You may be able to use your study budget for these courses, which is useful as the cost can add up to significant amounts of money.
■ Lecture courses are generally more suited for more senior doctors but may be interesting, particularly if in a field that you are interested in becoming a part of.

Attending specialty courses can be used to demonstrate your commitment to a particular field when it comes to job applications, so it is useful to find out what may be available at an early stage. There are many good courses run throughout the year at the Royal

Society of Medicine and the Royal Colleges (surgeons, physicians, anaesthetists, etc.), by *BMJ* Masterclasses and via local deaneries.

Professionalism

It may be the case that no one ever specifically teaches you how to be a professional. Don't worry if the transition from student to doctor is full of bumps and jolts – it certainly was for us. There isn't much mystery to being 'professional'; it's mostly about communicating well, building relationships and being responsible for what you say and do. However, this is no small thing to accomplish.

Communication

For an enjoyable job, good communication is essential. As a junior doctor, you may make about 10–15 phone calls for every patient you admit. You may interview up to 5000 people during the year. You will write volumes of notes that others will rely on and that might one day be used as evidence in court. You will physically touch thousands of people.

Although most medical schools do teach communication or relationship skills, you are still supposed to largely pick them up from your seniors. As you have probably already observed, many seniors are lacking in personal and communication skills. It pays to develop your own skills; they will save you bleeps, headaches, time and lawsuits. Over 90% of UK medical defence cases result from poor communication rather than from negligence. Many so-called personality clashes between healthcare professionals, patients and relatives can be solved by effective and imaginative communication:

1 It is really important and difficult to write legibly at 3 a.m. Write for others as you would have like to have things written for you. A fountain pen can force you to write legibly (or it can make things even worse!). Block capitals can be a good way to keep your writing legible if you have very messy writing.

2 Write your name and bleep number on ward boards. This is very helpful for the nursing staff if you are on call (e.g. 14 May cover: Jo Bloggs' bleep 1413). Never deliberately omit your bleep from the notes – the doctors who do this are unprofessional and potentially compromise their patients' care. It doesn't take many episodes of trying to get hold of a member of a different specialty who did not leave their contact details to understand the importance of this.

3 Let people know if you are distressed about something. Try not to transform grief or fatigue into defensive behaviour, such as silence or arrogance. People are usually pretty good at helping you out if they know what's up; you don't have to tell everyone but having a confidant such as your educational supervisor or a sympathetic senior can be invaluable and can help arrange cover if you need to attend a funeral or counselling.

4 We have all been shouted at unreasonably by colleagues at some time. Try not to take it to heart or to say something you will later regret. If they do have a legitimate point underlying their intemperance, learn the lesson and move on. If you experience sustained and unprofessional bullying from another member of staff (which does happen in hospitals), you should seek to stop it, either by assertively explaining to them that their behaviour is unacceptable (this may be easier said than done) or by taking the problem to a trusted senior or manager. The BMA helpline can assist too, for example, by helping to identify whom to take the case to next. Do not ignore it – you are a professional and do not deserve to be treated as such.

5 Most junior doctors lose their heads from time to time. Don't be afraid to say you're sorry. People usually respect apologies.

6 If conflicts arise, some useful tips include:

- Ask yourself, 'Are you sure you're right?'
- Does it matter?
- Try turning difficult questions back to the person asking them. For example, you can ask them: 'What makes you ask that question?'
- Try to appear calm, despite what you may feel inside.

7 There are many resources to help people understand choices about treatments more thoroughly, such as videos, pamphlets and online information. Contact a clinical nurse specialist, librarian or district health authority to find out if any are readily available.

8 Use an interpreter if necessary. Interpreters can usually be contacted through the switchboard for a telephone interpreter or can be booked by the ward clerk for a face-to-face session.

Consultants and senior registrars

■ Each consultant will have certain things they want to know about each patient (sometimes for no apparent reason). Your predecessor is usually a good source of this kind of information.

■ NEVER say you've done something when you haven't. It makes your team lose their trust in you and you may never get it back.

■ Impress your seniors by being straightforward and by knowing your patients well. This matters much more in your job than having read the latest *NEJM* issue. As the junior doctor, you are expected to have the most contact time with your patients; it can be very frustrating for your consultant to turn up to the ward round and ask a patient's blood results or social situation only to find that you haven't prepared this information in advance.

■ Try to know your patients as well as you can, but do not be too disheartened when it seems that your registrar or consultant effortlessly knows more about each patient than you do. Much of this is experience. However, it is also the case that whilst you are furiously looking for notes, your seniors have time to absorb information and think about the patients. They will also spend time that you are not aware of discussing patients with colleagues or relatives and in meetings/theatre/clinic. All these encounters are 'hidden' from you but give your colleagues information you do not have. Likewise, you will hold some information that your seniors do not; sharing this will invariably make you look good and will be appreciated by the team.

■ It takes time to learn 'what you need to know' for ward rounds and about each patient. Be tolerant with yourself – you are still learning.

GPs

You will talk and write to many GPs; some you will get to know quite well. The following are some recommendations from a number of GPs, including Joe Rosenthal, a GP who also teaches at the Royal Free Hospital in London:

1 Phone requests for admission:

- First check from your team if you can accept referrals. If not, politely redirect them to the correct person.
- Have paper and pen ready.
- Be polite.
- Listen first.
- Take down the following: name, age, problem, hospital number, GP name and number and expected time of admission.
- Ask for a list of the patient's medications, particularly if the patient may be confused.
- Inform casualty.

2 Phone the GP on discharge if the patient:

- Self-discharges
- Is in an unstable condition
- Has poor home circumstances
- Dies
- Needs an early review

Don't rely on the post! This can sometimes take weeks to reach a GP's desk.

3 Discharge letter. Complete *before* the patient leaves. Many are now electronic but ensure that it includes:

- Patient details
- Name of consultant
- Name of ward
- Diagnosis and important negative findings
- Treatment given
  - ○ Changes to regular medications
- Treatment on discharge
- Follow-up arrangements
- What the patient has been told
- Your name and bleep number

4 Think about the resources the GP has in his or her surgery. Try to avoid things like 'repeat CXR in 1 month' on the discharge form. The

GP is not an outpatient service and it may be much more difficult for them to arrange certain tests than it is for you. If there are loose ends requiring tests in future, set up a clinic appointment.

Nurses

It is crucial to get on with nurses, who are fantastic allies. They know most of what you need to know as a junior doctor and are usually keen and willing to teach you. Nurses are trained in a range of things that doctors aren't and vice versa, so the teams are complementary – remember this and use it to your advantage! Here are some hints for starters:

■ Always introduce yourself to nurses and other staff when you're new on a ward.

■ Always tidy up after yourself, especially your own sharps. Most needlestick injuries arise from sharps someone else did not clear up.

■ Don't expect nurses to do things they are not qualified to do. Nurses may have extended roles (such as IV drug administration) but they may not do it. It may be frustrating for you that a certain nurse cannot take blood or put in a catheter, but it is not their fault. Think how bad you would feel if your consultant lost their temper with you for something you could not do. Be careful about putting responsibility onto nurses; they do not have your training and you should not expect them to make the same judgements that you do. Also, remember that when making requests, nurses can be struck off much more easily than doctors.

■ Do unto nurses as they do to you. Make them cups of tea or coffee or offer to do an IV round if you're on the ward without much to do. This helps to create an easy, generous atmosphere on the ward, which makes coming to work much more fun.

■ To avoid heaps of bleeps, you can consider asking nurses to write down tasks and have one nurse bleep you with the list every couple of hours or so. Tell them you will return to do a round at a specific time (or at a particular hour – say, between 4 and 5 p.m.).

■ If you foresee problems with a patient overnight, discuss these with the nurses. Arrange 'bleep thresholds' for foreseeable problems. Instructions such as 'call me if his systolic falls below 100' may seem superfluous, but they suggest that you are on top of the problem and indicate your willingness to respond promptly. This reduces the frequency of those 'just thought you might like to know…' bleeps.

■ If multiple bleeps are a real problem, consider arranging a meeting with the medical or surgical manager and nursing staff to work out a better system. This is the sort of thing hospital managers are employed for. Talk to your senior if he or she is supportive. Try not to jump into this though if you are new to a job; often with a little time you will find that a system that seems strange or untenable actually works quite well. Frequent bleeps are often a symptom of nurses feeling under pressure or unsupported. It may also be that they are nervous about your accessibility. If you build relationships with them and they trust you to be there when there is a real problem then you will see the frequency of bleeps reduce dramatically.

■ If you have a plan in your head for a patient or can foresee a problem a patient might have (e.g. a delayed discharge date), let the nursing, social work and occupational therapy staff know so they can help you with it rather than having to nag you for information.

■ Write instructions to nurses in the medical notes, but also tell them. Ideally, it is best to have a senior nurse present when you do a ward round who can then hand over nursing tasks to their colleagues. If it is very important, then you can check later and reiterate it. Nurses have long lists of jobs to do, just like you do, and similarly, they can sometimes prioritize poorly or forget something that you have said.

■ Save time: get to know how team nursing works on your ward. Basically, team nursing means that nurses work in independent, often colour-coded teams, each of which looks after a certain number of patients. Do not try to elicit information about a 'red' patient from a 'green' nurse (see Team nursing). Also, don't be surprised if nurses assume that doctors work in a similar fashion – more junior staff may assume that only a certain number of the patients are 'yours'.

■ Nurses often work in three 8-hour shifts or sets of 12.5-hour shifts. Their rota is usually kept in the nurses' office. It may be helpful to know when a particular nurse will be available.

■ Try not to interrupt nurses when they are meeting for the shift 'report', on handover or on their breaks. Remember that breaks are sacred to nurses; if there is something urgent, then another nurse will always be covering their patients.

Helpful things to know about nurses

■ Nursing grades (varies between hospitals)

> Student nurse: attends university for 3–4 years (shorter for graduate programmes).
> Staff nurse: band 5 (1–4 are auxiliary nurses also known as healthcare assistants or HCAs).
> Senior staff nurses: band 5 or 6.
> Sisters/charge nurse: band 6 or 7.
> Nurse managers: bands 6–8.
> Modern matrons: bands 7 and 8.
> Lecturer practitioner: senior specialist nurse who teaches and advises more inexperienced staff.
> Nurse practitioners: gradually increasing in number but are still relatively thin on the ground in the United Kingdom. They are very experienced and are able to do a lot of what junior doctors do.

■ Nursing jargon

> Bank nurse is a nurse hired temporarily from a 'bank' agency, comparable to locums.
> Charge nurse is a male version of ward sister.
> Team nursing means that nurses work in colour-coded teams, each of which independently cares for different groups of patients. It means that nurses get to know their patients better. It also means that nurses may not know much about patients who aren't assigned to their team. If you want to know about a 'blue' patient, ask a 'blue-team' nurse.

> To 'special' is to provide intensive nursing for a seriously ill or agitated patient.
> Ward sister is the female version of charge nurse who may have overall responsibility for the patients.
> Modern matron, reintroduced by the government over the past few years in an attempt to return to traditional standards of cleanliness and care, is a senior nurse who oversees a department and is largely occupied with managerial and administrative duties.
> Back/late shift is the shift from approximately 2 to 9 p.m.
> Early shift is the shift from approximately 7 a.m. to 2 p.m.

■ Things nurses hate most

> Doctors treating them like second-class citizens.
> Doctors not answering bleeps reasonably quickly, so they have to wait by the phone for ages.
> Doctors leaving sharps and other rubbish around.
> Doctors not explaining things well to patients and not informing the nurse what they found out from the patient.

Patients

(See also Chapter 8, Breaking bad news.)
Listen to patients, even if you think their worries are trivial. Remember that you don't have to solve all their problems. Just listening can be a huge help:

■ If you do not have time to listen to a patient properly, either organize for someone else to listen (such as their nurse) or tell the patient that you will sit down with them later. Preferably give the patient a time and stick to it.

■ If you cannot make it back to talk to a patient, phone their nurse to tell the patient so they are not left waiting.

■ Avoid medical jargon when talking to patients. Even words you might assume are common parlance like abdomen are foreign to many patients; just try asking non-medics what a prostate is!

■ Give people information in bite-size chunks that they can manage. This is especially important for people who are anxious or when you are relaying frightening information.

■ Use conceptually clear diagrams wherever possible to explain yourself. Remember that anatomically correct diagrams may be more confusing than conceptually clear ones.

■ Be straightforward with patients. Answer questions honestly, even if it means saying that you don't know.

■ Do not be pushed into committing yourself to a diagnosis or prognosis if you do not have good evidence for it. Always offer to speak to your registrar or consultant if the patient requires further clarification regarding this.

Patients' families

Patients' families suffer terribly from lack of information from hospital staff. You can greatly alleviate this with minimal effort, and you will be showered with gratitude. If possible, take the patient's nurse with you to ensure continuity of care. There are two main problems you can easily help with: patient discharge and informing families about their relative.

Information about patient discharge

Making arrangements for home care can be a major ordeal, particularly for families where everyone works. You can make a big difference if you or the nurse can let the family know as soon as possible:

1 When (and if) the patient can go home and, if possible, if it is in the morning or afternoon. It may be possible for your patient to leave at a time that is convenient for family routines

2 Special instructions that the patient will need to follow at home and when they should go and see their GP

3 Drugs that will be needed and when in the near future

4 Who they can contact if something goes wrong

Hints

■ Find out the discharge procedure from nurses.

■ Be aware of hospital visiting hours so that you can tell families when patients are admitted. If they are not available during those times, a cursory phone call can go a long way to alleviate relatives' anxieties.

■ Liaise with nurses, social workers and occupational therapists, as they often have important information for patients and their families on discharge.

■ Remember that many people will not challenge a doctor and may endure a lot of hassle to do what you say, even when it makes no difference to the ward. If families are looking unhappy, ask them what's wrong. You may be able to help with little effort.

■ Imagine the patient was your relative and you had to look after them – what would you need to know?

■ Ask family members if they have any questions.

Information about what's wrong with the patient

(See Chapter 8, Breaking bad news.)
Your main duty is to care for the patient, not their family; you should get the patient's permission before divulging information to any family member. Taking time in a non-stressful environment to explain things to family members can be invaluable. Families remember how doctors explained things to them. Key features that we find make a difference include:

■ Take the family to a private room. This enables people to remember information and ask questions.

■ Try to get rid of your bleep. Hand it to a colleague.

■ Have all investigations and findings to hand. Be ready to answer lots of questions and be ready to admit uncertainty.

■ Write in the notes what you have told the family and tell the nursing staff; this is very important in cases with a poor prognosis.

■ Have tissues and cups of tea handy if breaking bad news.

■ If possible, collect all family members for one chat. Have the family nominate one family member to be the spokesperson. This is helpful in big families as it helps you avoid getting caught in the middle of family disputes and repeating yourself every time a family member turns up.

■ If the news is bad or unexpected, it may be courteous to ask your senior to see the family first.

Confidentiality

Breaches of confidentiality may be both unlawful and amount to professional misconduct, and you may be called upon to justify any such breach. Keeping confidentiality is not always as easy as it sounds – you may need to discuss patient histories with many people, both within the hospital and the community. The following guidelines should help you to keep legal confidentiality:

■ Refer to patients by name as little as possible.

■ Do not discuss confidential information with people over the phone unless you are certain of their identity and that they are authorized to receive the information.

■ Never discuss patients in public places, such as lifts and hospital canteens.

■ Never discuss anything with the press if approached. Refer immediately to your consultant or the hospital manager.

■ Refer police officers to your senior; do not feel pressured into discussing patients if you are unhappy.

■ Take care when discussing patients over the phone. Transfer ward calls to the doctors' office wherever possible. It is easy to find yourself shouting above the noise of a ward only to find that the entire ward can hear you.

■ Remember that curtains are not soundproof. If you have confidential or delicate

information to convey or obtain, consider taking the patient to a side room.

■ Do not talk about patients so that they may be identified outside of immediately relevant hospital settings. For example, don't tell your dinner guests stories about patients that they may recognize, even if you don't name them. It is better to avoid this kind of thing altogether, however entertaining it may be.

■ The MDU and MPS both have 24-hour advice lines if you are a member.

Exceptions to keeping confidentiality

There are common-sense exceptions to confidentiality, such as when you have good reason to believe that the patient is likely to cause death or serious harm to themselves or others. Sometimes, it may not be clear as to whether you should or shouldn't respect confidentiality. For example, if a patient admits a crime to you, should you tell anyone about it? As a general rule, if in doubt, you should:

■ Always ask your consultant for advice.

■ Document your decision and other relevant information in the notes to cover yourself in the event of a court case or complaint. Your medical defence insurer can advise you further if required.

Never promise absolute confidentiality.

References

1   Milne R., Chambers L. (1993) Assessing the scientific quality of review articles. *Journal of Epidemiology and Community Health* **47**, 169–170.

2   Breaking Bad News: Regional Guidelines from The National Council for Hospice and Palliative Care Services (2003). (Available at www.dhsspsni.gov.uk/breaking_bad_news.pdf)

Chapter 6
EMERGENCIES

This chapter covers the most common medical and surgical emergencies you are likely to see as a foundation doctor or whilst in A&E. We have provided common algorithms to follow, but each trust may have local policies on the intranet that you can also use.

Some common medical emergencies

1 Acute coronary syndrome
2 Stroke
3 Deep venous thrombosis (DVT) and pulmonary embolus (PE)
4 Haematemesis
5 Acute asthma
6 Acute pneumothorax
7 Anaphylaxis
8 Meningitis
9 Collapse or reduced mobility
10 Overdose

Acute coronary syndrome

This term covers a spectrum of disease, from unstable angina to an evolving myocardial infarction (MI).

The management will vary according to whether there is new left bundle branch block (LBBB) or ST elevation and according to the facilities available at your hospital. As usual assess A, B, C, D and E for each patient when they arrive, and treat life-threatening hypoxia or hypotension immediately.

If the patient is breathing spontaneously and maintaining their own airway, then the first step is generally to apply high-flow oxygen through a non-rebreathing mask. After establishing intravenous (IV) access, obtain a set of observations and give morphine for pain relief.

Take a focused history to elicit when the chest pain has started and pertinent cardiac risk factors:

- Previous MI or ischaemic heart disease
- Hypertension
- Diabetes mellitus
- Hypercholesterolaemia
- Smoking
- Family history

Important investigations include:

- Bloods for full blood count (FBC), urea and electrolytes (U+E), rise in troponin and clotting.
- An electrocardiogram (ECG) should be urgently performed to assess whether there is an indication for PCI or thrombolysis. The patient should be kept on continuous cardiac monitoring.

Figures 6.1 and 6.2 are provided as references to ensure that you don't miss a crucial step. They are taken from the NICE guidelines for STEMI and NSTEMI pathways. Your hospital will also have a local policy.

The Hands-on Guide to the Foundation Programme, Fifth Edition. Anna Donald, Michael Stein, Ciaran Scott Hill and Selina J Chavda.
© 2015 John Wiley & Sons, Ltd. Published 2015 by John Wiley & Sons, Ltd.

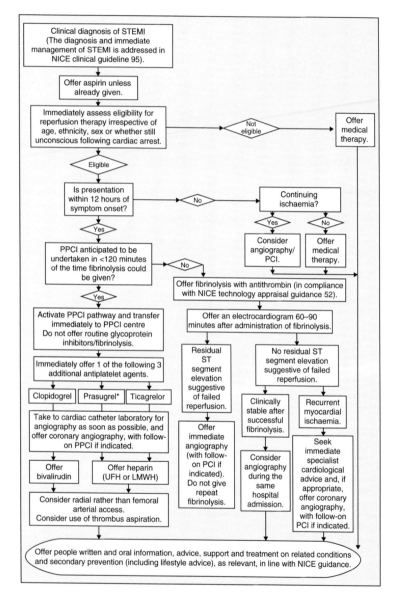

Figure 6.1 Acute MI (new ST elevation or new LBBB). National Institute for Health and Care Excellence (2013) Adapted from CG 167 Myocardial infarction with ST-segment elevation: the acute management of myocardial infarction with ST-segment elevation. Manchester: NICE. Available from http://guidance.nice.org.uk/CG167. Reproduced with permission.

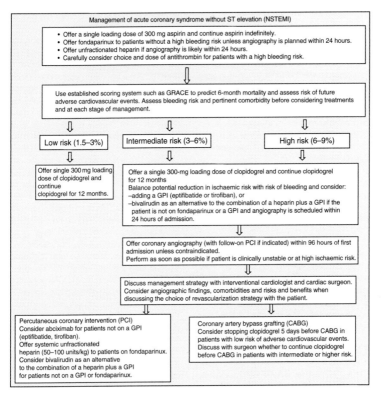

Figure 6.2 Acute coronary syndrome without ST elevation. National Institute for Health and Care Excellence (2010) Adapted from CG 94 Unstable angina and NSTEMI: the early management of unstable angina and non-ST-segment-elevation myocardial infarction. Manchester: NICE. Available from http://guidance.nice.org.uk/CG94. Reproduced with permission.

Stroke

Nationally, strokes are now dealt with at hospitals with hyper-acute stroke units (HASU) departments. Hospitals providing this service are able to administer thrombolysis as clinically indicated, and anyone who has had a suspected stroke should be taken there if any suggestive symptoms are present. These centres also run clinical trials, and so patients may have other treatments as part of a trial if they meet the selection criteria. Thrombolysis is currently indicated if onset of symptoms has occurred within four and a half hours of presentation.

It is unlikely that you will have to deal with a suspected acute stroke by yourself. However, there are always exceptions, in particular if a stroke has occurred but has not been recognized. It is therefore important to have a grasp of the initial emergency management and a knowledge of whom to contact when you suspect a stroke.

Start by making an initial assessment of the patient using an airway, breathing, circulation (ABC) approach. Provide any necessary urgent interventions such as oxygen and airway manoeuvres, IV fluids, controlling seizures and contacting intensive therapy unit (ITU) if the patient is likely to require intubation. Much of the medical management of a stroke is done after the patient reaches the ward, for example, organizing an echocardiogram and carotid Dopplers or starting anticoagulation. In A&E, assess the patient and then discuss with a senior colleague with a view to arranging imaging (CT head) and then considering transfer to a HASU. Once you have ruled out a bleed on CT, you can start 300 mg of aspirin, unless there are contraindications. Discuss with your senior or the stroke registrar on call if you are unsure.

If the patient's symptoms have resolved, this may suggest a transient ischaemic attack (TIA). You should perform an ABCD^2 score which predicts risk of a completed stroke over the coming days. A score of 4 or more indicates high risk of an early stroke. In addition, a person is at higher risk (even with a low score) if they have had 2 or more TIAs within 1 week (crescendo attacks). Those at high risk should be seen and assessed by a specialist within 24 hours, for example, in an outpatient TIA clinic the next day. If the score is ≤3 with no other episodes in the past week, they can be seen within 1 week. If the patient is on anticoagulation but has had symptoms of a TIA, they must have brain imaging immediately.

DVT and PE

Once you have reviewed a patient and suspect a DVT or PE, it is important to estimate the likelihood of these conditions. This will guide further investigations and management.

The pretest probability of a DVT is calculated using the Well's Score.

A score of ≥3 suggests high probability of DVT/PE, and so the patient should be treated. The same should be done with those patients with intermediate probability of DVT/PE. If they have a low likelihood, then a D-dimer test should be performed. Be wary of a raised D-dimer, as it is not specific for DVT and can be raised in a broad range of conditions including pregnancy, inflammation and malignancy. A negative D-dimer is a good way to exclude a DVT/PE, but if positive, you should treat and investigate.

Patients can generally be given LMWH injections at a treatment dose. This is calculated

according to their weight. Consult the *BNF* or your local hospital protocol for advice.

The USS scan can then be performed either the same day as an inpatient or if it is out of hours then urgently as an outpatient. If they do have a DVT and oral anticoagulation needs to be started, they should continue LMWH injections outside of hospital until their international normalized ratio (prothrombin ratio) reaches a therapeutic level. They will need to be taught how to inject, or they will need referral to district nurses.

Most PEs arise as a consequence of existing DVTs. Other possible sources include septic emboli from right-sided endocarditis or air, fluid, amniotic or fat emboli. Assess for risk factors (pregnancy/oral contraceptive pill/recent flights/immobilization in hospital/active malignancy/thrombophilia/recent surgery).

Once you have assessed the patient and ensured they are stable, perform the usual baseline tests including an arterial blood gas (ABG) and chest X-ray (CXR). Only perform a D-dimer test if the patient has a low probability of PE. If it is negative, you can reliably exclude PE. Imaging is usually a computerized tomography pulmonary angiogram (CTPA) and is now the recommended first-line imaging modality.

Thrombolysis is the treatment of choice for massive PE (i.e. where the PE has caused circulatory collapse). If it seems likely the patient may have a cardiac arrest, this can be given on clinical grounds alone. Otherwise, imaging (CTPA) should be arranged within 1 hour.

Haematemesis

Haematemesis can be a frightening prospect. You can do the best for your patient by following a series of important steps before definitive management, and control of bleeding is performed at endoscopy.

There are a number of causes of haematemesis. The following list gives the most common causes:

■ Peptic ulcer disease
■ Mallory–Weiss tears
■ Oesophagitis
■ Oesophageal varices

- Gastritis
- Malignancy
- Drugs such as non-steroidal anti-inflammatory drugs, anticoagulants and steroids

The patient may vomit fresh blood or 'coffee grounds'. There are a number of scoring systems for predicting mortality in upper GI bleeds, including the Rockall risk-scoring system and the Glasgow–Blatchford system for predicting those patients who are likely to need medical intervention.

When a patient presents in shock (tachycardic/hypotensive/oliguric), the following algorithm should be followed.

Initial management
- Protect airway to prevent aspiration – keep NBM.
- Insert two large-bore cannulae into each antecubital fossa.
- Take bloods to include coagulation screen, G and S, and crossmatch 4–6 units. Keep Hb > 8.
- Catheterize and monitor urine output (>30 ml/hour), and perform observations every 15 minutes.
- In patients with massive bleeding and shock, activate major haemorrhage protocol and transfuse O Rh-ve blood, clotting factors and platelets as advised by haematology.
- Notify surgical team of patients with severe bleeding in case of need for surgery.

⇩

If haemodynamically stable
- Give rapid fluids IV (N saline) until blood arrives, and then transfuse with blood.
- Correct coagulopathy with FFP and vitamin K.
- Give platelets if plt count <50 and actively bleeding.
- Give prothrombin complex to patients on warfarin and actively bleeding.

⇩

Endoscopy
- Perform endoscopy immediately if severe UGIB or within 24 hours for all other patients.
- Give PPIs (80 mg omeprazole/pantoprazole) post-endoscopy if signs of recent haemorrhage and non-variceal bleed.
- Send tissue samples for *H. pylori* (CLO test) if there is non-variceal bleed.
- Perform repeat endoscopy in patients who re-bleed after OGD, and consider interventional radiology or surgery as needed.
- If the cause of bleeding is varices, give terlipressin and broad-spectrum antibiotic cover.
- At endoscopy, variceal band ligation is performed.
- In uncontrollable variceal bleeding, consider TIPS procedure.
- Calculate Rockall score.

Consider following these steps with any reasonable suspicion of an upper GI bleed, as patients can continue to have occult bleeding and may deteriorate suddenly.

Acute asthma

An acute exacerbation of asthma can be very frightening for both the patient and the doctor. Patients can deteriorate quickly and so you need to instigate treatment quickly and recognize the near-fatal asthmatic exacerbation before it is too late. Escalate unwell patients quickly as they may need intubating and ITU care. The following guidelines are taken from the up-to-date BTS guidelines which can be found online at http://www.brit-thoracic.org.uk/Portals/0/Guidelines/AsthmaGuidelines/

Levels of asthma severity
Near-fatal asthma – Raised $PaCO_2$ and/or requiring mechanical ventilation with raised inflation pressures

Life-threatening asthma

Clinical signs	Objective investigations
Altered conscious level	PEF <33% best or predicted
Exhaustion	SpO$_2$ < 92%
Arrhythmia	PaO$_2$ < 8 kPa
Hypotension	Normal PaCO$_2$ (4.6–6.0 kPa)
Cyanosis	
Silent chest	
Poor respiratory effort	

Acute severe asthma

Any one of the following:

– PEF 33–50% best or predicted
– Respiratory rate ≥25 per minute
– Heart rate ≥110 per minute
– Inability to complete sentences in one breath

Brittle asthma

– Type 1: wide PEF variability (>40% diurnal variation for >50% of the time over a period >150 days) despite intense therapy
– Type 2: sudden severe attacks on a background of apparently well-controlled asthma

Take a brief history if you can regarding the triggers and number of hospital admissions including to ITU. Also assess for an infective exacerbation. Perform a focused examination also.

Investigations include:

● Bloods: FBC, U + E and C-reactive protein (CRP) in blood cultures if febrile
● ABG to assess for hypoxia and hypercapnia
● CXR for pneumothorax and signs of infection

Management includes:

1 High-flow oxygen.

2 Nebulizers driven on oxygen:

● Salbutamol 2.5–5 mg nebulizers
● Ipratropium bromide 500 mcg nebulizers (4–6 hourly)

Nebulizers can be given 'back to back' (i.e. one after another) if needed to try and improve wheeze.

3 Steroids: orally if the patient can swallow 40 mg prednisolone or 100–200 mg of IV hydrocortisone.

4 If there is no improvement, give 1.2–2 g IV magnesium sulphate. This decision is usually one that is discussed with a senior/specialist and requires cardiac monitoring.

5 Consider aminophylline if there is no improvement: load with 5 mg/kg if theophylline naive, and then use a maintenance dose of 500 mcg/kg/hour based on ideal body weight.

6 Inform ITU early if patient has life-threatening/ acute severe asthma or is deteriorating and not responding to medical therapy. Don't wait until they are peri-arrest to make this decision.

7 Routine use of antibiotics is not recommended, so only give them if you suspect an infective exacerbation (yellow/green sputum, fevers). Treat as per CAP guidelines (co-amoxiclav and clarithromycin should do the trick).

Acute pneumothorax

Pneumothorax is a diagnosis that isn't often seen but should never be forgotten. They commonly occur in young, tall, thin men spontaneously as a result of bullae rupturing. Common symptoms include sudden onset of breathlessness and pleuritic chest pain. Examination will show hyperresonance of percussion over the affected lung field and reduced breath sounds.

Investigations include:

● Bloods: FBC, U + E and coagulation
● ABG if concerned re hypoxia
● CXR

If you suspect a tension pneumothorax (i.e. one that is causing a significant impairment in respiratory or cardiovascular function), don't wait for a CXR – insert a large-bore cannula into the patient's second intercostal space, midclavicular line on the side of the suspected pneumothorax. Insert the needle all the way to the hilt. You should hear a hissing noise as the air escapes. It sounds scary, but you might save the patient's life and prevent them from arresting. It is worth noting that in many cases this method of decompression is inadequate. It is never a definitive treatment.

Treatment depends on age and co-morbidities. See the flow chart (Fig. 6.3) based on BTS guidelines.

Anaphylaxis

Anaphylaxis is a medical emergency. In true anaphylaxis, the patient will likely arrest unless they have adrenaline IM quickly. Anaphylaxis is a type I hypersensitivity reaction and is IgE mediated causing release of histamine and vasodilators. There are many precipitants including nuts, latex, fish, eggs and medications such as penicillins or contrast media. In some cases, however, no cause is found. Patients present with breathlessness, wheeze, tongue/lips swelling and periorbital oedema. Occasionally, patients may present in anaphylactic shock, with significant hypotension and tachycardia. If you suspect anaphylaxis, involve the anaesthetist early before the patient loses their airway – it is much easier to intubate an unobstructed airway.

If the cause is found, make sure the patient has advice on medic alert bracelets, avoiding the offending pathogen, and is taught how to use an EpiPen.

Investigations include:

• Bloods: can be done at the same time as gaining large-bore IV access but should not delay treatment. Serum tryptase can be helpful for purely academic purposes.

Treatment of anaphylaxis is simple:

1 Give high-flow oxygen and call the anaesthetist early. Intubate if needed. Do not force the patient to lie flat if they do not want to. This can trigger obstruction.

2 Give adrenaline IM 0.5 mg (0.5 ml of 1 in 1000) immediately and every 5 minutes until the anaphylaxis improves (BP improves,

tachycardia settles). By the time of the second dose, the anaesthetic team should be present. There is fear amongst juniors in initiating the adrenaline, but remember that if in doubt, then just give it. If the patient has anaphylaxis, the risk of harm is far greater from under-treatment than overtreatment.

3 Give IV fluids to support BP.

4 Give 10 mg of chlorpheniramine IV and 200 mg of hydrocortisone IV.

5 If a wheeze is present, treat as per acute asthma.

If the patient remains unstable/intubated, they will need transfer to ITU.

Meningitis

Meningitis is a medical condition that kills. It affects all ages and patients can become unwell very quickly. Symptoms include headaches, fevers (although in the elderly or immunocompromised there may not be a temperature spike), neck stiffness/meningism, photophobia and petechial non-blanching rash. Seizures and change in personality may suggest viral encephalitis.

Bacterial causes include meningococcus, pneumococcus and listeria.

Investigations include:

• Bloods: FBC, U+E, liver function tests (LFTs), CRP, coagulation, group and save (G&S), polymerase chain reaction (PCR) meningococcus and streptococcus, blood cultures and serology for Epstein–Barr virus, HIV and HSV

• Swabs: throat (viral and rectal)

• CT head looking for signs of raised intracranial pressure (ICP)

• Cerebrospinal fluid for protein, glucose, MC&S, gram stain, acid-fast bacillus and viral PCR (only perform lumbar puncture (LP) if there are no signs of raised ICP)

Treatment includes

1 IV ceftriaxone 2 g IV QDS, and if over 55 years old, add 2 g of ampicillin 4 hourly.

2 If concerned regarding encephalitis, add IV acicyclovir 10 mg/kg TDS.

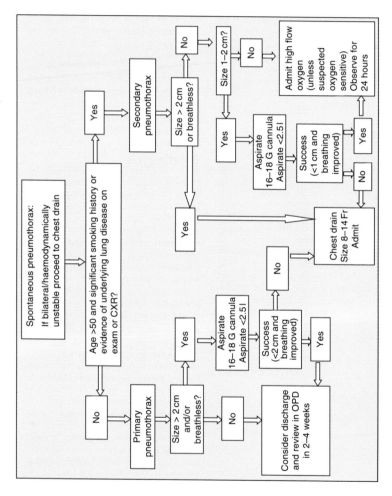

Figure 6.3 Management of acute pneumothorax as per BTS Guidelines. Reproduced with permission of British Thoracic Society and BMJ Publishing.

3 Steroids can be used in certain cases but should be discussed with the microbiologist before giving. It is generally indicated for pneumococcal meningitis and given in a dose of 0.15 mg/kg.

4 If there is any sign of raised ICP, call ITU immediately and the neurosurgeons. Only perform an LP if the CT head clearly excludes obstructive hydrocephalus or mass lesion (if in doubt, ask a radiologist/neurosurgeon), and give antibiotics urgently.

Collapse or reduced mobility

The potential causes of these problems are almost endless. Furthermore, as they are predominantly a problem in elderly patients with multiple co-morbidities, there is likely to be a number of factors playing a part in each individual patient. Often, such episodes are written off as a 'mechanical fall' or 'acopia'. These are not very helpful labels as they don't give any indication as to the underlying reasons for the collapse or reduction in mobility.

When faced with such a patient, first try to establish whether there has been any loss of consciousness. This can be much easier if there are witnesses accompanying the patient.

Syncope is defined as a transient loss of consciousness due to reduced cerebral perfusion. It can be broadly divided into cardiac and non-cardiac syncope.

Causes of cardiac syncope are:
- Peripheral factors causing hypotension: drugs/sepsis/posture.
- *Vasovagal syncope.*
- Vasovagal syncope is syncope secondary to stimulation of the vagal system due to factors such as pain or fear.

Cardiac syncope can be due to a number of conditions. These include aortic stenosis/arrhythmias/MI or ischaemia/structural diseases, such as cardiomyopathy.

The main differentials for syncope are seizures and metabolic disorders such as hypoglycaemia, uraemia or drug intoxication.

Take a careful history covering the circumstances of the fall, any associated symptoms or prodrome, previous falls and usual functional state. Carefully review medications especially in the elderly as antihypertensives and diuretics are the usual culprits. Check if the patient has been started on any new medication recently.

A thorough exam focusing on the cardiovascular, neurological and musculoskeletal systems is important. Consider all the co-morbidities and make a list of the most important contributing factors.

Investigations include:

- Blood glucose
- Basic bloods to look for infection: FBC and CRP (elderly patients can become confused when they have an infection, which makes them more prone to fall)
- Lying/standing BP
- ECG
- 24 hour tape
- Echocardiogram

Management depends on the underlying cause.

Overdose

There is obviously a huge variety of potential toxins which people can ingest, deliberately or otherwise. It is unrealistic to think that you will be up to date with the management of overdose of all medications and substances, although you will become familiar with paracetamol and salicylates.

The most important resource to be aware of is ToxBase, which is an online site that gives information on the treatment of overdose or accidental ingestion of most substances. Your A&E department will have an account, so make sure you find out the login details before you start.

Do not panic with overdose patients. There is usually more time than you think to sort them out and the vast majority have not taken devastating overdoses. Get senior medical assistance if the patient is in a critical condition. They may need transfer to ITU if they have a reduced **Glasgow Coma Scale** (GCS) or arrhythmias on their ECG.

In general

■ If in *any* doubt about how to treat someone, you can also phone the 24 hour National Poisons Information Service for more advice. You can also call the information services from ToxBase; they have a 24 hour on-call poisons expert to answer questions.

National Poisons Information Service
0844 892 0111 (www.toxbase.org)

■ The *BNF* has an excellent section on treatments for different substance overdoses at the beginning of the book (look under 'Poison' in the index).

Treating the patient

First, perform a brief initial assessment of the patient (ABC)

1 If the patient is unconscious, perform basic airway management and seek senior help urgently. If the GCS is falling or <8 or the respiratory rate is low, then consider early intubation. Call the anaesthetist early if this is the case. Check the airway for obstruction, dentures or vomit in any unresponsive patient.

2 Check for and treat hypoxia, hypotension and hypovolaemia. Also assess whether there is hypoglycaemia, hypothermia or arrhythmias.

Obtain a capillary blood glucose and ECG as well as basic observations. Consider doing a blood gas and, if necessary, a rectal temperature.

3 Secure IV access and take bloods (including paracetamol and salicylate levels as well as a clotting screen and LFTs). Paracetamol levels should be taken not less than 4 hours after ingestion, aspirin not less than 6 hours (longer may be necessary if the tablets have enteric coating). Every patient who states they have taken an overdose of any drug should have paracetamol and salicylate levels done routinely, as patients may conceal this or do not realize that the drugs they have taken contain these:

■ Lethal paracetamol overdoses may not become apparent for several days, when the person starts to become jaundiced or develop bleeding. The Parvolex treatment chart found in A&E, in the *BNF*, and on ToxBase is used to assess whether or not the patient needs treatment with a Parvolex infusion (N-acetylcysteine or 'NAC'). Take blood levels at least 4 hours after the patient has ingested the tablets.

■ If the level is *on or above* the line, the patient needs urgent treatment. Potential serious side effects of NAC include bronchospasm, hypoglycaemia, shock and vomiting. Glucose should be checked hourly. Newer guidelines suggest erring on the side of treatment if uncertain.

Guidance regarding paracetamol overdose

■ All patients with a timed plasma paracetamol level on or above a single treatment line joining points of 100 mg/l at 4 hours and 15 mg/l at 15 hours after ingestion should receive N-acetylcysteine (Parvolex or generics) based on the treatment nomogram (Fig. 6.4), regardless of risk factors for hepatotoxicity.

■ Intravenous N-acetylcysteine is the antidote to treat paracetamol overdose and is virtually 100% effective in preventing liver damage when given within 8 hours of the overdose. After this time, efficacy falls substantially and serious hepatotoxicity can occur. Where there is doubt over the timing of paracetamol ingestion including when ingestion has occurred over a period of 1 hour or more – 'staggered overdose' – N-acetylcysteine should *always* be given without delay (the nomogram should not be used).

■ Administer the initial dose of N-acetylcysteine as an infusion over 60 minutes to minimize the risk of common dose-related adverse reactions.

■ Hypersensitivity is no longer a contraindication to treatment with N-acetylcysteine.

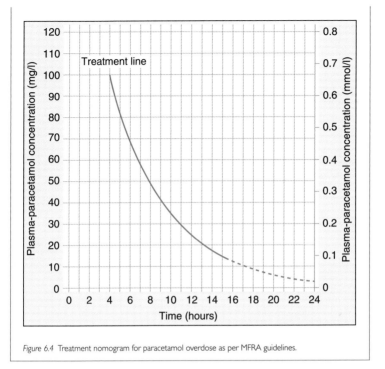

Figure 6.4 Treatment nomogram for paracetamol overdose as per MFRA guidelines.

■ Aspirin overdose initially causes a respiratory alkalosis due to direct stimulation of the respiratory centres. Patients then develop a metabolic acidosis, so serial ABGs should be performed if the overdose is significant. Features include tachypnoea, tachycardia and tinnitus.

Second, complete a more thorough history and examination

1 If possible, get a thorough history from the patient *as well as* from whoever is accompanying them. Try to ascertain:

- What precipitated the attempt
- Timing of the overdose and whether they used alcohol at the same time
- Previous attempts at overdose or other self-harm

- Premeditation of the overdose
- Any history of alcohol or drug abuse
- Any factors that make the attempt seem serious, such as a suicide note, or taking the overdose in a place where they were unlikely to be found
- Regret regarding the overdose and whether they would reattempt in the future

Building up such a picture can help you assess how likely the patient is to make another attempt at suicide. Risk factors include psychiatric disorders, physical illness, social isolation, unemployment and being male.

2 Examine the patient thoroughly.

3 Perform a mini-mental test score.

4 Discuss the patient with your senior regarding continuing supportive care and more definitive treatments. Additionally, you

will need to refer the patient to the psychiatrists. Patients are usually admitted under the medical team for a review by the mental health liaison team once they are medically well.

Surgery

The most common surgical emergencies you will encounter in A&E are:

Appendicitis
Cholecystitis
Bowel obstruction (large or small)
Leaking abdominal aortic aneurysm (AAA)
Renal colic (easily confused with AAA)
Ischaemic bowel
Ischaemic limb
Pancreatitis
PR bleeding

The good thing about all of these is that your role in the management is generally quite similar for each and involves recognizing the potential diagnosis, performing baseline investigations and initiating any non-surgical treatments such as antibiotics, pain relief and IV fluids. You should make the surgical team aware of the patient early on. If you think a person has a leaking AAA, do not wait until you have got the bloods and X-rays back before talking to someone!

On admission, you should:

1 Perform a focused history and examination.

2 Obtain baseline tests:

● Bloods: FBC/U&E/clotting/glucose/amylase/ CRP/G&S or crossmatch

● Urine: MSU + dipstick (consider pregnancy test if the patient is a young female with abdominal pain)

● ECG

● Radiology: abdominal X-ray (plain) (consider erect CXR if concerned about perforation)

3 Obtain IV access.

4 Write up IV fluids and regular medications on a drug chart.

You should ensure that patients have adequate pain relief. There is a common feeling that patients should not receive analgesia in case it masks any signs. This is never true:

● Diclofenac sodium (Voltarol) provides effective pain relief for renal colic. It can be given by rectal suppository or IM if the patient is vomiting/NBM.

● Occasionally, patients who are seeking opiates or a stay in hospital may fake surgical conditions. Look for needle marks, small pupils and odd histories. If you suspect a patient is faking pain, ask for senior advice. Although it may be undesirable to provide opiates for non-medical reasons, it is worse to fail to provide analgesia to someone who actually requires it. Bear in mind that if your patient is an opiate addict *and* has a real surgical condition, then they will need extra relief for severe pain.

Chapter 7
CARDIAC ARRESTS AND CRASH CALLS

You will almost certainly be a member of the hospital cardiac arrest team. If you are first on the scene, the absolute priority is to ensure adequate ventilation and perfusion – basic life support. It is one of the few occasions when a well-learnt plan of action is essential. Do not panic. Following the well-learnt advanced life support (ALS) algorithm is essential. For the most up-to-date information, please refer to the Resuscitation Council guidelines, available free at www.resus.org. uk. These are frequently updated and are fantastic learning tools.

Cardiac arrest calls

You do not have time to 'make a diagnosis'. Stay calm and then perform DR ABC:

1 Check for danger around the patient, and move yourself/the patient out of the way of harm.

2 Check if the patient is responsive by performing a 'squeeze, shake and shout'. This is exactly what it says on the tin. Squeeze the patient's shoulder, shake them to see if they wake up, and shout in their ears. If they are unresponsive, then:

• Shout for help – don't be shy!
• Turn the patient onto their back so that they are lying flat.
• Open the airway, and check that there is nothing obstructing the airway, like dentures, chewing gum, vomit, etc. Finger sweeps are out of vogue. If you need to use suction, do so, but only suction as far as you can see, that is, not down their airway. Once you are happy the airway is clear, perform a head tilt/chin lift.

Assess the patient's breathing (look/listen/feel for breathing/chest rise and fall for a maximum of 10 seconds.

The most up-to-date basic life support algorithm now in place does not ask people to assess for carotid pulses as it wastes time and proceeds straight to chest compressions. If the patient is making meaningful respiratory efforts, then opening the airway to avoid hypoxia is essential. It is a recognized fact that even well-trained doctors often cannot make an accurate assessment of whether a patient is in cardiac arrest or not. Agonal breathing (occasional gasps, slow, laboured or noisy breathing) is common in the early stages of cardiac arrest and is a sign of cardiac arrest and should not be confused as a sign of life/ circulation.

3 If you have confirmed cardiac arrest get help, preferably in the form of the resuscitation team. All UK hospitals should now use the standard 'crash call' number: 2222. You can ask someone else to do this whilst you remain with the patient, but remember that getting help is essential. State where you are (ward and bed number), that there is an adult cardiac arrest and that you require the adult cardiac arrest team.

4 Ensure that the airway is secure by using adjuncts such as oropharyngeal airways or nasopharyngeal airways if necessary; note that the former may trigger gagging or vomiting if the patient is not truly in cardiac arrest. Administer oxygen. You should only be inserting supraglottic airway devices or attempting tracheal intubation if you are specifically trained

The Hands-on Guide to the Foundation Programme, Fifth Edition. Anna Donald, Michael Stein, Ciaran Scott Hill and Selina J Chavda.
© 2015 John Wiley & Sons, Ltd. Published 2015 by John Wiley & Sons, Ltd.

to do so. It is definitely not the time to 'have a go'. The dangers to the patient of delays in chest compressions, failed intubations (particularly unrecognized) and laryngeal stimulation are huge. Any attempt must be confirmed by clinical examination and capnography.

5 Ensure someone, preferably two people working in rotations, commence adequate cardiopulmonary resuscitation (CPR, 30 chest compressions followed by 2 breaths). If you are on your own without a bag–valve–mask or oxygen, then focus on the chest compressions. These are your absolute priority. Maintaining a cardiac output is key in prolonging life, so compressions *must* be effective. Perform chest compressions at a rate of 100–120 beats per minute, at a depth of 5–6 cm.

6 Attach a defibrillator, ideally with a cardiac monitor. This should be done and defibrillation attempted (if indicated) within 3 minutes of the confirming arrest. If no cardiac trolley is readily available, a portable automated external defibrillator (AED) may be available. These AEDs provide voice prompts and are portable. Make sure the pads are applied properly and in the correct position. The pads have pictures printed on them to show you where to apply them. Ensure you have good contact with the chest. If necessary, remove chest hair. Do not stop chest compressions when applying the pads. If you are going to deliver a shock (in line with the Resuscitation Council guidance), then 'hands-off' time, that is, the pause between stopping compressions and delivering the shock, should be minimized to less than 5 seconds.

7 Attach cardiac monitoring and gain IV access.

8 Use the ALS algorithm in Figure 7.1, based on the new ALS guidelines by the Resuscitation Council (United Kingdom). We strongly recommend you read the guidelines in full (available from the Resuscitation Council (United Kingdom) website or the resuscitation officer in your hospital). This also contains guidance on how to proceed if you are fortunate enough to achieve return of spontaneous circulation (ROSC) in your patient.

Hints

1 Find out how the defibrillator works and learn the layout of your hospital's arrest trolley. Ensure you enrol on an intermediate life support or ALS course as soon as possible. If you do not know how to attach the defibrillators used in your hospital, you must learn how to do so as soon as possible.

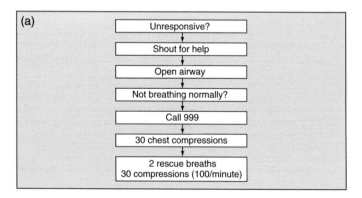

Figure 7.1 Protocol for (a) basic life support and (b) advanced life support (adults). Reproduced with the kind permission of the Resuscitation Council (UK).

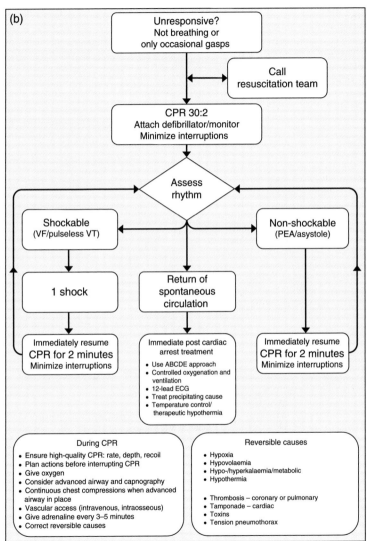

Figure 7.1 (continued)

2 Always wear gloves. Ideally, you should also use 'universal precautions'; these include a mask, eye shield and protective clothing. Be aware of sharps that may not have been disposed of properly, particularly those thrown on the floor.

3 Note the time of the crash call so you can keep track of how long the resuscitation has been in progress. If there are an adequate number of people nominate a scribe to note time and events.

4 The crash team will usually consist of a medical registrar, an anaesthetist, specialist trainees, and FY trainees, as well as nursing staff. It may feel chaotic but it is important that everyone has an allocated role (usually delineated by the team leader) to ensure the arrest call is run smoothly. As a junior, this may be in the form of performing compressions, scribing/keeping time, gaining venous access/bloods/arterial blood gases, giving drugs or tracking down the medical background. If you are unsure of your role, ask!

5 It is useful to know the patient's medical background although this is not a priority. Look for risk factors. The main causes of an arrest are divided into the '4 H's and 4T's':

- Hypovolaemia due to bleeding (e.g. oesophageal varices, recent surgery, bleeding disorder) or dehydration
- Hypo-/hyperkalaemia (e.g. anuric patient after major surgery, patient with severe renal impairment) and low glucose levels (always make sure a BM has been done)
- Hypoxia (e.g. due to choking)
- Hypothermia (remember the saying 'you're not dead until you're warm and dead')
- Tension pneumothorax (e.g. recent central line placement, chest drain, surgical procedures)
- Pericardial tamponade (e.g. recent chest trauma, recent MI, recent cardiothoracic surgery)
- Venous thromboembolism causing deep venous thrombosis or pulmonary embolus (e.g. major pelvic surgery or hip surgery)
- Toxins commonly due to drug overdose (e.g. dilated/constricted pupils, (intravenous drug user (IVDU) track marks, smell of alcohol)

The most common unexpected cardiac arrest calls in inpatients are due to pulmonary embolus and electrolyte imbalances. This is somewhat different to out-of-hospital cardiac arrests where primary cardiac causes predominate.

6 Cardiac arrest is traumatic for other patients on the ward. Use professional language and stay calm. Draw the curtains round the other patient cubicles if necessary.

7 After an unsuccessful arrest call, be sensitive to the fact that nurses and other doctors may have a close relationship with the patient and may be quite distressed by the death.

8 Always check to see if the patient has a 'not for resus in the event of cardiac arrest' form. This should be written clearly in the notes (see 'Do not resuscitate orders'). When in doubt, your duty is to attempt to save the patient's life, and so if there is any doubt, begin CPR.

9 If you are with a very unwell patient who you suspect might arrest in a few minutes, get help fast (e.g. getting your seniors or putting the call out). Many hospital switchboards can 'fast bleep' members of the cardiac arrest team to your location.

10 Cervical spine immobilization is only required in the context of trauma. Don't waste time with it in the context of a purely medical collapse.

'Do not resuscitate' orders

This is a complex area and a frequent cause of complaint and litigation. It is one of the most common reasons for the GMC to take doctors to task. Make sure you read the joint statement from the BMA and the Resuscitation Council (available at http://www.resus.org.uk/pages/dnar.pdf or from the BMA medical ethics department – tel. 020-7383-6286, email: ethics@bma.org.uk). The key points are as follows:

1 The decision not to resuscitate should only be considered when the likelihood of success is very small or if the patient does not wish to be resuscitated.

2 Your consultant is responsible for resuscitation status. Do not change a patient's resuscitation status (in either direction) without discussing the case with your senior. Only a registrar or above can sign the form. This must be countersigned by the consultant at the earliest possible opportunity and also by the nurse in charge. Always document the decision in the notes and state the rationale for the decision. Document the decision clearly – don't use codes like 'not for 2222' or not for arrest call.

3 Good communication is essential. All decisions should be discussed with the entire medical team, the nursing staff, the patient (providing he or she is mentally competent) and the family. This is now a requirement following a recent case in the media, and all DNAR discussions must be discussed with family members or the patient.

4 The decision should take into account the views of the patient, family, close friends and staff. Note that if a competent patient chooses to decline CPR, this decision must be upheld. However, patients cannot demand CPR against the opinion of the senior clinician; they are nevertheless entitled to a second opinion. If the patient lacks mental capacity or defers to the medical team, the consultant is responsible for the decision. Ultimately, decisions regarding CPR status are made by the medical team, but it is now necessary to involve the patient and family in the decision-making process.

5 If the patient has given an advance directive ('living will') whilst mentally competent, this must be followed, even if the patient is now mentally incompetent.

6 'Not for resus' does not preclude any measures short of CPR (this may have to be explained to the family). This is in contrast to patients who are being treated palliatively such as patients who are terminally ill or unlikely to survive and are believed to die over the next few days; these treatment plans are designed to ensure that patients are pain-free and comfortable at their time of death. Often, end-of-life medications are prescribed on the drug chart to prevent pain, nausea, respiratory secretions, agitation and restlessness.

7 Resuscitation status should be reviewed in the light of changes to clinical condition. The form has a section which states whether the DNAR order is indefinite or has a review date, when the order should be reviewed.

8 In the event of an arrest where the status is unclear, resuscitation should be attempted.

9 Documentation of discussions regarding CPR status in the medical notes is imperative, particularly those with relatives and patients.

10 Lastly, fill in the DNAR form as accurately as possible, and in as much detail as you can.

11 If in doubt about these guidelines, ring your defence union (they have a helpline for just such difficulties).

Chapter 8
COMMON CALLS

The Hands-on Guide to the Foundation Programme, Fifth Edition. Anna Donald, Michael Stein,
Ciaran Scott Hill and Selina J Chavda.
© 2015 John Wiley & Sons, Ltd. Published 2015 by John Wiley & Sons, Ltd.

This section provides help with problems you are likely to get bleeped for. In particular, it helps you to exclude serious conditions and to initiate basic mainstay management.

How to use this section

Like a recipe book, this section lists basic protocols for common calls. We recommend the following:

■ When first using the chapter, read the short blurb immediately beneath each call, which lists the most likely causes of each problem and things to watch out for. Differential diagnoses are listed in the way that makes them easiest to remember. Most of the time, this is in order of likelihood in the hospital setting.

■ Remember that unusual presentations of a common condition are more likely than common presentations of rare conditions. Always exclude serious conditions first rather than esoteric conditions. After all, common things are common.

To make this section easy to use in the middle of the night, we have kept abbreviations to a minimum.

Considerations for all ward calls

■ Never hesitate to call your seniors. It is their job to back you up. However, like everyone else, seniors do not like to feel dumped on. Unless it

is a dire emergency or you do not know what to do, make sure you have assessed the problem thoroughly and if possible make a provisional differential diagnosis and management plan. Performing a quick assessment of the airway, breathing and circulation (ABC) and doing basic investigations (e.g. electrocardiogram (ECG) and bloods in chest pain) will make your handover much more effective. Resist the temptation to call them as soon as you find a problem, unless it is immediately life-threatening. You may find that after you have assessed the patient, you do not feel the need to contact them immediately.

■ If you need help, always refer problems upwards (to seniors), not sideways (to other new doctors). No one will support you if things go wrong, and your only source of advice was someone at the same level as you.

■ Always examine patients in a good light even if it means switching on the main light.

■ Even in dire emergencies, act calmly and reassure the patient. If you need urgent senior help, stay with the patient and ask someone else to get hold of your senior. You can always fast bleep them if necessary or pull the crash bell to get help quickly.

■ Keep emergency routines fresh in your mind throughout the year. Patients can deteriorate when you least expect it, such as on rehabilitation wards.

■ After seeing patients, sit down with their notes and review their history to make sure you have not missed something, and document your findings clearly.

■ Whatever you are called for, don't forget to check the drug and fluid charts. A common error of junior doctors is not realizing that a patient's urine output is falling.

■ When tired, try not to argue with nursing or medical colleagues. If you feel you are being bleeped unnecessarily, take the matter up when you are well rested.

■ Do not be too hard on yourself if everything seems daunting. It is! Experience is the only way to develop good clinical judgement and familiarity with practical procedures. You will learn to cope; sometimes it just takes a little time.

Abdominal pain

Your priority is to exclude signs of peritonism and bowel obstruction. Common causes of non-acute abdominal pain, such as urinary tract infection (UTI), constipation and post-op pain, are not life-threatening but may require treatment.

When answering your bleep, ask:

■ For BP, pulse and temp
■ For a dipstick of the urine to look for signs of infection (nitrites, leucocytes and blood)
■ To keep the patient nil by mouth (NBM) until you review them

Differential diagnoses

■ Intestinal obstruction
■ Constipation
■ Adhesions
■ Hernia, volvulus and tumour
■ Peritonism
■ Inflammation/infection of any intra-abdominal organ (e.g. pancreatitis, cholecystitis, appendicitis)
■ Perforated viscus
■ Complications of pregnancy
■ Ruptured intra-abdominal organs (spleen)
■ Ruptured ectopic pregnancy (a life-threatening emergency)
■ Other gynaecological causes (ovarian torsion, tubo-ovarian abscess)
■ Leaking abdominal aortic aneurysm (a life-threatening emergency)
■ Intestinal infarction
■ Peptic ulceration/gastritis/severe oesophagitis

Extra-peritoneal causes include:

■ Urinary retention
■ UTI
■ Renal colic
■ Wound abscess
■ Basal pneumonia
■ Inferior myocardial infarction (MI) (often with associated nausea and vomiting (N&V), bradycardia and ECG changes in leads II, III and AVF)
■ Retroperitoneal bleed or abscess
■ Diabetic ketoacidosis (DKA) – check urinary ketones, BM and ABG for acid–base balance

---

On the ward

1 See the patient immediately. *If peri-arrest*, call for senior help and commence basic life support.

2 If the patient is stable, take a more thorough history and examine the patient. Don't forget to consider:

• Medical history: alcohol, diabetes, inflammatory bowel disease (IBD), ischaemic heart disease (IHD), recent procedures and previous surgery.

• Pain: localization and radiation, onset, character, relieving or aggravating factors and associated symptoms.

• Last menstrual period (LMP) and gynae history: previous peritonitis, pelvic surgery, pelvic inflammatory disease (PID), and previous ectopic pregnancy; intrauterine devices predispose to tubal pregnancy.

• *Per rectum* (PR) for melaena and constipation.
• *Exclude peritonism* and differentiate between localized or generalized peritonitis: fever, guarding, rebound tenderness and absent bowel sounds.
• *Exclude obstruction*: no flatus, no bowel motion, vomiting, cramping abdominal pain and abdominal distension. Check hernial orifices – this is vitally important and cannot be done reliably through clothing. Look for signs of ischaemia and necrosis.
3 Investigations to consider:
• Full blood count (FBC), clotting and G&S
• U&E, Ca^{2+}, amylase and glucose
• ABGs if acutely unwell or if you suspect pancreatitis, intestinal ischaemia or DKA (all cause a metabolic acidosis, as well as low pH, and the lactate will be raised).
• Radiology: erect chest X-ray (CXR) (free air under diaphragm, pneumonia) and supine/erect abdominal X-ray (AXR) (check for air–fluid levels, bowel distension, calcifications, air in biliary tree)
• ECG and troponin to exclude MI
• Midstream urine (MSU) for UTI (a common cause of abdominal pain in hospital) and urinary dipstick

Hints

■ Do not delay analgesia. Opiates do not mask the rigidity and rebound tenderness of peritonism.

■ Involve the surgical team early if necessary.

■ Gastritis and non-perforating peptic ulcers can cause severe epigastric pain but not true peritonism. The pain is usually relieved within minutes by antacids. Prescribe them IV.

■ Consider bowel infarction in patients who are acutely unwell with abdominal pain in the absence of peritonism. This is common in the elderly patient with atrial fibrillation (AF) who is not appropriately anticoagulated.

■ Free air under the diaphragm may persist for more than a week after abdominal surgery or laparoscopy, and in such a situation, it becomes an unreliable sign, so don't be fazed if you see it on a routine CXR!

Anaemia

You will usually be called by the lab for gross anaemia. In this case, your immediate concerns are to exclude bleeding. Chronic anaemia should always be investigated before transfusion unless the patient is acutely compromised, since donor blood may mask the cause (see Table 8.1). By far, the most common cause of anaemia in the United Kingdom (other than menorrhagia) is occult GI blood loss causing a microcytic iron deficiency anaemia.

Hints

■ Patients with chronic anaemia are particularly susceptible to heart failure following transfusion. Check for existing heart conditions, such as LV ejection fraction; discuss with your seniors first and transfuse them as slowly as possible. In those with heart failure or at risk of fluid overload, it may be necessary to give furosemide orally or IV with each unit. 20–40 mg per unit will usually suffice.

■ Be alert to mild anaemia when checking routine blood results. Slight Hb deficits are easy to miss and can be an early sign of serious disease.

■ Leukoerythroblastic anaemia means there are primitive red and white cells in the peripheral circulation. The patient may need a bone marrow biopsy and investigation for occult malignancy.

■ Consider intra- or retroperitoneal bleeding in acute anaemia and no external evidence of haemorrhage. Look for bruising in the flanks or around the umbilicus.

Table 8.1 Differential diagnoses of anaemia.

Low MCV (<96 fl)	Normal MCV (76–96 fl)	High MCV (>96 fl)
Iron deficiency	Acute blood loss	B_{12} or folate deficiency
Chronic bleeding (e.g. GI)	Haemolysis	Liver disease
Nutritional, that is, poor dietary intake of iron	Chronic infection or inflammation	Alcoholism
Thalassaemia (particularly if MCV is disproportionately low compared to Hb)	Anaemia of chronic disease	Marrow infiltration
Sideroblastic anaemia	Malignancy	Hypothyroidism
	Pregnancy	Reticulocytosis
	Chronic renal failure	Acquired sideroblastic anaemia
		Myelodysplastic syndromes
		Antifolate drugs (phenytoin)

On the ward

1 See the patient and assess the need for transfusion. Try to avoid transfusion until the diagnosis is clear, unless:
- Hb is dangerously low (<6 g/dl), although it is still usually possible to take samples for investigation prior to transfusion.
- The patient is symptomatic (feeling faint and having shortness of breath (SOB) at rest, tachycardia, angina and postural hypotension or has had serious acute blood loss).
- Where possible, avoid transfusions in patients with:
- Haemoglobinopathies, especially thalassaemia. They can usually cope with low Hb and are at risk of iron overload. Consult with your senior and a haematologist.
- B_{12} deficiency, as it may precipitate heart failure. Treat the B_{12} deficiency first, and check the folate also.

2 Take a history and examine the patient. Consider:
- Occult GI bleeding from malignancy – weight loss and change in bowel habit
- Menorrhagia
- Medication (non-steroidal anti-inflammatory drugs (NSAIDs), drugs causing haemolysis and marrow suppression)
- Recent procedures or operations
- Jaundice, skin rashes and lymph nodes
- Abdomen: splenomegaly and ascites
- PR and faecal occult blood (used for screening in the United Kingdom but not in hospital practice as it is non-specific)
- Cardiovascular system (CVS) – signs of infective endocarditis, prosthetic valves (can cause haemolytic anaemias) and flow murmurs (ESM over apex)
- Central nervous system (CNS) – signs of peripheral neuropathy or pseudodementia (B_{12} deficiency), rarely retinal haemorrhages

3 Investigations to consider:
- Repeat FBC and reticulocyte count
- G&S or crossmatch

- Iron studies (iron, ferritin, total iron binding capacity, transferrin saturation), B_{12}, folate and blood film
- U&E, liver function tests (LFTs), clotting screen to exclude disseminated intravascular coagulation (DIC)
- Lactate dehydrogenase, reticulocyte count and haptoglobin level are useful markers of haemolysis
- Other tests (e.g. bone marrow biopsy), according to the differential diagnoses

Arrhythmia

Whilst abnormalities in the heart rate and rhythm are relatively common and seldom life-threatening, never be afraid to call the crash team *before* the patient arrests! You are not expected to diagnose and manage arrhythmias without senior advice.

When answering your bleep
Ask nursing staff for pulse, BP and temp. Give O_2 if the patient is unwell, and if BP is dangerously low, consider IV fluids verbally.

ARRHYTHMIAS WHEN THE PULSE IS IRREGULAR WITH A NORMAL RATE
Atrial fibrillation (normal rate)
Wandering atrial pacemaker
Ventricular ectopics
Variable AV block

Hints

■ Measure and document both peripheral pulse rate and apex rate.
■ AF is associated with MI, IHD, mitral valve disease, thyroid disease, hypertension, pericarditis

---

On the ward (initial management for all arrhythmias)
1 See the patient. Check ABC. *If peri-arrest*, have someone call the crash team and commence cardiopulmonary resuscitation (CPR). Give 100% O_2, get nurses to attach a cardiac monitor, and put the chest pads on the patient.
2 If the patient is well and stable, take a brief history and examination. Consider:
- Cardiac symptoms (chest pain, palpitations, breathlessness, nausea, syncope, swollen ankles) and heart conditions (IHD, MI, valvular heart disease and rheumatic fever; previous episodes and management at the time).
- Pulse rate and rhythm.
- Circulatory status. Is the patient in shock (low BP, cold peripheries, sweaty)?
- Signs of cardiac failure (raised jugular venous pressure (JVP), peripheral oedema, basal inspiratory crackles and gallop rhythm – third and/or fourth heart sounds).
3 Do an ECG, and compare with previous ones. Continue to do serial ECGs.

On the ward
1 Severe symptoms are unusual. First do an ECG, then take a history and examine the patient. Atrial fibrillation and ectopics are common. Check the notes and find the most recent ECG for comparison. Is this a new problem?
2 In most cases, the arrhythmia is not significant. However, if the ECG reveals atrial fibrillation or multiple, frequent ectopics:
- Examine the patient for heart failure (raised JVP, basal crackles, swollen ankles) and mitral valve disease (murmurs, added sounds).
- Consider thyroid disease (check thyroid function tests (TFTs) and thyroid autoantibodies and look for thyroid acropachy, thyroid eye disease, goitre and pretibial myxoedema).

3 Investigations to consider:
- Emergency DC cardioversion. The key decision is rate versus rhythm.
- U&E, FBC, ESR and troponin.
- Serial ECGs.
- Consider T_4, TSH, digoxin levels and an echocardiogram.

4 Discuss further management with your senior.

5 If atrial fibrillation is compromising the patient, it may require immediate treatment with electrical or chemical control.

and other causes of a dilated atrium. Rarely, it is associated with atrial myxoma, infiltration, endocarditis and rheumatic fever. It is common following cardiac surgery, when it is usually temporary but may require short-term treatment with an anti arrhythmic like amiodarone. AF is common in patients with concurrent sepsis or electrolyte abnormalities and is more likely to resolve when these are corrected.

New-onset AF should usually be treated with anticoagulation. This may not be suitable in long-standing AF or in those with a high risk of falls, but it should always be considered, particularly in hospital where treatment-dose low molecular weight heparin (LMWH) (e.g. 1.5 mg/kg of enoxaparin) can easily be administered. To aid with decisions on anticoagulation, perform CHADSVASC and HASBLED scores on patient.

BRADYARRHYTHMIAS (ARRHYTHMIAS WITH A SLOW RATE)

Sinus bradycardia

Sudden stress, severe pain, post-systemic infection

Inferior MI: commonly results in first-degree AV block

AV heart block

Second-degree heart block: intermittent block with (Mobitz type I) or without (Mobitz type 2) an elongated PR interval

Third-degree heart block: complete heart block

Drugs: amiodarone, beta blockers and calcium channel blockers, digoxin

Faulty sinus node: sick sinus syndrome, infiltration, significant inferior MI

Hypothyroidism and hypothermia

Raised intracranial pressure (ICP)

Jaundice

On the ward

1 See the patient and assess ABC. Bradycardic arrhythmias can be serious. *If peri-arrest*, call the crash team and start CPR if necessary. Give 100% O_2.

2 If the patient is stable but symptomatic, inform your senior and:
- Consider urgent ECG and U&E. Put the patient on cardiac monitoring.
- Review all 'suspect' drugs.
- If symptomatic with sinus bradycardia or AV block, give atropine 0.6 mg IV (up to 3 mg in 24 hours). If bradycardia continues, get help. Discuss with cardiology regarding further management. Consider starting an adrenaline infusion 2–10 mcg/minute or transcutaneous pacing as a bridging measure whilst the patient waits for longer-term pacing. If this is necessary, call the anaesthetists as the patient may need sedation. Transcutaneous pacing in an awake patient is not ideal!
- Consider urgent digoxin levels.

3 If the patient is asymptomatic, do an ECG and discuss with your senior. Make sure they are on cardiac monitoring/telemetry.

Hints

■ A fourth heart sound with bradycardia is common following inferior MI.

TACHYARRHYTHMIAS (ARRHYTHMIAS WITH A FAST RATE)

■ Sinus tachycardia (regular rhythm, normal waveform)

■ Hypermetabolic states, for example, fever, anxiety, hyperthyroidism, anaemia, pain

■ Drugs, for example, digoxin, nitrates, nicotine, sympathomimetics, theophylline, salbutamol

■ Shock, sepsis or hypovolaemia of any cause

■ Heart failure

■ Supraventricular tachycardia

■ Atrial fibrillation with fast ventricular response (fast AF) (rhythm will be irregular)

■ Atrial flutter (has regular rhythm; often 300 atrial beats per minute, with a ventricular response at 150 bpm, that is, 1:2 conduction)

Atrial tachycardia (has regular rhythm)

■ WPW syndrome (rhythm is regular unless AF supervenes)

■ Nodal (junctional) (rhythm is regular)

■ Ventricular tachycardia

On the ward

1 See the patient. Assess ABC. *If peri-arrest*, call the crash team, request an urgent ECG and start CPR if necessary. Give 100% O_2.

2 If the patient is stable, do an urgent ECG and put patient on a cardiac monitor. Put the chest pads on the patient. On the basis of the ECG, decide if the patient has sinus tachycardia or an arrhythmia:

● If the ECG reveals a sinus tachycardia, treat the underlying condition.

● If the ECG reveals an arrhythmia, you need to differentiate between supraventricular tachycardia (SVT) and ventricular tachycardia (VT), which can be difficult. Seek senior advice if you are unsure.

Hints

■ Broad rule of thumb in discriminating between SVT and VT:

– SVTs have narrow complexes (<120 ms) and are not necessarily associated with serious underlying heart disease.

– VTs have broad complexes (>120 ms) and indicate serious underlying heart disease.

■ Carotid sinus massage can cause sinus arrest or strokes, especially in the elderly, or if the patient has had a recent MI or is digitalized. Use only if urgent action is required. Vagal manoeuvres are much better (Valsalva manoeuvre).

■ Atrial tachycardia with heart block is commonly associated with digoxin toxicity.

■ Discriminating VT from SVT with bundle branch block is not easy, and you should seek senior help. If the patient is compromised, treat as VT.

■ Whether the patient has a VT or SVT, you need to identify and treat the underlying cause, in addition to treating the arrhythmia (Tables 8.2a and 8.2b).

Calcium

Most labs report total serum Ca^{2+}, of which about half is bound to albumin. If the albumin levels are low, the lab result will underestimate total Ca^{2+}.

To calculate the corrected calcium, use the following formula:

$$\text{Corrected [Ca]} = \text{measured [Ca]} + \{(40 - [\text{albumin}]) \times 0.02\}$$

Alternatively, ask for an ionized Ca level which need not be adjusted for albumin (a special tube is required).

Table 8.2a Managing supraventricular tachycardias. If the patient has SVT and signs of compromise (hypotension, heart failure, impaired consciousness, or a heart rate of >200 bpm), get help fast. The patient may require 100–200 J of synchronized direct current (DC) cardioversion.

Atrial fibrillation	Non-AF SVT
■ Irregularly irregular pulse and no P waves on ECG	■ If the patient has SVT that is not AF, they may need immediate treatment, but discuss with your senior first ■ Regular rhythm narrow complex tachycardia
■ Most common type of SVT	■ Most SVTs respond to IV adenosine. Ensure that the patient is on a cardiac monitor and that a resus trolley is close to hand. Inject 6 mg adenosine with a flush rapidly into a large peripheral or central vein. If there is no response after 1–2 minutes, give 12 mg and then a further 12 mg if necessary. Expect facial flushing, nausea and transient breathlessness. Warn the patient of transient chest pain when you inject the adenosine
■ First-line treatments of acute fast AF are rate control (with metoprolol or digoxin) or rhythm control (with amiodarone or synchronized cardioversion)	■ Adenosine cannot be given to patients with asthma. In this case, use verapamil
■ Metoprolol controls the ventricular rate, but does not resolve the fibrillation. Amiodarone can restore the rhythm but requires large-vessel IV access (central line). Amiodarone requires a loading dose. Amiodarone cannot be given peripherally	■ Record a rhythm strip before, during and after each dose of adenosine ■ Once the underlying rhythm is elicited, treat accordingly ■ If the patient becomes compromised in anyway, shock with DC cardioversion, and then load with amiodarone

Table 8.2b Management of ventricular tachycardias.

- ■ Treat pulseless VT in the same way that you would VF – commence CPR
- ■ Sustained VT usually precipitates shock unless treated with monophasic DC cardioversion (200–360 J), so seek urgent senior help
- ■ If haemodynamically unstable, treat with synchronized DC shock, and then load with IV amiodarone
- ■ If haemodynamically stable, correct low K and Mg, and load with amiodarone.
- ■ Avoid amiodarone in patients with long QT syndrome
- ■ Investigations to consider:

U&E for K, Ca, Mg, troponin, FBC if acutely unwell

- ■ Consider in the future the need for ICDs and long-term oral amiodarone

Hypercalcaemia

On the wards, this is often spurious and an incidental finding. However, true hypercalcaemia needs to be corrected. Rarely, it requires urgent treatment.

Differential diagnoses

■ Spurious: tourniquet left on too long or blood taken from the drip arm

■ Hyperparathyroidism (primary and tertiary)
■ Malignancy: bony metastases, myeloma and paraneoplastic syndrome
■ Drugs: thiazide diuretics, excessive ingestion of Ca^{2+}-containing antacids and excessive vitamin D intake
■ Rarer causes: granulomatous diseases (e.g. sarcoid, TB) and endocrinopathies

On the ward

1 See the patient. Check that the result reflects true hypercalcaemia. In hospital, hypercalcaemia is frequently 'spurious', due to dehydration, venous stasis, taking blood from an infusion arm or abnormal albumin. However, a corrected Ca^{2+} of above 3.5 mmol/l requires treatment.

2 Exclude acute symptoms that require urgent treatment (anorexia, vomiting, abdominal pain, impaired mental state, dehydration). If acutely symptomatic:

● Seek senior advice.
● Consider saline diuresis, 3–6 l normal saline/24 hours IV depending on LVEF and furosemide 40–120 mg 2–4-hourly according to response. A central venous pressure (CVP) and urinary catheters are useful to monitor fluid balance (a catheter is also kinder if the patient has difficulty getting to the loo).
● Avoid phosphates until Ca^{2+} levels are normal or risk deposition of Ca^{2+} phosphate ('metastatic Ca/Pi deposition').
● Consider hydrocortisone (especially useful in malignancy, sarcoid and vitamin D intoxication), calcitonin or mithramycin therapy.
● Pamidronate is also useful in hypercalcaemia secondary to bony metastases.

3 If the patient has true hypercalcaemia but is not acutely unwell:

● If dehydrated, request that the patient drink enough fluid to maintain a urine output of about 2–3 l/day. If very dehydrated or unable to drink, consider IV fluids – normal saline is best.
● Investigate the cause of hypercalcaemia, exclude renal impairment and correct abnormal K and Mg levels.

4 Investigations to consider:

● U&E, ESR, phosphate, alk phos and Mg^{2+}.
● ECG. Review CXR for lung malignancy (squamous cell lung Ca produces parathyroid hormone (PTH)-related peptide causing hypercalcaemia).
● Consider plasma Igs, serum and urine electrophoresis, urinary Bence-Jones protein, skeletal survey, bone marrow biopsy (myeloma investigations) and PTH levels.

Hypocalcaemia

Like hypercalcaemia, hypocalcaemia can be spurious and may be caused by acute hyperventilation. Hypocalcaemia is rarely an emergency, unless Ca^{2+} is <1.5 mmol/l (risking laryngospasm).

Differential diagnoses

■ Spurious (low albumin as in malnutrition or chronic malabsorption, blood taken from drip arm)
■ Acute hyperventilation
■ Pancreatitis

■ Hypoparathyroidism – thyroid surgery or neck irradiation
■ On TPN without adequate Ca^{2+}

■ Vitamin D deficiency – malabsorption, renal disease, phenytoin or phenobarbitone
■ Excessive ingestion of phosphate

On the ward

1 Assess the severity of the patient's condition. Check that the result is not spurious. Look for peripheral or oral paraesthesia, carpopedal spasm, Chvostek's sign (tapping over the facial nerve induces facial twitch), confusion and tetany.

2 If hypocalcaemia is symptomatic or Ca^{2+} <1.5 mmol/l, seek immediate senior advice and institute treatment to prevent laryngospasm. Give 10% calcium gluconate 10–20 ml in 50–100 ml 5% dextrose over 5 minutes (not faster), followed by 1–2 mg/kg/hour IV for 6–12 hours according to response. Correct Mg^{2+} deficiency and measure phosphate. If the phosphate is high, discuss with senior. The patient may need phosphate binders and slow correction of Ca^{2+}, as too rapid correction can result in metastatic deposition of calcium phosphate.

3 Asymptomatic hypocalcaemia (Ca >1.75 mmol/l) does not require immediate treatment. Give oral supplements (2–4 g daily in divided doses) that contain cholecalciferol.

4 Investigations to consider:
● U&E, albumin, Mg^{2+} and phosphate
● Amylase, PTH and vitamin D levels

Chest pain

Chest pain always requires urgent attention. Whilst angina, oesophagitis, oesophageal spasm, and musculoskeletal pain are the most common causes of chest pain, never forget pulmonary embolus in the hospital setting.

When answering your bleep

Ask the ward staff to:

■ Perform an ECG.
■ Repeat the vital signs.
■ If the patient has a history of IHD, prescribe sublingual glyceryl trinitrate (GTN) two puffs over the phone. Aim for sats >94%, but take care in patients with chronic obstructive pulmonary disease (COPD).

Differential diagnoses (*do not miss these!)
Cardiac
■ Angina (IHD, LVH/HOCM)
■ Acute MI*
■ Pericarditis or myocarditis, including post-MI Dressler's syndrome
Lung/pleura
■ Pulmonary embolus*
■ Pneumothorax*
■ Pleurisy/pneumonia
Aorta
■ Dissection*
■ Aneurysm
GIT
■ Oesophageal spasm
■ Oesophagitis/gastritis
■ Pancreatitis, cholecystitis and peptic ulcer disease/perforation

---

On the ward

1 Assess the patient. *If peri-arrest*, get help (e.g. crash team) and institute emergency treatment:
● 100% O_2 via a non-rebreathing mask
● IV access
● Urgent U&E, FBC, troponin and ABGs
● Serial ECGs and cardiac monitoring
● Urgent mobile CXR

2 If the patient is stable, take a thorough history and examination. Do not forget:
- Temperature, BP, pulse and circulation (well perfused or cold and clammy?)
- The key to the diagnosis is the history. Specifically:
(a) Ask about the pain. Have they had this pain before? Do they have known IHD, risk factors for cardiac disease or oesophagitis/oesophageal spasm? Does the pain feel anginal? Is it relieved by GTN? What are the relieving or precipitating factors (exercise, posture or food)? Pain lasting less than 30 seconds, stabbing or sharp in quality and highly localized is unlikely to be due to ischaemia.
(b) Any N&V (common with MI), recent falls or trauma?
- Listen for pleural and pericardial rubs (often missed).
- If there are odd chest noises and hyperresonance, think of pneumothorax. Always check for tracheal deviation (tension pneumothorax).
3 Investigations to consider:
- ECG ± CXR.
- IV access if you suspect an MI.
- Repeat ECG in 1–2 hours (there may be no ECG changes in an early MI).
- U&E, troponin, FBC, clotting and G&S, if anticoagulation or surgery is likely.
- Blood gases in PE.
- D-dimers are sensitive but not specific for emboli. They are good as rule-out tests, so if the D-dimer level is low, the chance of an embolism is very low (reassuring). However, if the level is high, it could be an embolus or just as easily a different diagnosis such as infection, inflammation, malignancy or pregnancy. Very high levels can suggest DIC.
4 Discuss with your senior.

Others

■ Shingles
■ Costochondritis
■ Rib or vertebral collapse

Hints

■ Pain radiating to either arm, neck or jaw suggests cardiac ischaemia. Pain radiating to the back could be a dissection. Check BP in both arms.

■ Sublingual GTN will often provide immediate relief of angina and is a useful diagnostic aid. It also relieves oesophageal spasm, but over a few minutes.

■ Oesophageal spasm or severe anxiety sometimes causes ischaemia-like changes on the ECG. Seek advice if unsure.

■ A tachycardic patient may also show rate-related ischaemic changes but these do not normally occur with a simple sinus tachycardia. Slowing the rate should reverse the changes.

Confusion

Beware of unexpected confusion in patients. In particular, hypoxia is common but easily missed in the elderly. Never assume disorientation or dementia without first excluding serious medical causes and ascertaining the patient's usual mental state.

When answering your bleep

■ Ask for a ward capillary blood glucose test ('BM stick' – this stands for **Boehringer Mannheim,** the old name for **Roche Diagnostics**).
■ Temp, BP, pulse and urine dipstick.
■ Pulse oximetry if available.

Differential diagnoses

'DIM TOP' (Mike's South African acronym!):

■ **D**rugs (especially sedatives and analgesics like opiates, anticonvulsants)

■ **I**nfection (anywhere, commonly UTI and pneumonia)
■ **M**etabolic (hypoglycaemia, Na, K, Ca, liver failure, uraemia)
■ **T**rauma (concussion, subdural haematoma)
■ **T**oxins (alcohol withdrawal, drugs, others)
■ **O**xygen deficit/hypoxia (pneumonia, pulmonary oedema, PE, respiratory depression (opiates), anaemia)
■ **P**ain and discomfort (any cause, including urinary/faecal retention)
■ **P**sychiatric/dementia
■ **P**erfusion abnormalities (stroke, transient ischaemic attack (TIA), nonconvulsive status)
■ **P**ost-op confusion (hypoxia, urinary retention, infection, drugs, abnormal electrolytes, pain, blood loss, disorientation, alcohol withdrawal)

On the ward

1 Assess the patient's general condition and vital signs. If the patient is very agitated or violent, get help from nurses and security team. Consider sedation but be careful. Please check with a senior if you are considering sedation. If you do sedate a confused patient with any history of trauma, you are obliged to CT them – try and agree this with radiology before the sedation!

2 If the patient is stable, take a history and examination. Don't forget to:

● Specifically exclude cardiac and respiratory distress. Consider pulse oximeter readings, ABGs and CXR. Hypoxia is a surprisingly common cause of confusion that is easily missed.
● Perform a mini-mental test score. Is the patient truly confused or just disoriented, in pain or angry?
● Ask about recent falls, funny turns or previous strokes/TIAs. Is the patient in atrial fibrillation or do they have a patent foramen ovale or carotid artery disease?
● Check possible infection sites (IV lines, UTI, chest, surgical wounds) and palpate for a full bladder or packed colon (urinary retention and constipation are common causes of confusion).
● Look at both fundi for papilloedema – a hard sign of raised ICP (e.g. in subdural haematoma) – and assess the CNS for localizing signs (inc. pupil reactions). Pupils are often naturally asymmetrical (anisocoria or Adie's pupil), but in the context of confusion or neurology, this cannot be assumed.
● Check drug and fluid charts and review the medical background.

3 Ask the nursing staff or a relative about the patient's usual mental state. Is this a new occurrence? What is their baseline cognition?

4 Investigations to consider:
● U&E, glucose, FBC and ESR and ABGs
● Blood cultures
● LFTs (including clotting)
● Plasma Ca^{2+} in patients with malignancy
● MSU
● ECG
● CXR and CT head

Hints

■ Nurse the patient in a moderately lit room and minimize noise. Give repeated reassurance to the patient. A well-loved family member or a familiar nurse caring for the patient is invaluable.
■ Consider nursing the patient on a mattress on the floor. Some hospitals have special 'soft-walled' beds. Bed rails and 'hand ties' are regarded by most nursing staff as unnecessary and potentially dangerous. Physical restraint is rarely used in the United Kingdom.
■ Soft music, surrounding the patient with pictures of family.
■ Secure NG tubes and IV lines with bandages. It is occasionally necessary to put mittens on the patient's hands.

■ If you have excluded serious causes, consider short-term sedation with a benzodiazepine (lorazepam 0.5–1 mg IM, repeated after 4 hours if necessary). Use with caution in the elderly.

Alternatives include:

− Haloperidol 5–10 mg IM or PO. (Avoid in elderly patients. Haloperidol is useful in the more acute setting. Have a resus trolley to hand. You may need to wait 10–20 minutes for the drug to take effect.)

− In alcoholic patients, consider clomethiazole instead.

− ALWAYS DISCUSS WITH A SENIOR PRIOR TO USING SEDATION

■ You may not find any cause for the patient's confusion. Patients may simply be disoriented from a change in environment; but make sure you exclude serious medical causes first. Clear, repeated explanation about where the patient is and why can be helpful, as is a small map showing where the toilets are and how to call for nursing assistance.

Constipation

Constipation is common in hospital due to immobility, drugs and having to use a bedpan. Remember that it is a symptom and not a diagnosis. It is better to treat the cause than to blindly prescribe laxatives. Constipation is more common in the elderly and often missed.

Always be alert to obstruction. Post-op ileus is common, usually resolves by itself and should never be treated with laxatives!

Differential diagnoses

Poor (low roughage) diet and dehydration
Immobility
Drugs
● Ca^{2+}-based drugs (e.g. antacids, and calcium channel blockers)
● Ferrous sulphate
● Opiates
● Tricyclic antidepressants
● Anticholinergics
● Diuretics (furosemide)
Embarrassment at using a bedpan
GI tract
● Pain (anal fissures, haemorrhoids, rectal prolapse, recent surgery)
● IBS
● Obstruction (acute and subacute) from any cause especially tumours, strictures, diverticulosis
● Ileus (pseudo-obstruction)
Metabolic
● Endocrine − hypothyroidism, hypercalcaemia or hypokalaemia
Neurological
● Spinal cord compression/lesions/trauma
● Hirschsprung's disease
● Chagas disease
● Diabetic neuropathy

On the ward
1 See the patient. Exclude:
● Intestinal obstruction. If present, you must exclude a tumour and other sinister causes like strangulated hernias.
● IBD. This can cause constipation; never prescribe laxatives in these patients without first consulting your senior.
● Pain/embarrassment which inhibits straining. Have they had recent surgery? In certain surgeries (like cardiothoracic), it is important that patients do not strain for prolonged periods.
2 Take a brief history and examination. Don't forget:
● To ask the patient how often they usually open their bowels.
● PR (faecal impaction, anal fissure). It is essential that you perform a PR − much serious pathology can be missed if this is omitted.
● Drug and fluid charts.
3 Investigations are seldom necessary but consider:
● K^+, Ca^{2+} and FBC

- T4 and TSH if you suspect hypothyroidism
- Sigmoidoscopy or colonoscopy if malignancy is suspected

4 Management. For simple constipation:

- Ensure adequate hydration, encourage more roughage, and mobilize if possible.
- Bulk-forming agents: Bran cereals or ispaghula husk (Fybogel).
- Stool softeners: docusate sodium 200 mg PO BD (cheap) or lactulose 15 ml PO BD (expensive).
- Stimulants: senna or bisacodyl. Glycerine suppositories if NBM. Co-danthrusate (danthron docusate) is effective but reserved for very elderly or terminally ill patients due to risk of danthron-induced tumours.
- Enemas, for example, phosphate enema 100 ml PR.

5 Consider prophylaxis for patients at risk of constipation (bedridden, e.g. post-op and stroke patients or patients on regular opiates).

Diarrhoea

By far the most common cause in hospitals is drugs (antibiotics and laxatives), but infection should always be excluded. Less common but important to consider is constipation with overflow. In all cases, the patient may need to be rehydrated.

Differential diagnoses

- Anxiety
- Drugs: laxatives, broad-spectrum antibiotics, or antacids containing Mg sulphate and also cimetidine, colchicine, cytotoxic agents, digoxin or thiazide diuretics
- Intestinal obstruction with overflow (neoplasm)
- Faecal impaction with overflow, especially in elderly patients
- Infection: *Clostridium difficile* or *Norovirus*
- IBD, other causes of intra-abdominal inflammation, ischaemia, etc.
- Hyperthyroidism

On the ward

1 Exclude dehydration (BP lying and sitting for postural drop, JVP, mucous membranes). Also check renal function.

2 Directed history and examination:
- Risk for intra-abdominal sepsis (recent surgery, diverticular disease), IBD or immunocompromise (including HIV)
- N&V, blood or mucus PR
- Peritonism or impaction
- Drug chart for new drugs, laxatives, antibiotics

3 If the patient is otherwise well and an infective cause is unlikely with no evidence of colitis or intra-abdominal mischief, send a stool sample for MC&S and consider an antidiarrhoeal agent like loperamide when cultures are negative.

4 If the patient has systemic signs or is taking antibiotics:
- Take a fresh stool specimen for MC&S and **C. difficile** toxin.
- Bloody diarrhoea (dysentery) can be caused by polyps, ischaemic or pseudomembranous colitis, cancer, IBD or infection with shigella, campylobacter, salmonella or haemorrhagic forms of *Escherichia coli*. Take a history of foreign travel.

• Consider sigmoidoscopy and biopsy if the patient has bloody diarrhoea or the stool culture is negative.

5 Further investigations to consider:

• U&E FBC to check white cell count (WCC), amylase (pancreatitis) and coeliac serology/jejunal biopsy if there are signs of malabsorption and TFTs if thyrotoxicosis is suspected.

• Electron microscopy (EM) of stool specimen for viral infection (SSRVs) and stool polymerase chain reaction (PCR).

• Stool culture for ova, cysts and parasites – this usually requires a 'hot' stool.

• Inflammatory markers (C-reactive protein (CRP) and erythrocyte sedimentation rate (ESR)) especially if the patient has known IBD.

• Special cultures/stains in immunocompromised patients for cryptosporidia, mycobacteria, etc.

• Plain AXR (to look for colonic distension and obstruction) if the patient has pain or known IBD.

6 Irrespective of the cause, you must ensure adequate hydration:

• Oral rehydration regime (see *British National Formulary* (*BNF*) – oral rehydration).

• IV fluids if severe or the patient cannot drink.

Hints

■ Barrier nursing is advisable until infection is ruled out.

■ Wash your hands with water and soap between patients.

■ Be wary of diarrhoea in patients on steroids. Their abdomens may be 'silent' despite serious intra-abdominal mischief.

■ If no cause is found, then consider referral to a gastroenterology specialist. There are numerous rarer causes of diarrhoea including carcinoid syndrome, VIPoma, amyloidosis, Addison's disease, laxative abuse, lactose intolerance and tropical sprue that may need to be excluded.

Electrocardiograms

Do not get too worried about interpreting ECGs during your first job. Whilst the range of potential anomalies is bewildering at first, practice really does make perfect and junior doctors are only expected to diagnose a handful of important conditions. For a more complete guide, consult Hampton's *ECG Made Easy* and *ECG in Practice*. Whatever the ECG diagnosis, remember to treat the patient, not the ECG!

Common ECG diagnoses

■ Atrial fibrillation (no P waves, rate can be fast or normal)

■ Recent or past MI

■ Third-degree heart block (no relationship between P waves and QRS complexes)

■ Ventricular tachycardia

Basic ECG parameters to consider

■ Rate: 60–90 bpm (lower in athletes).

■ Rhythm: irregular or regular.

■ Axis: normal, from −30° (aVL) to +120° (III) (some use from 0° to 90°).

■ P waves: present/absent before each QRS complex?

■ PR interval (start of P wave to start of QRS): constant? Normal interval is 120–200 ms (3–5 small squares).

■ QRS interval: up to 120 ms (three small squares) is 'narrow complex' and represents normal conduction system. If greater than this or 'wide complex', then the origin of the rhythm is likely to be ventricular unless there is bundle branch block. Check height of the R waves. Are Q waves present?

■ ST segment: isoelectric (i.e. on segment, baseline is the line between the T wave and the P wave) – raised if ST elevation (STEMI) and depressed if ST depression (ischaemia, digoxin toxicity).

■ T waves: upright or inverted/flipped (ischaemia) – tented in hyperkalaemia and flattened in hypokalaemia.

If the ECG is abnormal, consider each parameter systematically:

Abnormal rate and rhythm

Atrial tachycardia

- Rate >100/minute
- Narrow QRS (<120ms) (except in SVT with BBB or WPW syndrome)
- P wave abnormal (shape, size, upside down, swallowed by QRS)

Sinus arrhythmia

- Normal P waves, QRS complexes and rate.
- Regularly irregular. Rate varies with breathing (variation in cardiac output related to venous return as a result of altered intrathoracic pressures).

Atrial fibrillation

- No P waves
- Irregularly irregular narrow QRS complexes

Atrial flutter

- Sawtooth baseline of atrial depolarization.
- Regular QRS complexes. Often the 'saw' to QRS is regular and constant at 2:1, 3:1 or 4:1.

AV nodal rhythm

- Narrow QRS complex.
- P waves hidden within the QRS complex or just preceding it (very short PR interval). P waves may be inverted.

Ventricular tachycardia

- Wide QRS (>120ms) and rate >150/minute.
- Abnormal T waves.
- P waves are often absent or may have no relationship to QRS complexes. Regular rate.

Note: If there is a rapid QRS rate without P waves, a wide QRS (>120ms), this indicates VT (unless there is pre-existing BBB), whereas a narrow QRS (<120ms) indicates AV nodal tachycardia.

Calculating the axis

1 If the QRS is predominantly positive (i.e. the deflection of the QRS complex is upwards) in I and II, the axis is normal.

2 If the QRS in lead I is negative and III is positive, the axis is to the right 'ar**R**iving together'.

3 If the QRS in lead I is positive and II and III are negative, the axis is to the left '**L**eaving each other'.

4 Alternatively find a lead in which the QRS complexes have equal positive and negative deflections. The axis lies 90° to that lead.

5 To determine the actual axis, see Figure 8.1.

P waves

1 Indicate atrial depolarization and are best seen in leads II and V_1.

2 Large left atrium (p. mitrale): bifid and wide (>110ms) – P wave in II and biphasic in V_1.

3 Large right atrium (p. pulmonale): peaked P waves (>2.5mm).

4 No P waves: atrial fibrillation.

5 Negative P wave in I is either dextrocardia if QRS complexes become smaller from V_{1-6} OR 'technical' (due to lead misplacement) if there is normal R wave progression from V_{1-6}.

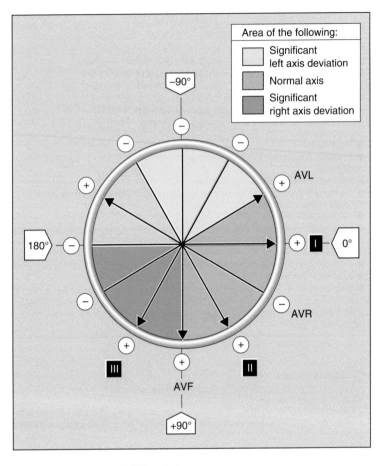

Figure 8.1 Determining the axis for ECG examination.

PR interval

Delay indicates abnormal AV conduction.

Second-degree heart block type 2 and third-degree heart block require a permanent pacemaker due to the risk of degenerating into complete heart block and asystole:

1 First-degree HB: prolonged PR interval (>200ms) in each cycle but all P waves conducted.

2 Second-degree HB:

• Type I: progressive lengthening of the PR interval and then followed by a non-conducted P wave is called the Wenckebach phenomenon (type I).

• Type II: some P waves are not followed by a QRS complex. May find 2 (or 3) P waves before a QRS complex, that is, 2:1 (or 3:1) block.

3 Third-degree HB: no relationship between P waves and QRS complexes, ventricular escape rhythm <50/minute and QRS usually wide.

4 A consistently short PR interval indicates conduction down accessory pathways (e.g. WPW). May be associated with 'slurred' upstroke of the QRS.

QRS complexes

Wide complexes (>120 ms) indicate abnormal ventricular depolarization, occurring in VT, ventricular extra-systoles, complete heart block or bundle branch block:

1 Ventricular extra-systoles: no P wave, *early* QRS and abnormally shaped QRS complex and abnormal T wave. Next P wave is 'on time'. Isolated extra-systoles are a common normal finding (particularly in young, fit people). A *late* QRS is not an extra-systole but instead a 'rescue beat'. They are not normally of concern unless there is structural heart disease or post-infarction when they are associated with increased risk of death.

2 Left bundle branch block (LBBB): RSR 'W' pattern in V_1 and 'M' pattern in V_6. Inverted T waves in I, aVL, V_{5-6} (remember the mnemonic 'WiLLiaM'). The presence of LBBB may mask underlying infarction. Once you have identified an LBBB, further comment is generally unreliable. It is associated with acute MI, aortic valve disease, cardiomyopathy and may be seen after cardiac surgery.

3 Right bundle branch block (RBBB): RSR 'M' pattern in V_1 and 'W' pattern in V_6. Inverted T waves in V_1–V_3 and deep and wide S wave in V_6 (remember the mnemonic 'MaRroW'). Often a normal variant but can be associated with IHD, acute massive PE or cardiomyopathy.

4 Ventricular strain: inverted T waves and depressed ST segments in the appropriate chest leads (V_1–V_3 for RV and V_4–V_6 for LV).

5 RVH: R wave larger than S wave in V_1 and no RBBB and deep S in V_6. Sometimes, there is right axis deviation and 'p. pulmonale'. NB: a dominant R in V_1 is seen in posterior infarction with RBBB.

6 LVH: the Framingham voltage criteria is R wave in V_6 >25 mm in height OR combined voltage of R wave in V_6 and S wave in V_1 >35 mm in height. There is occasionally an associated left axis deviation. Causes of LVH include heart failure and outflow disorders including aortic stenosis (AS) and hypertrophic obstructive cardiomyopathy (HOCM).

ST segment and T waves

1 Depressed ST segments: ischaemia, digoxin toxicity ('inverted tick' ST depression and inverted T waves in V_5–V_6) and posterior MI.

2 Elevated ST segments (always serious): infarction, coronary artery spasm (variant angina), pericarditis/myocarditis (saddle-shaped ST segments in all leads), ventricular aneurysm and posterior ischaemia.

3 T wave inversion is often non-specific but in the context of chest pain points to critical ischaemia. Widespread T wave inversion is seen in massive cerebral events like subarachnoid haemorrhage and Friedreich's ataxia-associated cardiomyopathy.

Table 8.3 Diagnosing infarction sites by ECG changes.

Site of infarction	Changes seen in leads
Anterior	$V_1–V_4$
Septal	$V_2–V_4$
Lateral	I, aVL, $V_5–V_6$
Inferior	II, III and aVF
True posterior	Dominant R in V_1 (exclude RV strain and RBBB) $\pm$ ST depression in $V_1–V_2$

Important ECG abnormalities to recognize

Myocardial infarction

Sequence of changes (see Table 8.3):

1 At first, the ECG may be normal.

2 Within 6 hours, tall T waves and raised ST segments are evident.

3 Within 24 hours, T waves invert and ST segments normalize.

4 After 24 hours, Q waves are evident and ST segments are normal.

NB: T wave inversion may or may not persist. Q waves persist. Once Q waves appear, little revascularization therapy can be performed.

Pulmonary embolism

There are often no ECG changes:

1 Sinus tachycardia.

2 Evidence of RV strain/hypertrophy

3 Right axis deviation.

4 RBBB.

5 Deep S in I, Q wave in V3, inverted T in V3 ('SI, Q3, T3'). A rare sign.

Hyperkalaemia

1 Tented 'tall' T waves.

2 Small or absent P waves.

3 Widened QRS complexes (this is with severe hyperkalaemia and eventually 'stretches out' into torsades de pointes VT or VF).

4 No ST segment.

5 Note that if there is **hypo**kalaemia, there will be an absent/flattened T waves, prominent U waves, prolonged PR interval and ST depression.

Finally, before making any diagnosis on the basis of an ECG remember to first check the patient (and that the ECG is from the correct patient!). Second, check the ECG leads and attachments. Third, check the calibration (is the trace running at the correct rate and voltage?).

Eye complaints

Except for the simplest problems, junior doctors are not generally expected to diagnose or treat eye diseases. Do not be afraid to seek an ophthalmological opinion.

The acute red eye

Differential diagnoses: conjunctivitis, foreign body, corneal ulceration or herpes keratitis, acute glaucoma and acute iritis

---

On the ward

1 Take a brief history and examination. Don't forget:
- Clinical background, especially diabetes and other systemic diseases
- Visual acuity and discharge
- Pupils: shape and direct and consensual responses
- Ophthalmoscopy to assess red reflex (normal in conjunctivitis and simple foreign body) and fundus

2 Unless the cause is obvious, notify your senior and seek ophthalmological opinion. If you suspect conjunctivitis, take swabs for MC&S, and viral PCR if you are concerned about herpes keratitis

- If the problem is unilateral, ask about previous history of shingles (look for periocular vesicles) or iritis (which often recurs in the fellow eye). Conjunctivitis or ulceration can also be unilateral.
- Exclude conjunctivitis: the eye usually feels itchy, gritty and teary. Vision, pupillary responses and red reflex are all normal. Purulent discharge suggests bacterial conjunctivitis, whereas sticky white discharge may be associated with allergic conjunctivitis. Look at the pattern of redness/injection. Intensity of injection around the periphery suggests conjunctival inflammation, whereas injection around the cornea suggests corneal or intra-ocular inflammation.
- Exclude acute glaucoma: the eye is red and painful, the pupil is hazy and fixed, and the patient sees halos around lights. Seek urgent ophthalmological assistance – this is a medical emergency as the patient may lose their sight if you do no act quickly.
3 Exclude a foreign body: there is a history of trauma. Foreign bodies are sometimes hidden under the inside of the upper lid. Invert the upper lid over a small spatula (cotton bud or orange stick). Bear in mind that the sensation of having a foreign body in the eye can also be caused by corneal ulcers and acute keratitis. Refer to ophthalmology urgently if you suspect a complex foreign body, as it may be difficult to remove non-surgically.

Sudden loss of vision in one or both eyes

This is always an emergency. Seek immediate ophthalmological advice. Differential diagnoses are acute glaucoma, central retinal artery or vein occlusion, amaurosis fugax (retinal artery stroke/TIA), optic neuritis, retinal detachment, severe hyperglycaemia and temporal arteritis.

Floaters

Floaters are usually condensations of vitreous, but can be blood, bits of retina or inflammatory cells. They are normal with increasing age, but if they have appeared recently or suddenly, seek an ophthalmological opinion.

Falls

Whilst most falls in hospital are trivial, they are a common cause of fracture in the elderly. You need to sign an incident/

Datix form when called to investigate a 'fall'.

When answering your bleep

Consider asking for a ward glucose test and baseline observations including lying and standing BP.

Differential diagnoses

■ Simple accident (slippery floor, disorientation)
■ Poor vision (no glasses, cataracts)
■ Drowsiness from drugs, especially sedatives and recent anaesthesia
■ Loss of consciousness: TIA, fit, vasovagal, postural hypotension, cough/micturition syncope, arrhythmias/MI AS, hypoglycaemia and symptomatic anaemia
■ Poor motor function/balance: generalized weakness, frailty, Parkinson's or cerebellar disease and peripheral sensory/motor neuropathy

On the ward
1 See the patient.
2 Ask the patient what happened. Don't forget:
- Temp, pulse and BP, including postural drop.
- Consciousness level and mini-mental test score if appropriate.
- Skin for bruising, bleeding, cuts and fractures.

- Bone tenderness for fractures. Especially look for hip, wrist and scaphoid fractures. Examine the skull carefully if the patient has hit their head. If there are signs of head injury or drowsiness, consider a CT head.
- Drug and fluid charts (sedatives, hypoglycaemic agents, vasodilators (especially ACE inhibitors and alpha blockers) anti-arrhythmics).

3 Investigations to consider:

- U&E, FBC (looking particularly for raised WCC and low Hb) and glucose.
- MSU.
- ECG.
- The patient may need cardiac investigations later (e.g. ECHO, 24 hour tape).

4 Fill in an incident form (ask the nurses for one).

5 Write in the patient's notes. Include:

- Time and date.
- Brief history of accident.
- Brief examination findings – do a neuro exam to include pupillary reactions.
- That you signed an incident form.

6 Ask the nurses to continue to do regular neuro observations and to contact you if the patient's condition deteriorates.

7 Think about causes for the fall. Plan with the nurses how to prevent future accidents.

Hints

■ Many falls are caused by patients being in an alien environment, particularly in elderly patients with poor righting reflexes. To prevent future falls, show patients the call button and remind them that they need to call the nurse for toilet assistance after anaesthetics or sedatives.

■ Fractures or simple bruising in the elderly can lead to substantial blood loss. Check limbs for occult fractures.

■ Sudden loss of consciousness is most commonly caused by fainting, postural hypotension and arrhythmia. MIs and TIAs rarely present with syncope alone.

Fever

In hospital, fever is most commonly due to infection, blood transfusions and drugs.

On the ward

1 See the patient. Check temperature, pulse and BP. Fever above 40 °C requires urgent action. If there any signs of shock (tachycardia, hypotension with warm peripheries), ensure large-bore IV access and commence aggressive IV fluid resuscitation. Take blood cultures (at least two sets). Discuss IV broad-spectrum antibiotic cover with your senior urgently.

2 Exclude immunosuppression. Check the patient's history, latest WCC and glucose. In all cases, look for infection site.

3 Try to localize the source of infection. Ask about:

- Abdominal pain, cough and sputum, diarrhoea, dysuria/frequency, prosthesis/heart valves, rashes, rigors/chills
- Recent surgery or invasive procedure
- Recent sexual contacts and travel abroad (TB, malaria, amoebiasis)
- Drugs

Common sites for infection:

- Chest, wound/line sites (cannula/PICC Lines) and bladder.
- Skin and leg ulcers.

- ENT (remember ears). Check for meningism and photophobia.
- IV lines, catheters and drains – how long have these been in place?
- Do not forget to examine the genitalia, do a PR (ischiorectal/prostatic abscess), and consider *per vaginum* (PV exam) (PID). Check joints for tenderness and swelling (septic arthritis).

4 Check the legs for DVTs.
5 Investigations to consider:
- Urine dipstick and MSU
- FBC (for white cell differential), U&E, CRP, LFTs, ESR and blood gases or pulse oximetry if you suspect a PE or pneumonia
- Blood cultures peripherally and from lines
- Other cultures (sputum, stool, CSF, wound swabs, catheter tips)
- Radiology (CXR, AXR, sinus X-ray, US, CT scan, ECHO)
- Serology
6 Management. Take cultures and decide whether to start antibiotics straight away:
- You should start antibiotics if the patient is immunocompromised or diabetic as these patients can deteriorate rapidly.
- Conservative management is usually appropriate for patients in the following circumstances, if their temp is <38.5 °C:
- Up to 24 hours post-op or following invasive procedures.
- Following blood transfusion (see Blood transfusions).
- If antibiotics are started in the past 24 hours.
- Paracetamol (1 g 4–6 hourly) is a good antipyretic. Give IV if necessary. For fevers above 40 °C, prescribe tepid sponging and fanning as well.
- If SBE is a possibility, you need to take three sets of blood cultures from different sites and at different times (3–6 hours apart). Do not start antibiotics before consulting with your senior, as starting antibiotics before a diagnosis is confirmed may prevent isolation of an organism which makes effective treatment much more difficult.
- Remember to make best use of your microbiology department. They are usually eager to help you, and there is a 24-hour on-call cover.

Differential diagnosis

Think of 5 Ws: wind (i.e. respiratory), wound (including lines), water (urine), walking (deep venous thrombosis (DVT)) and wonder drugs

■ Infection, especially UTI, phlebitis/cellulitis, pneumonia and gastrointestinal infections causing diarrhoea. More common in diabetics – check feet for ulcers and lacerations as portal of entry and between toes for fungal infections

■ Drug induced: antibiotics, allopurinol, and ibuprofen
■ Common during blood transfusions
■ Thrombosis and secondary infarction: DVT, PE, MI and ischaemic bowel
■ Tumours
■ Alcohol withdrawal
■ Hyperthyroidism
■ Inflammatory and vasculitides, especially IBD and rheumatoid arthritis
■ Post-surgery

Table 8.4 Common post-operative causes of fever.

Days 1–2	Days 2–4	Days 5–10
Atelectasis ± LRTI	DVT	As for days 1–4
Aspiration pneumonia	Pulmonary embolism	Deep abscess formation
UTI	Wound infection	

The immunocompromised patient with fever

A patient is defined as immunocompromised if they have WCC $<2 \times 10^9/l$ and an absolute neutrophil count $<1 \times 10^9/l$ (neutropenia), are HIV positive with a low CD4 count or are on high-dose steroids or other immunosuppressants (chemotherapy, DMARDs, immunomodulatory drugs).

On the ward

1 Take a quick history and examination remembering:
- The patient can have weird organisms (bacterial, viral, fungal, protozoa) in weird places, including the CNS.
- Check *all* orifices.
- They can deteriorate rapidly (within hours). Seek senior advice early.

2 Investigations:
- Culture everything!
- If there is a central line, take peripheral and central blood cultures (include a culture from each lumen of triple lumen cannulae).
- Take stool, urine, sputum, MSU and wound swabs, including from around the entry site of indwelling IV lines.
- Consider removing lines and culturing the tips (cut using sterile technique – sterile scissors and gloves – and send to microbiology in a sterile container). Discuss with senior before removing any line you cannot easily replace!
- Recheck FBC for neutrophil count, platelets and Hb.
- U&E and glucose. Consider amylase, G&S, clotting, ESR, CRP.
- CXR (mobile).
- Specimen for serology if patient is new.

3 Start broad-spectrum antibiotics once cultures are taken. Check the latest protocol with a microbiologist. Oncology and haematology units usually have a written management protocol available. An aminoglycoside plus a beta-lactam, with or without extra anaerobic cover (metronidazole), is usual. Add flucloxacillin/teicoplanin if a staphylococcal wound or line infection is likely.

Fits

Your aim is to prevent the patient from harming themselves and to end the fit as soon as possible. Most fits last less than 5 minutes and do not require active treatment, but prolonged fits require urgent treatment to prevent hypoxia and brain damage. The longer a seizure persists the harder it usually is to terminate.

When answering your bleep

■ Ask the ward to do a blood glucose. Instruct the nurses if necessary to put out a crash call.
■ Proceed immediately to the ward.

Differential diagnoses

■ Epilepsy (this diagnosis requires at least two fits; this can be triggered by omitted anti-epileptic doses)
■ Drug or alcohol withdrawal
■ Hypoxia (fever in children)
■ Stroke/subarachnoid haemorrhage/subdural
■ Tumours (either primary malignancy or more commonly metastases)
■ Infection or inflammation of the brain and meninges
■ Metabolic causes: hypoglycaemia or hyperglycaemia, deranged Ca^{2+}, Mg^{2+}, Na^+, thyroxine, urea and bilirubin (liver/renal failure)
■ Drug overdose: tricyclics, phenothiazines, and amphetamines
■ Non-epileptic seizures (pseudo-seizures)

On the ward

1 Place the patient in the recovery position. Protect the patient's head with a pillow.

2 Do not forcibly restrain the patient:

- Give 100% O_2 by face mask and insert an oral airway if possible, but never force one. Call the anaesthetist early to get an airway.
- Establish IV access.
- For adults, give 2–4 mg lorazepam (IV bolus) or rectal diazepam (5–10 mg) if IV access is impossible. If the fit does not terminate within 5 minutes of IV therapy, repeat IV lorazepam 2 mg.
- If not already done, check blood glucose with blood glucose stick. If the patient is hypoglycaemic (glucose <2.5), give 50 ml of 50% dextrose IV immediately. Flush the line with saline as concentrated dextrose is highly irritant to veins. Alternatively give glucagon (1–2 mg IM or SC). Set up maintenance IV fluids containing dextrose (10% dextrose is good for this purpose).

3 If the patient is still fitting, call your senior. Meanwhile, if the patient is not already dosed with it, give phenytoin 1000–1500 mg (15–18 mg/kg) IV slowly (not exceeding 50 mg/minute). Watch for hypotension. If the patient has been taking phenytoin, the next step is phenobarbitone (15 mg/kg IV or IM slowly up to 100 mg/minute) – but get senior advice first. The patient may need ventilation. The final step in termination is general anaesthesia.

4 Once the fit has terminated:

- Examine the patient for localizing CNS signs and evidence of raised ICP (check fundi, BP and pulse).
- The patient will probably be drowsy (post-ictal).
- Consider consequences for the patient's driving licence.

5 Investigations to consider:

- FBC, U&E (Na is very important as hyponatraemia is a cause of fits), blood glucose, Ca^{2+} and Mg^{2+}.
- ABGs
- Blood cultures if febrile
- CXR
- CT scan if the cause is unclear and there are localizing neurological signs
- LP if suspected bacterial meningitis (exclude a space-occupying lesion first with CT; LP in the presence of an obstructed CSF flow can cause coning)
- Toxicology screen if indicated by the history
- Blood for anticonvulsant levels (some hospitals can do these within an hour)

Hints

■ If you arrive after the patient has stopped fitting but it sounds like a typical grand mal seizure, discuss prophylaxis with your seniors. If known epileptic, consider why they fitted now: Does it fit with their usual pattern of seizures? Is there an intercurrent infection? Are they known to have alcohol excess? Is there poor adherence to treatment? Drug levels will give you the answer to this.

■ If you suspect malnourishment or chronic alcohol abuse, give Pabrinex IV prior to any dextrose or IV fluids.

Intravenous fluids

IV fluid prescribing is really simple provided that you keep an eye out for the cardinal sins of IV hydration:

1 Overhydration, risking heart failure

2 Electrolyte imbalance, especially Na^+ and K^+

3 Phlebitis

4 Unnecessary and expensive if the patient can drink!

How to prescribe IV fluids

1 Decide on the daily volume of fluid required:
- Look at the fluid chart each day to make sure that you are keeping up with daily losses. Remember that in addition to recorded losses (urine, faeces, vomit), people lose 500 ml/24 hours in insensible losses.
- The average person needs 3 l/24 hours (each litre given 8 hourly).

2 Decide on which fluid(s) to use:
- Most patients can be given a daily total of 2–3 l of fluid in ratio of 2 l of 5% dextrose water to 1 l of normal (0.9%) saline. These should contain a total of 40 mmol of K^+ and 60–120 mmol Na^+ in 24 hours. This is typically written up as shown in Table 8.5.

3 Exceptions:
- Replace saline with dextrose water in patients with liver failure or ascites (the overactive renin–aldosterone system in these patients tends to retain salt).
- Avoid dextrose water in patients recovering from DKA or with hyponatraemia.
- Potassium imbalance is easy to achieve with IV fluids – and easy to correct. Measure electrolytes daily and adjust the K^+ accordingly.
- Hyponatraemia is a common and potentially lethal complication of IV hydration. If the patient's Na^+ falls below 135 mmol/l, the first step is to reduce the total IV fluid load and substitute dextrose with normal saline.

Table 8.5 Example of typical fluid chart.

Date	Fluid	Added drugs	Rate	Volume	Signature
01/05/14	Normal saline	+20 mmol KCl	125 ml/hour	1000 ml	J. Bloggs
01/05/14	5% dextrose		125 ml/hour	1000 ml	J. Bloggs
01/05/14	5% dextrose	+20 mmol KCl	125 ml/hour	1000 ml	J. Bloggs

Table 8.6 A rough guide to the electrolyte content and daily production of body fluids.

Fluid	Na^+ (mmol)	Cl^- (mmol)	K^+ (mmol)	HCO_3^- (mmol)	Daily volume (ml)
Sweat	50	40	5	~	Variable
Gastric	60–100	100	10	~	1500–2000
Bile	140	100	15–30	15–30	200–800
Pancreatic	140	75	5	70–120	200–800
Ileal	140	100	5	15–30	2000–3000
Diarrhoea	50	40	35	45	Variable

Hints

■ At least daily, examine elderly patients for signs of fluid overload (raised JVP, peripheral oedema, bibasal crepitations, tachypnoea, reduced saturations) and reduce fluids if necessary. Check the fluid charts and request daily weighing.

■ See Table 8.6 for a rough guide to body fluid content.

Upper gastrointestinal bleeds

Patients with UGIB can deteriorate rapidly, and small bleeds can herald major bleeds.

Whilst answering your bleep
Ask for BP and pulse to be taken as you head for the ward. If your nurses can get large-bore IV access, then ask them to do so and draw bloods including a group and save.

On the ward
The basic approach for all upper GI bleeds is the same:
1 See the patient. Wear universal precautions and then assess the severity of the bleed.
2 If the patient is hypovolaemic or at high risk for a major bleed, then they will require urgent treatment. To assess for severe hypovolaemia, check the BP, pulse and JVP (pulse >100/minute, sweaty and pale, cold peripheries, postural drop >20mmHg and JVP imperceptible when lying at 30° or less).
3 Treat on the basis of clinical findings. Remember that a small initial fall in Hb could be associated with a massive life-threatening bleed. Acute bleeds do not immediately alter Hb.

High-risk and hypovolaemic patients
If the patient is hypovolaemic or a high-risk patient:
1 Notify your senior immediately.
2 If hypotensive, give 100% O_2 and lower the patient's head.
3 Insert two large-bore cannulae (one in either arm), even if the patient's bleeding seems to have stopped.
4 If pulse >100 bpm or there are other signs of a major bleed, give 500 ml of crystalloid stat and repeat if necessary whilst waiting for blood.
5 Urgently crossmatch 4–6 units of blood. Use O-negative blood if the patient is still unstable after 1.5 l of fluid and a crossmatch is not available.
6 Do FBC and clotting studies. Transfuse until haemodynamically stable; 80% of bleeds stop spontaneously but 20% re-bleed. Correct any clotting abnormalities.
7 Insert urinary catheter. Monitor urine output hourly.
8 Consider inserting a CVP line, especially if the patient has a cardiac history or difficult venous access (consult your senior).
9 If the patient is anticoagulated at the time of the bleed, anticoagulation will need to be reversed. Discuss with your senior as to the best drug and dose to use.

Further investigations and ongoing medical management (discuss with your senior)
1 U&E. Bear in mind that urea is often raised due to blood in the gut, so look at the creatinine to assess renal status.
2 ECG and CXR in high-risk patients to look for aspiration and perforation.
3 Give IV pantoprazole (80mg over 1 hour) followed by a continuous infusion of 8mg/hour for 72 hours. Administration is only evidence based if given for recurrent bleeding ulcers post-endoscopy.
4 Monitor pulse, BP and urine output hourly until stable. Slow the rate of a blood transfusion once the pulse is less than 90 bpm and BP systolic is greater than 100mmHg. Ask to be called if there are signs of:
• Re-bleed
• Further haematemesis or melaena
• Increasing pulse rate (by more than 10 bpm)
• Systolic BP dropping by more than 10mmHg
• Urine output being less than 0.5 ml/kg/hour
• The patient becoming confused

5 Repeat clotting studies if patient has had more than 4 units transfused. You may need to give FFP.

6 Repeat FBC daily. Transfuse if Hb less than 8 g/dl or if symptomatic so that Hb > 10 g/dl.

7 Daily FBC and U&E. Repeat G&S if necessary (if previous sample was used up).

8 Ensure 2 units of packed red cells are available for 48 hours after haemostasis.

9 Keep the patient NBM for 12 hours (longer if surgery is likely) and for at least 8 hours before endoscopy.

10 Ensure that the patient is on the next endoscopy list (usually the following morning).

11 Discuss high-risk patients with the surgical team, in case the patient deteriorates.

Low-risk patients

If after initial assessment the patient is well and at low risk of bleeding (e.g. only coffee-ground vomitus, no melaena, normal pulse, BP and JVP, warm peripheries):

• Take a history and examination to exclude the risk of a big bleed.

• Insert a large cannula and consider repeating a FBC and G&S.

• Inform your senior.

• Ask the nurses to monitor vital signs.

• Most patients will require no further action.

Hints

■ Confirm with the patient that they have had true haematemesis, not haemoptysis or an occult nose bleed.

■ Vomitus can look like coffee grounds and contain small amounts of blood if the patient has not eaten for several days.

■ In acute bleeds, the reported Hb lags approximately 12 hours behind the actual red cell loss – be guided by the clinical signs.

■ Calculate the patient's Rockall score.

Lower gastrointestinal bleeds

Major lower GI bleeds, usually heralded by fresh or altered blood PR, are much less common in the hospital setting than upper GI bleeds. If called for a lower GI bleed, first exclude local causes such as piles and fissures. Follow the protocol for upper GI bleeds, with the possible addition of an urgent sigmoidoscopy.

Glucose

Whilst *hyper*glycaemia is rarely an emergency, patients can die or suffer brain damage from *hypo*glycaemia, so they need urgent attention.

Hyperglycaemia is commonly caused in diabetics by acute illness, corticosteroid treatment and test error. In non-diabetics it may be caused by blood taken from a drip arm, from latent carbohydrate intolerance which may be unmasked by sepsis, acute stress (e.g. MI) and steroids, and from laboratory error. Hyperosmolar complications take days to develop, whilst DKA and hyperosmolar hyperglycaemic state (HHS) have a dramatic clinical presentation:

On the ward

Hypoglycaemia is usually caused by oral hypoglycaemic agents and poor insulin control:

1 See the patient. If they are alert and well, repeat the blood glucose stick and take a sample for an urgent glucose test from the laboratory. Give them a concentrated sugar drink, such as sweet tea, or Hypostop and some biscuits.

2 If the patient cannot drink or is unconscious, administer 50 ml of 50% dextrose IV immediately. Flush the vein with 50 ml of saline or give 1 mg glucagon SC/IM. Most wards have a 'Hypostop box' on the crash trolley that contains Hypostop and glucagon.

3 Check recent insulin or oral hypoglycaemic doses. Adjust as necessary. Consider other, much rarer, causes of hypoglycaemia in the hospital setting, including liver failure and acute alcohol consumption.

4 Ask the nurse to repeat ward glucose readings. If the patient was semi-conscious or unconscious, repeat at least hourly until stable. Ask to be called if ward glucose readings are lower than 5 or more than 11 mmol/l.

5 If the patient has overdosed on long-acting insulin or oral hypoglycaemic agent, set up a 10% dextrose drip and adjust rate according to blood glucose readings (4–6 hourly once fully conscious and readings normal). Keep running for at least 48 hours.

1 See the patient. Repeat blood glucose stick and also send blood for urgent biochemistry glucose analysis.

2 Check urinary ketones. If these are positive, do an ABG and manage as DKA. If negative and the lab glucose result is greater than 22 mmol/l, the diagnosis is more likely to be HHS – give IV fluids and discuss with your senior.

Hints
■ Laboratory venous blood glucose results are often around 10% higher and more accurate than finger-prick assays.

■ Type II diabetes may require insulin for control during acute illness. Do not be afraid to give if indicated. You can prescribe PRN Actrapid 4–6 units SC on the PRN side of the drug chart and document that it is to be given if the BM is greater than 25.

Haematuria

In the hospital setting, haematuria is commonly caused by UTI or traumatic catheterization. However, haematuria may be the first sign of serious renal tract disease, such as tumour, stones or renal parenchymal disease (see Table 8.7).

On the ward
1 Exclude vaginal or anorectal bleeding.
2 Test for UTI: send an MSU and repeat the dipstick (look for protein, leukocytes and nitrites). If symptomatic, treat for UTI once the MSU is sent.
3 If a UTI is unlikely or the patient is unwell, discuss with your senior. Consider further investigations in light of the clinical context:
• Urine cytology and microscopy to look for casts.
• FBC, ESR, CRP and U&E.
• AXR for calculi and urogram or CT KUB.
• Repeat urinary dipstick daily until diagnosis is clear.

Table 8.7 Differential diagnoses of haematuria (consider the anatomy of the renal tract).

Renal parenchyma	Renal tract	Extra-renal (systemic)
■ Glomerulonephritis	■ UTI	■ Bleeding diathesis
■ Cystic disease	■ Trauma (e.g. catheters)	■ Vasculitis (e.g. SLE)
■ Tumours	■ Calculi	■ Malignant hypertension
■ Analgesic nephropathy	■ Prostatic disease	■ Emboli
■ Tuberculosis	■ Tumours	■ Sickle cell disease
	■ Bladder inflammation (e.g. infection)	

Hints

■ Urinary catheters can cause slight haematuria and usually do not require active treatment unless infection or non-trivial trauma is present. Some haematuria after catheterizing patients in acute urinary retention, due to bladder decompression, is normal.

■ If the urinary dipstick reveals significant proteinuria (2+ or more), renal parenchymal disease is likely. Commence a 24 hour urine collection to measure protein and creatinine clearance, and send urine for a urinary protein–creatinine ratio.

■ If no red cells are seen on microscopy despite significant dipstick-positive haematuria, consider haemolysis, myoglobinuria (rare) and rhabdomyolysis (do a serum CK).

■ Anticoagulation within the therapeutic range rarely causes haematuria but may unmask renal tract pathology.

Headaches

Tension headaches are common in hospital. The key to the diagnosis is the history.

Differential diagnoses and key symptoms

■ Tension headache: no associated symptoms. Pain can be severe, usually symmetrical and band-like. Often associated with stress and anxiety.

■ Migraine: usually history of previous episodes. Severe, throbbing pain which may be unilateral or asymmetric. May have prodromal symptoms (visual symptoms such as flashing lights, tunnel vision, cranial nerve deficit rarely lasting more than 1 hour; N&V, photophobia/phonophobia). Classic history makes the diagnosis, but exclude other causes if patient is drowsy and has neurological deficit or visual symptoms.

■ A variant is cluster headaches: unilateral pain becomes severe around one eye which becomes red, swollen and watery. Episodes last up to 1 hour and can occur several times a day. The pain can be excruciating.

■ Medication misuse headaches – patients commonly on mixed analgesics (co-codamol) often containing opiates. Withdraw analgesia to cure headache. Rebound headaches are common.

■ Sinusitis: dull, unilateral or central frontal headache, worse on leaning forwards/looking down and local tenderness.

■ Drug induced: especially nitrates, digoxin, tricyclic antidepressants and benzodiazepines

■ Meningitis and encephalitis: photophobia, stiff neck, ± fever and rash. Requires urgent LP (if no signs of raised ICP or focal neurology) and antibiotics/ acyclovir. Get senior help urgently.

■ Subarachnoid haemorrhage: sudden onset of severe headache (like an explosion in the back of the head) and meningism. Occasional atypical history (small leaks) mimicking meningitis. CT scan ± LP (showing red cells uniformly spread throughout the CSF in all bottles).

■ Raised ICP: present on waking, often associated with vomiting. May have blurred vision, raised BP and slow pulse. Fundi show papilloedema.

■ Brain abscess: non-specific pain, temperatures, change in personality if frontal lobe, may have seizures and may spread from ear infection. Diagnosis requires index of suspicion and CT. A raised CRP in this context should not be ignored.

■ Hypertensive encephalopathy: always markedly elevated BP (diastolic >130 mmHg) and other signs of malignant hypertension.

■ Subdural haematoma: alcoholic, anticoagulants and head trauma. Suspect in the elderly who have had a fall, with new-onset confusion or hemiplegia.

■ Acute glaucoma: usually presents with a dull pain behind the eyes which the patient may describe as a headache. There may be an arcuate scotoma. Urgent ophthalmology referral required.

■ Temporal arteritis: patient >50 years old. Subacute onset of frontal headache. Commonly associated with fever, malaise, myalgia, weight loss, jaw claudication, unilateral blindness or other visual disturbances (indicating imminent occlusion of the ophthalmic artery). A typical history, tender temporal arteries and a markedly raised ESR establish the diagnosis. Temporal artery biopsy should be undertaken but may be negative due to skip lesions. Do not withhold treatment for biopsy.

■ Trigeminal neuralgia – intense stabbing pain in the distribution of the trigeminal nerve. Typically unilateral and often triggered by the cold, shaving and eating.

On the ward

1 See the patient. Briefly exclude emergencies.

2 Perform a history and examination. Ask the patient if he or she has had similar headaches before. If history is typical for tension headache or migraine and if there is no evidence of fever, stiff neck, raised ICP or temporal artery tenderness, then prescribe analgesia (see the succeeding text). If, however, the headache is persistent, you should:

• Examine the pupils and (raised ICP), ENT (otitis media, sinusitis), CNS (especially cranial nerves) and gait (if history is suggestive of space-occupying lesion).

3 Investigations to consider: if the history is typical for a tension headache or migraine and there are no sinister signs, then no investigations are necessary. Otherwise, consider:

• ESR and CRP

• LP and CT scan and then LP

• Temporal artery biopsy

4 Treatment: once the rare but serious causes are excluded, mild–moderate cases can be managed with 1 g of paracetamol 4–6 hourly PRN. 10 mg metoclopramide IV is also shown to be very effective in acute migraine as it counteracts the effects of acute gastric stasis. If the patient is already on paracetamol, try ibuprofen (400 mg QDS) unless NSAIDs are contraindicated. The next line of therapy is triptans – these are usually started in specialist clinics. Migraine prophylaxis includes propranolol titrated up from 20 mg.

Hints

■ Always consider meningitis in patients with fever and headache, although any febrile illness may have an associated throbbing headache.

■ The scalp may be tender with tension headaches, migraine, temporal arteritis or shingles.

■ Be alert to depression in patients with recurrent tension headaches or migraines.

Hypertension

Hypertension is common but rarely requires treatment in the middle of the night unless there is evidence of heart failure, malignant hypertension or severe renal disease.

On the ward

1 Recheck BP and pulse. Use a manual sphygmomanometer if needed. Note previous readings. Make sure you use a big enough manometer cuff if the patient has large arms. Exclude:

• Heart failure: raised JVP, basal crackles, swollen ankles and enlarged liver.

• Malignant hypertension: headache, confusion or depressed level of consciousness and deteriorating vision. Perform fundoscopy to check for fresh retinal haemorrhages and dipstick urine for haematuria/proteinuria.

- Renal failure: check urine output and recent creatinine result.
2 If there is heart failure, malignant hypertension or renal failure, start to treat the cause and call the medical registrar for further management.
3 Otherwise, an elevated BP alone is seldom an indication for treatment. However, if the diastolic BP is greater than 130mmHg, put the patient to bed and prescribe a calcium channel blocker and aim to reduce the blood pressure slowly over 2–3 days. Nifedipine can cause a dramatic fall in BP, so avoid if possible. Call your senior if there is no response within 2 hours. Amlodipine 5mg as a stat dose is usually first line.
4 If the patient is in pain or anxious (common causes of elevated systolic pressure), provide analgesia and reassurance as appropriate.

Perioperative hypertension

Pre-op hypertension: Most anaesthetists will not anaesthetize a patient with a diastolic BP >100mmHg. Discuss prescribing 10mg of nifedipine PO or further sedation with the anaesthetist or your senior. Five milligrams SL nifedipine will reduce the blood pressure within 5 minutes and may be repeated. Ensure the anaesthetist is aware of the problem. They may prefer to manage the patient with IV labetalol. Note that many analgesic drugs vasodilate and cause a drop in blood pressure after induction. *Post-op hypertension* is often related to pain and will settle with adequate analgesia. If persistent, discuss with your senior.

Hints

■ Do not treat hypertension for at least 48 hours following a stroke. Dropping the BP under these circumstances can cause brain damage due to infarction and loss of the ischaemic penumbra.

■ Raised ICP can cause hypertension and bradycardia (Cushing's reflex).

Hypotension

Hypotension is a common call, particularly post-op. Hypotension is seldom an emergency, but whilst on the phone, ask how far the BP has fallen. A fall in systolic BP of >20mmHg is significant and >40mmHg (or systolic BP <80mmHg) is an emergency. Trends are more important than absolute values.

Differential diagnoses

■ Hypovolaemia (bleeding, dehydration)
■ Low peripheral resistance (post-general anaesthetic, infection, vasovagal, anaphylaxis, drugs: ACE inhibitors, nitrates, antihypertensives)
■ Poor cardiac function (arrhythmia, CCF, PE, tamponade, acute MI, valve failure, myocarditis, cardiomyopathy)

On the ward
1 See the patient and repeat the BP, manually if needed. If well but feeling faint, vasovagal or drug causes (including general anaesthesia) are likely. Drop the patient's head and raise the legs. Check the drug chart and do an ECG.
2 If unwell, feel their peripheries.
- If the patient has cold, clammy peripheries, consider:
  – Hypovolaemia (bleeding or dehydrated: JVP down)
  – Cardiac causes (MI, heart failure or arrhythmia: may have raised JVP. Check for irregular pulse, basal crepitations, history of IHD and chest pain)
  – PE (raised JVP, short of breath. Check for DVT, often no signs)
  – Anaphylaxis (wheezy, short of breath, new drug started)

- If the patient has warm peripheries, consider sepsis (JVP variable, fever). Check for source of infection (chest, abdomen, urine, skin, cannulae, surgical wounds). Exclude immunocompromise. Note that in some patients, severe sepsis may cause circulatory shutdown (cold peripheries) without going through a stage of vasodilatation.

3 Treat according to the cause.

- If hypovolaemic:

– Place the patient's head down.
– Insert large-bore IV cannulae. Give rapid IV fluid.
– Give face-mask O_2 100% (at least in the short term).
– Catheterize and monitor urine output.
– If hypovolaemic secondary to blood loss, replace with blood.

- If cardiac causes are most likely:

– The patient may go into shock. Get senior help and do an ECG stat.
– Give face-mask O_2 100%.
– Sit the patient up.
– Arrange for a mobile erect CXR.

If septic:

– Insert large-bore IV access, rapid IV fluids.
– Give face-mask O_2 100%.
– Blood cultures (two times) are mandatory, FBC and U&E.
– Consult your senior urgently before giving broad-spectrum antibiotics.

- Less common causes:

– PE. Do urgent ECG, CXR and ABGs. Discuss anticoagulation with your senior. If haemodynamically unstable, they may need thrombolysis.
– Anaphylaxis. Give 100% O_2, adrenaline 0.5 ml of a 1:1000 solution IM, salbutamol 5 mg nebulizer if wheezy, hydrocortisone 100–200 mg IV and chlorpheniramine 10 mg IV. Repeat IM adrenaline every 5 minutes until BP recovers.
– Consider adrenal insufficiency, especially if the patient is on steroids or has a history of Addison's disease. Give hydrocortisone 100 mg IV (to cover the added stress of illness irrespective of the cause).

4 If you feel out of your depth, call for senior help immediately. Most often the cause is obvious, but if not, do the following until help arrives:

- IV access.
- Face-mask O_2.
- ECG and mobile CXR.
- Bloods: FBC and clotting screen (INR and APTT), U&E, glucose, G&S (crossmatch if suspect bleeding), ABGs or at least pulse oximeter and blood cultures.
- Monitor urine output and consider catheterization.

Hints

■ Post-op falls with hypotension are common and often due to opiate analgesia. If the patient is otherwise well with no evidence of bleeding, ask the nurses to continue to monitor the temp, BP and pulse and to call you if the patient becomes unwell or the BP substantially dips from its post-op plateau. The BP should rise as the anaesthesia wears off.

■ Bradycardia suggests a vasovagal or arrhythmias (e.g. complete heart block unless the patient is on beta blockers or has raised ICP).

■ If the patient is hypovolaemic, but there is no evidence of dehydration or bleeding, consider an occult bleed. Risk factors for occult bleeding include NSAIDs, stress ulceration, recent instrumentation/surgery and hidden fractures (especially in the elderly).

Insomnia

Avoid prescribing sleeping tablets without first considering why the patient cannot sleep. Provided the patient does not take them home and develop dependency, short-acting sleeping tablets can be helpful. Zopiclone 3.75 mg at night is a good starting dose.

Differential diagnoses and suggested management

1 Noise, light or too much daytime sleep. These are the most common causes of insomnia in hospital and often the hardest to fix. Common-sense suggestions include:

• Suggesting that the patient need not worry about not sleeping at night. If they really need to sleep, they will.
• Avoiding stimulants before bedtime, such as cigarettes, tea or coffee.
• Wearing ear plugs and an eye visor.
• Minimizing noise from monitors.

2 Pain:

• Analgesia will facilitate sleep better than sleeping tablets.

3 Confusion, excessive anxiety or irritation and depression:

• Do not sedate the patient without excluding medical causes.
• Depression is common in hospital patients. Be wary of inducing benzodiazepine addiction in such patients (who may be especially vulnerable). Seek psychiatric advice if in doubt.

4 Disturbed sleep pattern due to frequency of micturition, orthopnoea or paroxysmal nocturnal dyspnoea:

• The patient may need better control of left ventricular failure (LVF). Avoid prescribing diuretics close to bedtime.

5 Disturbance in regular medication and bedtime habits:

• Often patients take an over-the-counter 'sleeping remedy' at home or have a supply of sleeping tablets which are not included in the general practitioner's (GP's) letter. The patient may not inform you about them unless specifically asked and may suffer rebound insomnia in hospital.

Management with benzodiazepines

Benzodiazepines (e.g. zopiclone 3.75–7.5 mg at night) are the mainstay of therapy for insomnia, but some patients cannot tolerate them. Amitriptyline 25–50 mg nocte is useful when neuropathic pain accompanies sleep disturbance. Use lower doses of all sedatives in the elderly (consult the *BNF*). Beware co-prescribing with opiates.

If you prescribe a sedative, tell the patient to call the nursing staff if they need the toilet. Sedatives in an unfamiliar environment can cause falls.

Itching

Except in the unusual event of anaphylaxis, itching is rarely serious. Exclude simple dermatological problems before considering symptomatic treatment if the patient has skin lesions or a rash.

Differential diagnoses (if no visible skin lesions or rash)

• Dry skin
• Drugs or allergies
• Jaundice
• Fe deficiency anaemia
• Hyperthyroidism
• Diabetes
• Early shingles
• Infestations (scabies, lice)
• Rarities: polycythaemia rubra vera (myeloproliferative diseases) and Hodgkin's lymphoma
• Late renal failure

On the ward

1 Check the patient's skin for rashes or lesions.

2 If there are no visible skin lesions, by far the most common cause of itching is dry skin, followed by drug reactions. Try to identify and replace the drug (seek pharmacological advice if unsure). Treat with emollient lotions after bathing (e.g. Dermol lotion, Aqueous cream). Use cold compresses and moisturizers such as E45 for localized itching. Advise minimal use of soap and shampoo. Prescribe soap substitutes, such as Dermol 500, for the patient to use when bathing.

3 If you are called at night and the patient is well, it is reasonable to treat symptomatically. Choose a sedating antihistamine at night (e.g. chlorpheniramine 4 mg TDS) or a non-sedating one if preferred (e.g. cetirizine 10 mg OD).

Hints

Scabies is common and can cause intense itching anywhere on the body, except the head. The S-shaped burrows are easy to miss – look carefully around the itching site, particularly along the fingers and in the interdigital webs. Consult the *BNF* for treatment of scabies and other infestations. Clothes and bedding need to be washed in a hot wash. Check with nurses that other nearby patients and relatives (or staff!) are not similarly infested. Put the patient in a side room, ensure that they are treated promptly, and inform them that although the scabies is treated, the itching can persist for many weeks after.

Major trauma

It is unlikely that you will ever be solely responsible for patients with major trauma. However, if you are first to arrive at a trauma scene, it is worth having a mental plan of action. This is a simple format based on the advanced trauma life support (ATLS) protocol and is intended for initiating management of the person until senior help arrives. The main thing to remember is to get help fast from someone who knows what they are doing.

On the ward (or A&E)

1 Do not be distracted by gruesome injuries. Start with a primary survey (ABC) whilst senior help arrives. If you have time before the patient arrives, then don universal precautions and prepare the equipment you think will be necessary (airway adjuncts, cannulae and fluids, defibrillator and pads, etc.). If there is massive haemorrhage, then apply direct pressure to the wound.

2 Airway and cervical spine control: maintaining a clear airway is absolutely vital. Without this, everything else is futile. Clear the airway of any blood, teeth and foreign bodies. Do not move the neck more than necessary; get someone to hold the neck still until a hard collar can be placed. Intubation requires skill, and in addition to moving the cervical spine, it can cause cardiovascular instability and actually compromise oxygenation if performed incorrectly. This is therefore best left to those who have specific training. It is often best to start with an oropharyngeal airway and bag–valve–mask ventilation if the patient is obtunded. If they are biting down or coughing on the oral airway, it should be removed to stop them from vomiting. Traditional teaching is to avoid nasopharyngeal airways in the trauma situation, especially if they have facial trauma. However, unless they have large amounts of facial trauma, it is unlikely to be detrimental and may allow oxygenation that is otherwise not possible.

3 Breathing and oxygenation: give 100% oxygen (by non-rebreathing bag) and check if the patient is breathing. If not, start basic life support.

4 Circulation and haemorrhage control: check for a carotid pulse and start basic life support. Get good IV intravenous access (2× green cannula or ideally larger) but do not give fluids unless systolic blood pressure is less than 90 mmHg as this may unnecessarily dislodge any clots that are preventing exsanguination. Obtain baseline bloods including a clotting and group and save, in case the patient has internal bleeding or needs to go to theatre. An ABG/VBG is helpful. In the case of a traumatic cardiac arrest (penetrating or blunt), the cause may be due to hypovolaemia or a tamponade. In these circumstances, chest compressions and defibrillation will not be effective. However, it is not detrimental so it is standard practice to follow standard ALS/ATLS protocols until expert help arrives. If the cause is a haemopneumothorax, then needle decompression may buy time until formal thoracostomy/chest drain insertion can be performed.

Hints

■ Once senior help arrives, continue with a specific task (e.g. IV access) and watch how the trauma team works. This is the best way to get experience.

■ Consider an ATLS course, particularly if you intend to pursue a career in trauma or surgery.

Minor trauma

Do not feel embarrassed about asking for help with minor injuries; the variety can make them more challenging than you might imagine. Despite this, you will learn quickly and common sense usually prevails. The most common minor injury results from falls in hospital. When answering your bleep, ask for:

■ BP and pulse
■ Any analgesia the patient has received

On the ward

1 Start by assessing airway, breathing and circulation.

2 When seeing the patient, ask about likely causes.

3 Give analgesia if the patient is in pain. Paracetamol or ibuprofen is usually adequate.

4 Things to consider with any injury are:

● Skin break: a plaster or dressing is adequate in most cases. If there is a laceration, clean the wound with sterile water or normal saline. If the skin edges are opposed to each other and are not likely to be displaced, leave well alone. Otherwise steri-strips or sutures may be necessary. This may need specialist input if on the face.

● Soft tissue injury: analgesia and rest are sufficient. For limbs or joints, consider resting the joint acutely, ice, splint and elevation. Advise early mobility of the affected area once swelling subsides.

● Fracture: if there is bony tenderness, perform a plain X-ray of the area. Two views are more useful than one. If there is a fracture, call the orthopaedic team for advice.

● Organ injury: if concerned, reassess airway, breathing and circulation, and seek urgent senior help.

Hints

● The best person to ask about minor injuries is usually a senior nurse. They will be able to give you advice on management.

● Fracture clinics are useful places to send well patients with fractures for follow-up after discharge.

● 'Ottawa rule' for ankle injuries states that there is usually no need to perform an X-ray on an ankle if:

○ The person is weight-bearing after the injury and can weight-bear for two steps.

Table 8.8 Differential diagnoses to a moribund patient (acronym: CASH).

Chest	Abdomen	Systemic	Head
■ Pulmonary oedema	■ Haemorrhage	■ Drug overdose (e.g. opiates)	■ CVA
■ MI	■ Perforated bowel or viscus	■ Hypothermia	■ Post-ictal
■ Arrhythmias	■ Pancreatitis	■ Septicaemia	■ Hydrocephalus
■ Pneumonia	■ Ruptured or leaking AAA	■ Hypoglycaemia	■ SAH
■ Asthma		■ Anaphylaxis	
■ Pulmonary embolus		■ Major electrolyte derangement	
■ Dissecting aneurysm			
■ Pneumothorax			

o No tenderness over the posterior or tip of the medial malleolus.

o No tenderness over the posterior or tip of the lateral malleolus.

o No tenderness over the calcaneum or navicular.

o No tenderness over the base of the 5th metatarsal.

o No tenderness of the proximal fibula.

Document these when tested and lower your threshold for reattenders.

The moribund patient

If you are called to see a 'peri-arrest' patient, don't panic. You usually have more time than you think. The priority is to buy time by supporting the vital functions whilst getting basic background information and examining as you go. Call your senior early and do not be afraid to call the crash team before the patient arrests. This is often advised but rarely undertaken. Think CASH! (Table 8.8) Stay calm and remain polite; if the doctor panics, so will everyone else.

On the ward

1 See the patient urgently. Check their ABC:
- Airway clear? Y/N
- Breathing? Y/N; trachea central? bilateral breath sounds?
- Circulation – pulse? Y/N; if Y, BP?

2 Bring (or get somebody to bring) the crash trolley to hand and to call the crash team if an arrest looks imminent.

3 Give high-flow O_2 (15 l via non-rebreathing mask).

4 Establish large-bore IV access: 16G if possible. Don't rush. Consider inserting two cannulae at separate sites.

5 If BP <80 mmHg, consider starting rapid IV fluids unless a cardiac cause is probable.

6 Whilst the infusion is being set up, quickly assess preceding symptoms, past medical history (PMH) and current medications. Examine the chest and heart.

7 If a cardiac cause is likely:
- Do an ECG and request a mobile CXR. Do not delay treatment.

● Pulmonary oedema, arrhythmias or MI are the most likely causes. Consider pericardial tamponade.

8 Exclude hypoglycaemia or opiate overdose:

● If blood glucose is less than 2.5 mmol/l, give 50 ml of 50% glucose IV (flush vein with saline afterwards) or 1 mg glucagon IV/IM/SC.

● Note the size of the pupils. Give naloxone 400–800 µg IV if the patient has pinpoint pupils and is on opiates. Repeat if necessary.

9 Listen to the chest. If markedly tachypnoeic in the absence of pulmonary oedema or pneumothorax, consider PE.

10 Feel the peripheries. If the patient has warm peripheries with hypotension, consider sepsis.

11 Consider anaphylaxis:

● New drug started recently, hypotensive, SOB, wheezy, swollen lips/eyelids and urticarial rash.

● Give 100% O_2, adrenaline 0.5 mg (i.e. 0.5 ml of a 1:1000 solution) IM, salbutamol 5 mg nebulizer, hydrocortisone 100 mg IV, chlorpheniramine 10 mg IV and aggressive IV fluid resuscitation. Give adrenaline every 5 minutes until BP recovers.

If the cause is not clear, do a brief neurological examination: level of consciousness (Glasgow Coma Scale), pupil and eye movements, limb tone, reflexes and plantars. Consider occult bleeding, post-ictal states and meningitis or encephalitis. Seek senior advice.

12 Urgent investigations:

● ECG.

● FBC and INR, U&E, CRP, glucose and amylase.

● ABGs.

● Mobile CXR, as erect as possible to check for free air under the diaphragm. View carefully for a pneumothorax, which is often missed in a panic.

Hints

■ Metabolic acidosis, confirmed by an ABG, can cause compensatory tachypnoea. If the patient has metabolic acidosis and hypotension, consider sepsis, ischaemic bowel, perforated viscus, pancreatitis and acute kidney injury.

Nausea and vomiting

Any acute illness can cause non-specific N&V. Be wary, however, of prescribing anti-emetics without also investigating the cause. If the patient is distressed, it is reasonable to give an anti-emetic before examining them.

Differential diagnoses

1 Surgical conditions

● Intestinal obstruction and peritonitis
● Acute cholecystitis
● Paralytic ileus

2 Medical causes

● Local causes
– Oesophagitis
– Gastritis
– Gastroenteritis
– Peptic ulcer
– Pyloric stenosis
● Central causes
– Raised ICP
– Migraine
– Brainstem lesions
– Meniere's disease
– Labyrinthitis
● Systemic causes
– Infection (UTI, pneumonia, gastroenteritis)
– Metabolic (organ failure, DKA, Addison's, MI, electrolyte imbalance – Na^+, K^+, Ca^{2+})
– Drug reactions (opiates, digoxin, NSAIDs, dopamine agonists, chemotherapy)

3 Special causes

● Pregnancy
● Bulimia/anorexia

On the ward

1 Exclude severe dehydration (BP sitting and lying, tachycardia).

2 Rule out common surgical conditions – intestinal obstruction and peritonism.

3 Think about medical causes as in the aforementioned.

4 Special considerations:

- Is the patient pregnant? Do a urinary pregnancy test, and consider serum beta-human chorionic gonadotrophin (bHCG) levels.
- In the elderly, an inferior acute MI can present with N&V in the absence of pain. Do ECG and serial cardiac enzymes.

5 When there is no obvious cause after history and examination:

- If the patient had a single episode of vomiting without associated symptoms or signs, ask the nurses to observe the patient and monitor temp, BP, pulse and urine output. Dipstick the urine to exclude UTI, especially in the elderly.
- If N&V persists or there is systemic upset, consider FBC, U&E and CRP.

6 Further investigations to consider include:

- Ca^{2+}, Mg^{2+}, phosphate and amylase
- ABGs if with severe vomiting to look for a metabolic alkalosis

7 Management options to control symptoms: the two most commonly used drugs are cyclizine 50 mg PO/IV/IM and metoclopramide 10 mg IM or IV (caution in young women due to risk of dystonic reactions like an oculogyric crisis). Alternatives include:

- Domperidone: 10–30 mg PR.
- 5-HT3 antagonists (e.g. ondansetron, granisetron) are very effective but are expensive and usually reserved for chemotherapy-induced N&V.

Oxygen therapy

Methods of oxygen delivery

Face masks (e.g. system 22 or Ventimasks) are good for acute situation. Controlled percentage face masks control the amount of O_2 the patient receives and are graded 24, 28, 35, 40 and 60%. You need to adjust the O_2 flow rate at the wall or cylinder, according to the rate printed on the mask – usually about 2 l/minute for 24% masks and 15 l/minute for 60% masks. It takes at least 15–20 minutes for blood gases to equilibrate after changing the percentage of inspired O_2. This is **not** a reason to delay giving oxygen; there is no justification in removing a patient from oxygen for a 'baseline' ABG. It is hypoxia that kills, not hypercapnia, so high-flow O_2 in an acute situation is appropriate and then weaned down.

Nasal specs are useful if the patient cannot tolerate a face mask and for longer-term O_2 therapy. It is difficult to regulate O_2 delivery with nasal specs, so regular blood gas checks may be necessary. For standard-size specs, a flow rate of 4–6 l/minute is usual for achieving an inspired O_2 percentage of 30–40%.

For patients with COPD

Under normal conditions, the concentration of CO_2 in the blood is the primary stimulus of the respiratory drive. Some patients with severe COPD become insensitive to CO_2 levels and are dependent on low O_2 levels (mild hypoxia) to maintain their respiratory effort. If you give too much O_2, the hypoxic stimulus is lost and they will hypoventilate, leading to CO_2 retention (hypercarbia). This can cause CO_2 narcosis and ultimately death.

Therefore, when non-emergency O_2 therapy is required in patients with COPD:

1 Start with a 24% face mask and re-measure the ABGs after 30 minutes to 1 hour to

ensure that the CO_2 levels are not rising. You need to find a level that achieves a fine balance between improving oxygenation and keeping the CO_2 at a safe level. Ask for senior advice if the CO_2 level rises >1.5 kPa above the previous ABG level or rises above 8 kPa.

2 If the CO_2 level does not rise but hypoxia is still a problem, increase the oxygen to 28% then 35%, etc., repeating the ABGs 30 minutes to 1 hour after each change.

3 If you cannot increase the percentage O_2, despite persisting hypoxia, because of hypercapnia, mechanical ventilation may be necessary. Bipap is a common choice of non-invasive ventilation in type 2 respiratory failure, but patients may need to go to a high dependency unit to receive this. Discuss with your senior urgently if you think the patient requires this.

Hints

■ Use a humidifier with O_2 if possible.
■ Patients may be left on O_2 for longer than necessary. Always ask whether or not they really need it, as the face mask and straps are uncomfortable.
■ Strictly, you are supposed to prescribe O_2 therapy on the drug chart.

Pulse oximetry

Pulse oximetry measures the percentage of blood O_2 saturation. It is not a direct assay of PaO_2 or $PaCO_2$. It is not as trustworthy as arterial blood gases, particularly in COPD patients, as they may retain CO_2 in spite of reasonable percentage O_2 saturation. Also, pulse oximetry may not detect low PaO_2 due to the steep sigmoid curve of the O_2 saturation curve. If in doubt, do ABGs.

Phlebitis

Phlebitis is indicated by pain and redness at IV sites and is prevented by changing the IV site every 2–3 days. Phlebitis can easily become a cellulitis, so take care. On your ward round,

regularly assess all lines and decide if they need to be in. If not, remove them.

Management

1 Remove the cannula and apply heat (e.g. damp, warm towel).

2 Elevate the limb.

3 Give mild analgesia if the site is very painful (e.g. paracetamol 1 g QDS or consider NSAIDs if young and no history of renal impairment).

4 Suppurative phlebitis is more worrying (pus at the IV entry site, induration, fever and enlarged draining lymph nodes). Try to express some pus and send a swab to microbiology for urgent MC&S. Prescribe IV antibiotics to cover **Staphylococcus aureus**. If the patient is well, flucloxacillin alone may suffice. The addition of penicillin may be needed or clindamycin. Discuss local protocols with a microbiologist. Surgical drainage is occasionally required.

Potassium

Hyperkalaemia

K^+ greater than 6.5 mmol/l needs urgent treatment, but exclude false-positives from old or haemolysed samples or if taken from drip arm. Repeat the sample if in doubt. In the hospital setting, by far the most common cause of hyperkalaemia is drugs or renal failure. Differential diagnoses are:

■ K^+ sparing diuretics – spironolactone and amiloride (beware: if these are given with ACE inhibitors, rapid fatal rises in potassium can occur)
■ ACE inhibitors
■ Excessive K^+ supplements, orally or IV
■ Metabolic acidosis
■ Acute renal failure
■ Diabetic ketoacidosis
■ Cell lysis – tumour lysis syndrome
■ Massive tissue trauma/blood transfusion
■ Mineralocorticoid deficiency
■ Addison's disease

On the ward
1 See the patient. Repeat K+ on a VBG and lab bloods. Check their renal function (U&E). In the meantime, if the initial K+ was greater than 6.5 mmol/l:
2 Do an ECG urgently.
3 Get IV access and give calcium gluconate (or chloride) 10 ml of a 10% solution IV over 10 minutes.
4 If acidotic on ABG, discuss with your senior. The use of bicarbonate (100 ml of a 4.2% solution) is highly controversial, and not usually used.
5 Give 10 units of Actrapid insulin with 50 ml of 50% dextrose IV infusion (insulin drives K+ back into cells).
6 Consider calcium resonium 15 g 6–8 hourly PO or 30 g PR if with long-standing hyperkalaemia. As this causes severe constipation, give laxatives concurrently.
7 Salbutamol nebulizers can also help as a short-term fix.

Hypokalaemia

In the hospital setting, hypokalaemia is usually caused by diuretics, inappropriate replacement fluids or taking blood from the drip arm. Differential diagnoses are:

■ Inadequate potassium replacement in IV fluids
■ Renal losses
■ Diuretics
■ Other drugs – amphotericin B, carbenicillin and ticarcillin
■ Excess mineralocorticoid (tumours or Conn's syndrome)
■ Cushing's syndrome/steroids/ACTH
■ GI tract losses: diarrhoea/vomiting/intestinal fistulae/villous adenoma
■ Intracellular potassium shifts
■ Insulin administration
■ Purgative abuse

On the ward
1 See the patient. If the K+ is less than 2.5 mmol/l or less than 3.0 and the patient is taking digoxin, you need to replace K+ urgently, as there is a risk of arrhythmias:
• Give 20 mmol/hour KCl at a concentration not exceeding 40 mmol/l. Concentrated K+ damages peripheral veins. Never give bolus KCl, which can cause fatal arrhythmias.
• Do an urgent ECG. Consider cardiac monitoring.
• Monitor K+ 4 hourly until stable.
2 2 If the K+ is between 2.5 and 3.0 mmol/l:
• Oral replacement therapy is usually sufficient. However, if the patient is at risk for arrhythmias, give cautious IV therapy (10–15 mmol/hour).
3 If the K+ is greater than 3.0 mmol/l:
• Give oral replacement therapy unless the patient is NBM or vomiting. Prescribe 80–120 mmol K+ in divided doses per day. There is a wide range of pills with varying amounts of K+ in each. You can also advise the patient to eat K+-containing foods.
4 Investigations to consider:
• Monitor K+ every 1–2 days.
• Consider measuring Mg. Hypomagnesaemia may cause hypokalaemia refractory to therapy.

Hints

■ Avoid slow-K non-effervescent tablets, as they cause severe oesophageal and gastric irritation. Use the horrible tasting, but more effective, soluble effervescent tablets or syrups. To make more palatable, mix with orange juice or squash.

■ In patients with normal renal function, it is difficult to overdose with oral K^+. However, DO NOT give K^+ if the patient is oliguric. Consult your senior.

■ Low plasma bicarbonate levels suggest that the patient has long-standing, intracellular K^+ depletion. K^+ replacement can take days.

■ Contrary to popular belief, hypokalaemia secondary to vomiting is due to metabolic alkalosis.

■ Be careful in prescribing long-term oral K^+ supplements for patients to take home due to risk of hyperkalaemia. It is usually wise to limit to take outs (TTOs) to 3 days with GP review.

Rashes and skin lesions

The algorithm below is designed to help you make an initial diagnosis of the patient's rash or skin lesion. By far, the most common cause of new rashes in hospital is drug reactions, but psoriasis, shingles, eczema and other skin conditions can all flare up with the stress of illness. Dermatologists are usually helpful and keen for referrals. Seek their advice.

Questions to ask

1 Are the lesions filled with fluid?
● No → go to the next question.
● Clear fluid → (1)
● Pus → (2)
2 Are the lesions coloured but not red?
  Yellow → (3)
  White → (4)
  Brown → (5)
  Skin coloured → (6)
3 If the lesions are red, are they scaling?
● No scaling:

– Macular/flat → (7)
– Papular/ → (8)
– Scaling:
– No epithelial → (9)
– Epithelial → (10)

Disease categories 1–10

1 Vesiculobullous diseases:

● Vesicles – herpes simplex/shingles/chicken pox/scabies/dermatitis herpetiformis/dyshidrosis
● Bullae – pemphigus/pemphigoid/bullous impetigo/erythema multiforme bullosum

2 Pustular diseases – acne/folliculitis/rosacea/Pustular psoriasis

3 Yellow lesions: xanthelasma/necrobiosis lipoidicum

4 White lesions: tinea versicolor/pityriasis alba/vitiligo

5 Brown lesions:

● Macules – freckles/lentigines
● Papules and nodules – junctional or compound naevi/melanoma/seborrhoeic keratoses
● Patches and plaques – café-au-lait spots/giant pigmented hairy naevus

6 Skin coloured papules and nodules:

● Rough surface – warts/actinic keratoses/squamous cell carcinoma

• Smooth surface – condylomata acuminata/basal cell carcinoma/epidermoid cysts/lipomas/molluscum contagiosum

7 Vascular reactions:

• Blanching lesions – macular and diffuse erythema (toxic erythema, e.g. skin rash of viral illness, and toxic epidermal necrolysis, a medical emergency)/urticaria/erythema multiforme/erythema nodosum

• Non-blanching (purpuric) lesions – vasculitides

8 Inflammatory papules and nodules:

• Papules – insect bites/pompholyx/pyogenic granulomas/cherry angiomas/granuloma annulare

• Nodules – furunculosis ± cellulitis

9 Papulosquamous diseases:

• Plaque formation – psoriasis/lupus erythematosus/mycosis fungoides/tinea corporis/tinea cruris/tinea pedis

• Predominantly papular – lichen planus/secondary syphilis/pityriasis rosea

10 Eczematous reactions: atopic dermatitis/dyshidrotic eczema/contact dermatitis

Diagnosing skin tumours

■ Melanoma

• Itching/crusting/bleeding/change in size, shape or colour of mole/irregular contours/variegated colour/weight loss/satellite lesions

■ Basal cell carcinoma

• Pearly nodule/ulcer with prominent blood vessels

■ Squamous cell carcinoma

• Non-healing/crusting ulcer with rolled edge

Hints

■ Generalized erythematous rash (or blistering) and fever should ring alarm bells as they may be associated with serious bacterial infections (e.g. streptococcal and staphylococcal toxic shock syndrome).

■ Take very seriously any new rash in people who are immunocompromised (e.g. HIV, high-dose chemotherapy, leukaemia), as this could herald fatal sepsis.

■ Similarly, take seriously a new rash in people taking medication that may cause agranulocytosis (e.g. ticlopidine or carbimazole).

Shortness of breath

When answering your bleep
Ask the nurse to assess the respiratory rate, pulse, BP and, if possible, peak flows if asthmatic and pulse oximetry readings.

Differential diagnoses

■ Acute LVF (flash pulmonary oedema)
■ Asthma
■ Pulmonary embolus
■ Pneumonia
■ Pneumothorax
■ COPD exacerbated by acute illness

Rarely
■ Pericardial tamponade
■ Anaphylaxis

On the ward

1 See the patient. Check the temperature, BP and pulse and assess for respiratory distress (respiratory rate >30/minute ± cyanosis) and hypotension.

2 If the patient is hypotensive, consider acute MI, large PE, tension pneumothorax, pericardial tamponade and anaphylaxis. Lower the patient's head and institute emergency treatment. Get senior assistance

3 If the patient is markedly tachypnoeic or cyanosed:

• Give high-flow O_2 even if the patient has COPD.

• Exclude pneumothorax with auscultation and percussion of the precordium.

• Give salbutamol 5 mg stat using a nebulizer if wheezy. Repeat as necessary.

• Examine quickly for acute pulmonary oedema (JVP, basal crackles or effusion). If present, sit the patient up, and give furosemide 40–80 mg IV, diamorphine 2.5–5 mg IV slowly and an anti-emetic (e.g. metoclopramide 10mg IV/IM). Consider MI or arrhythmia and do an urgent ECG.

- Request an urgent mobile CXR.
- Do ABGs.
- Notify your senior: get help early if the patient is deteriorating.
- Important note: if you cannot distinguish between early pulmonary oedema, asthma or pneumonia (often difficult to differentiate), treat for all three. If there are no signs of heart failure or asthma, consider pulmonary embolus. Give treatment-dose LMWH if in doubt and confirm the diagnosis later.

4 If the patient is not acutely distressed: take a full history and examination. Do not forget to ask about new-onset pleuritic chest pain or acute non-traumatic leg swelling, history of asthma or IHD and any recent changes in medication. Consider the differential diagnosis and treat accordingly.

5 Investigations to consider:

- FBC, U&E and CRP
- ABGs
- CXR (expiratory to show a pneumothorax better)
- ECG
- Urgent ECHO or FAST scan if you suspect tamponade

Hints

■ A good way to assess respiratory rate is to breathe with the patient, as this also reveals abnormal breathing rhythms (not all dyspnoeic patients are tachypnoeic).

■ Patients at risk for pneumothorax include those with a central line, pneumonia, COPD or asthma.

■ Psychogenic SOB (hyperventilation) is suggested by peri-oral tingling, pins and needles; carpopedal spasm; and especially alkalosis on ABGs. Treat by having the patient breathe into a paper bag.

■ A fever suggests infection, but also consider PE or MI.

■ Check for pulsus paradoxus (drop in BP of greater than 10mmHg on inspiration), which suggests severe asthma, pericardial constriction or tamponade.

■ If possible, take an ABG sample before starting the patient on O_2. Do not delay oxygen for an ABG.

The sick patient

The following is a checklist of things that you should consider when seeing any patient who is very unwell (modify in light of the specific system involved):

1 What are the temp, BP, pulse, oxygen saturations and respiratory rates?

2 Are ABC adequate?

3 Does the patient need the following?

- Analgesia
- ABGs or pulse oximetry
- Baseline bloods
- CXR (mobile)
- ECG/cardiac monitor
- IV access
- IV fluids
- O_2
- Senior opinion
- Urinary catheter

Sodium

Hyponatraemia

Mild to moderate hyponatraemia is common in hospital due to excess IV (hypotonic) fluids. Hyponatraemia usually develops over days; cautious replacement of Na^+ should be observed. More urgent treatment is required if there are neurological symptoms which range from lethargy to severe confusion, seizures or coma, but symptoms should not be ascribed to hyponatraemia immediately if the serum Na^+ is >125mmol/l.

Differential diagnoses

■ Overhydration with IV fluids
■ Renal/metabolic – nephrotic syndrome, Addison's disease, interstitial renal disease/nephritic syndrome, *SIADH*, diarrhoea, vomiting and small bowel obstruction
■ Malignancy
■ Drugs – chlorpropamide, haloperidol and thiazide diuretics
■ Chest – infection and CCF
■ Cirrhosis
■ Severe hypothyroidism
■ Burns

On the ward

1 See the patient and assess their fluid balance (JVP, fluid chart, chest).
● If dehydrated, measure urinary Na^+:

– If urinary Na^+ >20 mmol/l with hyponatraemia, consider renal causes.
– If urinary Na^+ <20 mmol/l, consider other causes.

● If not dehydrated, is the patient oedematous?

– If yes, volume overload is likely. Exclude nephrotic syndrome, CCF, cirrhosis and severe hypothyroidism.
– If no, but the urine is concentrated (urine osmolality >500 mmol/kg or high specific gravity), SIADH is most likely. Look for the cause.

2 Investigations to consider:
● Urinary Na^+, urine and plasma osmolality, U&E and liver chemistry
● CXR

3 Management: treat underlying cause. Urgent Na^+ replacement may be required if patient is severely symptomatic and Na^+ <125 mmol/l. Seek expert guidance.
● If hyponatraemia is mild with no symptoms and the patient is not dehydrated, treat by restricting fluid only. Start with 1.5 l/day, and reduce by 50 ml/day if there is no improvement.
● If the patient is dehydrated with normal renal function, give 0.9% saline.
● Beware of correcting hyponatraemia too rapidly. This can cause central pontine myelinolysis with irreversible brain damage and locked-in syndrome. IV hypertonic saline is rarely required unless the patient is fitting or unconscious.

Hints

■ Hyponatraemia due to ectopic antidiuretic hormone secretion may be the first sign of a small-cell carcinoma of the lung.
■ SIADH can only be diagnosed if the patient is hyponatraemic and the urine Na >20 mmol/l and osmolality >500 mmol/kg, with a plasma Na <125 mmol/l or plasma osmolality <260 mmol/kg.

■ Mild hyponatraemia is frequently seen in severely ill patients but rarely needs treatment.

Transfusions

Whilst blood transfusions are common in hospital, always be alert to transfusion reactions.

Blood transfusions

For chronic stable anaemia

These patients have had a low Hb for a long time. Provided that there has been no additional acute fall in Hb, transfusion is not urgent and is seldom needed in the middle of the night. Ensure any blood tests (FBC, iron studies, B_{12} and folate, blood film, Hb electrophoresis) have been sent before transfusion. Transfusion should be slow to avoid causing heart failure:

1 Estimate the red cell deficit (1 unit of packed cells raises the Hb by 1 g/dl).

2 In general:

- Transfuse the patient to >8 g/dl if they have a reversible cause of anaemia.
- Transfuse to >10 g/dl if they have an irreversible cause of anaemia (e.g. myelodysplasia) or as per the haematologists request.
- In patients having radiotherapy for malignancy, keep Hb >12 g/dl.

3 Check the patient's pulse, BP, JVP and chest for basal crackles as a baseline before transfusing.

4 The rate of transfusion will depend on the clinical setting and the presence or absence of heart disease:

- Transfuse slowly (each unit over 3–4 hours) in the elderly.
- Give furosemide 20–40 mg PO before the first unit and then with each bag if you are concerned about heart failure.
- If the patient becomes fluid overloaded, give furosemide (frusemide) 40 mg IV as a stat dose (do not mix in with the bag of blood). Repeat as necessary.

5 If the patient has had a previous transfusion reaction, give hydrocortisone (100 mg IV) and chlorpheniramine (chlorphenamine) (10 mg IV) before the transfusion. This is often necessary in patients who have had multiple transfusions.

Hints

■ Do not transfuse blood through lines used for solutions containing dextrose, as this causes red cells to clump.

■ Blood is usually given via a special giving set which should be available on the wards.

In the acute setting

1 Estimate how many units of blood the patient will need. In the acute setting, the Hb level lags the actual red cell loss by 12–24 hours. Crossmatch units as needed (4–6 units in an acute GI bleed). In an emergency situation, you can use 'flying squad' or O-negative blood. If a patient is acutely haemorrhaging, you can activate the major haemorrhage protocol pathway, so you can urgently get blood, FFP and cryoprecipitate to your location.

2 Packed cells have few clotting factors and platelets. Therefore, for transfusions of more than 4 units, check the INR and APTT, and add 2 units of FFP for every 4 units of packed cells. You may need cryoprecipitate also. Always discuss with the haematology team.

Hints

■ In acute and subacute bleeds, the mean cell volume (MCV) is normal.

■ Remember hidden fractures in the elderly. The thigh can conceal 2 l of blood. Similarly, always think of retroperitoneal bleeds if the Hb is dropping with no obvious external losses.

Platelet transfusions

Indications

■ Platelet count $<20 \times 10^9/l$ or $<40 \times 10^9/l$, and the patient is at risk of bleeding (e.g. going for major surgery)

■ Thrombocytopenia or dysfunctional platelets with active bleeding

To order platelets, you only need to know the patient's blood group; a crossmatch is not necessary. If the patient has had a previous platelet transfusion reaction (common), administer hydrocortisone (100 mg IV) and chlorpheniramine (chlorphenamine) (10 mg IV) before the transfusion. If the patient's platelets are not incrementing, discuss human leukocyte antigen-matched platelets with the haematologist (they are very expensive).

Transfusion reactions

■ *Slow rising fever <40°C*

A fever of <40°C is very common during transfusions. Slow the transfusion and give paracetamol (1 g 6 hourly) if the patient is otherwise well.

■ *Severe transfusion reaction*

If the patient has a rapid temp spike >39°C at the beginning of a transfusion, temp >40°C at any time, an urticarial rash, wheezing and hypotension (anaphylaxis):

1 Stop the transfusion immediately. Send the bag and line to the lab for analysis.

2 Give the patient hydrocortisone 200 mg IV and chlorpheniramine (chlorphenamine) 10 mg IV stat.

3 If the patient deteriorates or becomes hypotensive, give 0.5–1.0 ml of a 1:1000 solution of adrenaline IM.

4 Monitor closely (risk of shock and acute renal failure).

5 Repeat bloods from patient after event.

Hints

Platelet clumping often leads to erroneously low platelet counts. You can ask the haematologist to confirm an unexpectedly low count by manual differentiation or blood film.

Urine: Low output (oliguria/anuria)

Oliguria is defined as a urine output of less than 500 ml in 24 hours. The minimum urine output is 0.5 ml/kg/hour (35 ml/hour in a 70 kg patient). Urgent assessment is required for an output of less than 20 ml/hour, for a daily output of less than 500 ml or for painful urinary retention (see Table 8.9).

Hints

■ Remember to alter the doses of renally excreted drugs if the patient has prolonged oliguria. Patients with peripheral oedema may still be hypovolaemic.

■ Never use K^+-containing solutions for fluid challenges, as the impaired kidney may not be able to clear K^+.

Table 8.9 Differential diagnoses of oliguria/anuria.

Pre-renal	Renal	Post-renal
Hypovolaemia/hypotension	Nephrotoxic drugs	Blocked catheter
■ Occult bleed	■ Aminoglycosides	■ Urinary retention
■ Dehydration	■ IV contrast dyes	■ Prostate enlargement
■ Cardiac failure	■ Penicillins	■ Tumour
	■ Sulphonamides	■ Idiopathic
Apparent hypovolaemia	■ NSAIDs	■ Stones
■ 'Leaky capillaries'		
■ Septicaemia	■ Systemic diseases	
■ Pancreatitis	■ SLE	
■ Post-major surgery	■ Malignant hypertension	
■ CCF, liver failure	■ Interstitial nephritis	
Renal artery occlusion		
■ Emboli		
■ Aortic dissection		

On the ward

1 Check first for post-renal causes as these are most common:

• Palpate the patient's abdomen for a distended bladder. Catheterize if the patient is in urinary retention. This can easily be confirmed at the bedside with a bladder scan. Remember to do a PR in men and PV in woman once the bladder is relieved, to exclude prostatic disease and pelvic masses. If a prostate-specific antigen (PSA) is needed, then this should be taken before rectal examination, as rectal examination stimulates the prostate to produce PSA, causing a falsely raised reading.

• If the patient is already catheterized, ask the nurse to flush the catheter.

2 Check for hypovolaemia and sepsis:

• Check BP, pulse, temp and JVP.

• Assess fluid balance.

• Consider sepsis.

• If the patient is hypovolaemic, challenge with 500 ml IV normal saline over 30 minutes or gelofusine 250 ml stat. If there is no urinary response, recheck their JVP and repeat the fluid challenge if it is low. In patients with poor cardiac function, give 200 ml challenges of crystalloid.

3 Check for CCF:

• Oliguria indicates very poor cardiac output. Management should be discussed with your senior.

4 If you are unsure of the cause, get senior advice and do the following urgently:

• U&E. A creatinine–urea ratio of less than 10:1 (i.e. urea disproportionately raised) suggests a pre-renal cause.

• Urinary Na^+. A urinary Na^+ of less than 15 mmol/l suggests pre-renal causes; more than 20 mmol/l suggests renal causes.

• Urine microscopy.

■ In a patient with oliguria or anuria (with a near-empty bladder), catheters can be very uncomfortable. This is relieved by a bladder washout.

■ If a catheterized patient has passed absolutely no urine for many hours, the most likely cause is a blocked catheter. If a washout does not clear the catheter, try replacing with a new catheter. Clot retention is often a common cause of blocked catheters and may require a three-way catheter to be inserted. Discuss with the urologist for further advice.

Basic emergency routine

■ If the patient is in peri-arrest, get help fast and don't hesitate to call the crash team. Check ABC.

■ Briefly check for the 6 Hs:

1 Hypoglycaemia

2 Hypotension

3 Hypothermia

4 Hypovolaemia

5 Hypoxia

6 Arrhythmias (heart)

Check the BP (lying and sitting if possible) and JVP, look for cyanosis, and measure the respiratory rate. Do a blood glucose, ECG and pulse oximeter reading; check temperature; and consider doing a blood gas:

■ Ensure good IV access, take baseline bloods, and consider a catheter and O_2. Monitor the patient's condition (quarter to half-hourly observations, ECG monitor, urine output) and do baseline investigations.

■ If the patient is well or stable, you have time for a more thorough history and examination. Before ordering new tests in the middle of the night, look at recent baseline tests and consider how new information will change management. If a test is not urgent but you don't want to forget it, write the card for the morning and write it in the notes.

Obstetrics and gynaecology calls

Talking to the patient

Many gynaecology patients will be shy and embarrassed about their symptoms. They will base their behaviour on yours. If you are uncomfortable, they will be too, and this will make history taking and dealing with the problem much more difficult. History taking should also expand on the previous gynaecological and obstetric history. This should focus on:

1 Previous pregnancies and details (e.g. full term, type of birth (vaginal vs. caesarean section), miscarriages and terminations (medical vs. surgical)).

2 LMP and cycle information, that is, how long they bleed for and number of days between cycles.

3 Date of last cervical smear and any previous abnormalities.

4 Any previous gynaecological problems and treatments.

5 Sexual history – ask directly whether they are sexually active, if they have a casual or regular partner, what type of contraception they use and about any sexually transmitted diseases. Patients will not volunteer information if you don't ask!

• Find out what the patient has come to see you about, and always check if they have questions or worries. Don't forget to ask if pregnancy is planned. If not, ask her how she feels about it and who is entitled to know. Document this in the notes.

• Listen to the patient. Female patients with pelvic pain will often get mislabelled as gynaecology patients. Keep an open mind. Appendicitis referred as an ectopic pregnancy is common, as is PID.

• If taking GP referrals, always take clear details and think where and when is best to see the patient. Remember about any early pregnancy clinic (EPC) and genitourinary medicine (GUM) clinic, if appropriate. All patients should have a urinary pregnancy test before being referred to you.

• Be specific about details of the presenting complaint, especially with PV bleeding (e.g. is it definitely vaginal or could it be rectal? Is the blood just on wiping or on underwear? Needing to wear a pad? If so, how many? Any clots? Any flooding? Any offensive smelling discharge?).

• Take accurate PMH to assess suitability for theatre if necessary.

• Certain words are prone to being misunderstood by non-medical people, for example, many patients think all ovarian cysts or breast lumps are the same as cancer.

• Routine pre-op clerking is similar to any surgical pre-clerking. Patients tend to be younger than surgical patients so pregnancy and fertility are important issues. Always send a group and screen, FBC, urea and electrolytes and clotting if the patient is going to theatre.

Gynaecological examination

Examining the abdomen

■ Before you examine the patient, make sure you have a private area. Most A&E departments have a separate room for this very reason. Have a chaperone and document their presence. Make sure you have everything you need (e.g. swabs, slides) before you start, so you do not leave the patient half naked.

■ When examining the abdomen, don't forget surgical and medical conditions. If the patient has RIF tenderness, don't forget appendicitis. If the patient is post-operative, check for bowel sounds to exclude obstruction. Similarly suprapubic pain could be a UTI.

■ Urinalysis is an easy test and can provide important clues.

■ Listen to the ward sister or midwife. They are very experienced.

Bimanual (vaginal) examination

■ Many patients will not know what to expect. Explain what you are going to do beforehand and what the patient should expect to feel. Talk to the patient whilst you are examining her and tell her what you are doing.

■ The cervix takes practice to feel. The cervix can be tender so warn the patient that it might hurt before you test for cervical excitation (pain in the adnexae when the cervix is moved to one side).

■ Both adnexae need to be examined and this often requires quite firm pressure. Once experienced, you will be able to feel the ovaries. Warn the patient beforehand.

Using the speculum

■ Warm the speculum under warm water first if it is metal.

■ Use a lot of lubricant on the speculum.

■ Use a smaller speculum in post-menopausal women, as there will likely be some degree of atrophy, and extra lubricant.

■ It is easier to assess a cervical os with a speculum. Cervixes are in different positions in every person, so it will take a bit of practice to learn where to look and how to position the instrument. If the cervix is posterior, try using a larger speculum. Getting the patient to put her hands under her bottom can help to bring the cervix into view. Alternatively, use a Sims' speculum, with the patient lying on her side.

■ Do not rush. Never force the speculum. If the patient is in pain, be prepared to try a smaller speculum or abandon the procedure. Ask for senior help if in doubt.

■ Observe for any discharge; you will soon learn to distinguish different types and learn what is normal. It is good practice to take triple swabs (high vaginal, low vaginal and endocervical) for all patients whilst the speculum is in. When you withdraw the speculum, keep looking for abnormalities, particularly on the walls of the vaginal vault; not all will be visible with the speculum in.

Obstetric examination

■ Precise measurements are necessary. Use a tape measure to measure symphysis–fundal height.

■ Remember that medical and surgical conditions do not have classical presentation in pregnancy. Have a low threshold for suspicion for other pathologies. WCCs are raised in pregnancy, so it is not a useful marker.

■ Listen for foetal heart or use a Doppler probe if available. Foetal heart sounds should be audible after 13–15 weeks' gestation. Reassure the patient that in early pregnancy, it may not be detectable. The foetal pulse is much faster than the maternal pulse.

■ Before you perform a vaginal examination on any person of more than 20 weeks' gestation, check the placental position on the 20-week ultrasound scan to exclude placenta praevia (especially crucial if presenting with PV bleeding). Speak to your senior if no scan is available as rupture of a praevia can be catastrophic for both mum and baby.

■ Take triple swabs. Candidal infection is common in pregnancy. Remember that infection can cause uterine irritability and therefore induce (preterm) labour.

■ Speculum examination can also be used to assess for preterm rupture of membranes. A pool of liquor may be seen in the posterior fornix or liquor coming through the open os.

Being a male

Being a man in a woman's world can be a very disconcerting, intimidating experience. It is ridden with medico-legal hazards and cultural obstacles, but it can be extremely rewarding to view life on the other side:

■ Always be sensitive to the patient's feelings, wishes and privacy. It is best to offer to speak to the patient without the presence of relatives or partners.

■ Always ask permission before examining (or even touching) the patient. At each stage of examining a patient (i.e. normal physical, breast, genitalia, vaginal, rectal), check with them before proceeding. Cover up parts you have already examined.

■ Have a neutral chaperone (preferably of the same gender as the patient) with you. Do not rely on relatives. Document who was there by name and title and that you gained consent

■ It is advisable not to try any humour and to always remain professional at all times.

■ Although most of the above tips are directed at male doctors, they also apply to female doctors (including the need for a chaperone).

Common gynaecological calls

Gynaecological problems should be considered when investigating common symptoms such as abdominal pain and anaemia. If you are confronted with a complex gynaecological or obstetric problem, refer to the specialists.

Vaginal bleeding

Menstrual bleeding is common in hospital, but if the patient is post-menopausal or the bleeding is abnormal, carcinoma of the cervix and uterus must be excluded. Differential diagnoses include:

■ Menstrual bleeding (illness can cause abnormal periods).

■ Break through bleed on the oral contraceptive pill, especially if the patient is taking antibiotics.

■ PID, especially if intrauterine contraceptive device is in situ.

■ Fibroids or endometriosis.

■ Tumours (e.g. cervical or uterine).

■ Threatened miscarriage or ectopic pregnancy – the latter is a diagnosis you cannot afford to miss. In abdominal pain, *always* do a pregnancy test.

On the ward

■ Confirm that bleeding is vaginal, not rectal, and that this is different to normal menses.

■ Exclude pregnancy-related bleeding (ask about the LMP, contraceptive use and recent sexual history). Always think of pregnancy in pre-menopausal women. Send urine for bHCG if in doubt.

■ Consider PID, especially if with low-grade fever or tender abdomen. Do a PV examination for pelvic tenderness, and take triple swabs.

■ Get a gynaecological referral if the patient is post-menopausal or premenopausal with persistent bleeding and no obvious cause.

■ Investigations to consider:

- HPV smear
- High vaginal swab
- FBC, clotting studies and ESR/CRP

Hints

Anticoagulation does not cause abnormal PV bleeding but may unmask mucosal defects or tumours.

Dysmenorrhoea

This is a common and painful problem for menstruating women.

On the ward

■ Differentiate the pain from other causes of lower abdominal pain. Most women will recognize period pain.

■ Mefenamic acid 500 mg TDS or ibuprofen 400 mg TDS is useful. Co-codamol and codeine are alternatives. A hot water bottle also helps. Avoid stronger opiates.

Termination of pregnancy

As a junior doctor, you may be asked to be involved with terminations of pregnancy (TOPs) in the following scenarios:

1 Counselling patients in clinic which will include taking consent and prescribing the agents for a medical TOP

2 Assisting in theatre

3 Dealing with any immediate or delayed complications of TOP

If you have any moral objections, you should make them known to your consultant at the beginning of the job, and you will not be expected to be involved. However, whatever your ethical beliefs, it will be expected that you will deal with any patient who is unwell after a TOP and refer them to someone else should a pregnant patient want advice on TOP.

General tips

■ Although a delicate issue, if the patient is underaged you should try to ascertain the age of the father as there may be child protection issues for the patient, which you have a duty to report. Inform your senior if this is the case.

■ Always discuss contraception – most forms of hormonal contraception should be started on the day of the TOP.

■ If unsure of gestation, get an ultrasound scan. The TOP may not be legal.

■ It is normal for a pregnancy test to remain positive for up to 2 weeks post-TOP. But if bHCG levels are persistently positive, this could imply retained products.

Chapter 9
DEATH AND DYING

Terminal care

About 65% of people die in hospital in the United Kingdom, and as the population's mean age continues to increase, the total number will rise. Caring for dying people is stressful, particularly as a junior doctor. Evidence suggests that junior doctors come to terms with mortality at a much younger age than most people.

There are five elements to good end-of-life care: communication, pain control, symptom control, good prescribing knowledge and self-care. The last element is often forgotten but is as important as the others.

Communication

Breaking bad news

Breaking bad news is difficult but important. Contrary to popular opinion, people remember how bad news was given to them. Whilst every situation demands a unique approach, the following may be helpful:

■ If you are uncertain about how to start, talk to the patient's nurse. It is generally a good idea to ask nurses what they think the patient knows before seeing the patient. Take a nurse with you to the bedside.
■ If the patient would prefer, ask them to have family present. This will save you breaking the news twice and allow questions to be asked together.
■ If possible, take the patient to a private room to tell them bad news.
■ Have tissues handy.
■ Hand your bleep to a colleague for at least 15–20 minutes.

■ If you are unsure about how to proceed, it can be helpful to ask the patient 'What do you know so far?'
■ Do not be afraid to give information. People almost always want more information than doctors give them.
■ Watch and listen to the patient carefully for clues about how much information they want. It is acceptable to ask the patient 'how much do you want to know?' If the patient is shocked by the diagnosis, they may not take all the information at once, so you may need to repeat it either later in the conversation or at a later date.

> **Useful questions to assess how much someone wants to hear**
> 1 What have you been told?
> 2 Are you the sort of person who wants to know exactly what's going on?
> 3 Would you like me to tell you the full details of the diagnosis/results/treatment options?
> 4 How much do you want to know about what is going on?
> 5 Do you want me to go on?

■ Tell the truth and answer questions directly when asked (the patient may have been waiting

The Hands-on Guide to the Foundation Programme, Fifth Edition. Anna Donald, Michael Stein, Ciaran Scott Hill and Selina J Chavda.
© 2015 John Wiley & Sons, Ltd. Published 2015 by John Wiley & Sons, Ltd.

. Be ready to answer
to admit uncertainty.
g, even in the face of
e with honest uncer-
tions and findings to
explain them to the
e the medical notes in
ss-refer as needed.
jargon.

■ Write down relevant information to give to the patient, and consider drawing diagrams to explain what you are saying more clearly (about 60% of spoken information is lost). If it is a new diagnosis, patient information leaflets on the condition can be helpful in consolidating the information you have given them.

■ Break down the information into chunks and ask the patient to repeat what you have explained to them if necessary.

■ Ask the patient to write down questions they might have over the next few days. Give them your name or that of a colleague so that they can contact a doctor if they need to.

■ Find out if the patient wants you to break the news to their relatives. If the patient's relatives are present at the time then give them space to answer questions also, and ensure they have contact details for a member of your team also. Make sure the patient has given consent for you to discuss the details of the case with their relatives.

■ Make an appointment if necessary with the senior members of the team at a later date.

■ Write in the notes what you have told the patient. This saves embarrassment for the team and sets a baseline for future explanations.

■ It is very important to communicate to the nurses what you have told the patient. They can follow up with further information and support.

■ Consider other people who can help with breaking bad news: other doctors, nurses, chaplain or religious support worker (about 25% of families in the United Kingdom accept chaplaincy support), general practitioner (GP), nurse, police, social worker or support groups. The inpatient palliative care team is an excellent resource and is very helpful in a multitude of situations ranging from breaking bad news to symptom control.

Ongoing communication with dying patients

■ Pay a quick visit to the patient's bedside the next day (or at night if you're on call). Ask them how they're feeling and if they have any questions. This will help put the patient at ease.

■ Pain causes fear and anxiety, which may lead to the patient being withdrawn or aggressive. Often patients can be quite reticent about talking about pain or discomfort. Reassure them that pain can be controlled. There is no reason that your patients should be in pain (this is a common misconception for patients – particularly many stoic elderly patients who feel they should just 'grin and bear it'). Dealing with pain is one of the most important contributions you can make to a dying patient.

■ If someone's English is poor, ask the nurses or switchboard to help you to book an interpreter. There is also a telephone interpreter service now widely available that can be used 24 hours a day.

■ Be aware of functional symptoms, such as headaches and insomnia, which are best treated with reassurance, although it is important to make sure there are no real medical causes for the symptoms. A direct approach is usually the best one. A colleague once had a patient who had 22 symptoms in 24 hours. The patient had been told that she had metastatic cancer that week. The doctor asked her outright 'How are you coping with the spread of your cancer?' She burst into tears and told her she was terrified of dying.

■ Maintaining continuity of care, despite ward staff changes, is especially important for dying patients. Tell patients and relatives that you are going home for the weekend or on holiday, when you will be back and the name of the doctor who will replace you.

■ Elisabeth Kubler-Ross suggested five stages of dying in her 1969 book *On Death and Dying*. These were denial, anger, bargaining, depression and acceptance. Pitch your information and communication to wherever the person is today.

■ Do not be surprised by dying patients' aggressive or abnormal behaviour. This is when they need acceptance the most. Do your best not to take it personally – and check that there is no physical cause (e.g. pain, hypoxia, constipation, etc.). Managing dying patients is not easy; it is a difficult skill and you are unlikely to always say the right thing.

■ Many dying people say that the most hurtful and distressing thing for them is avoidance and silence. Although it is often hard to do, allow patients to discuss dying with you openly. You may be the only person they feel able to talk to frankly.

Five questions to ask dying patients

1 What have they most enjoyed in their life? Ask them to describe it to you.

2 What would they like someone to hear that they have never said?

3 What would they most like to say to people they love that they have never said? Ask them if there is any way they can communicate this (e.g. write a card, phone them from the ward, ask them to visit, relay a message).

4 What are they most frightened of? You may be able to reassure them about pain and symptom control. Many patients can just be afraid of death. Listening to their fears can be equally therapeutic.

5 What do patients need to do (in practical terms) before they die? Talk to support staff (nurses, Macmillan nurses, palliative care team members, social workers) and relatives about making this happen. These can include financial matters or writing wills. It is very difficult for people to do things from a hospital bed. Remember that some industrial diseases are eligible for financial support and that this is dated from the time of application, for example, Mesothelioma (call the Department for Work and Pensions Benefit Enquiry Line on 0800 822 200).

■ Look patients in the eye when you talk to them.

■ Find out what their expectations are, and if they have any specific wishes about their death.

Hint

Breaking bad news is inherent to being a doctor. The importance of breaking bad news well is reflected by most medical schools in their curriculums. Regardless, it is a skill we can always improve upon. The *BMJ* has published several articles on this topic including a Learning Module 'Breaking Bad News to Patients and Relatives' that we would recommend completing.

Difficult situations

■ Try turning difficult questions for you back to the patient. For example, you can ask them: 'What makes you ask that question?' Ultimately, honesty in the face of difficult questions is the best policy. Offer to ask a senior to come and answer questions you cannot (but it is usually unwise to guarantee they will come). Never lie or make up information; it is easy to lose the trust of your patient at this crucial time in the course of their illness.

■ If family members make it clear to you that they don't want the patient to know that they are going to die, ask your senior, palliative care team or nurses for help. The relatives are not your primary responsibility, although obviously you have to work with them. You can point out that it is your duty to inform patients of their condition unless it will cause them undue harm, this is rarely the case. It is often worth speaking to the relatives separately to find out why they do not want this information passed on to the patient. More often than not, situations can be resolved with good communication.

■ If you disagree with the amount/content of information given to a patient by your seniors it is generally unwise to directly contradict them. Try talking to them to establish why they have made that decision. You can also consult colleagues (and if the situation is more serious, then your medical defence organization) if you are uncomfortable with the way a situation is being managed.

■ Write down relatives' concerns in the patient's notes. Documentation is key.

Mistakes we've made: Avoid them!

■ Do not underestimate how much caring for dying patients can affect you. Take time to reflect on your feelings, and if necessary speak to fellow colleagues about how you are feeling.

■ Write things down and draw clear diagrams for patients to look at after you've gone. Patient information leaflets are very helpful at explaining conditions, treatments, etc.

■ Do not leave patients waiting. If you promise to return, do so. People stay awake waiting for doctors to return. If you can't visit when you said that you will then call the ward and ask for the patient to be informed that you will be late, and when you will come instead.

■ Never give the patient the impression that the medical staff have given up on them. Someone can always be present to help deal with their symptoms. Statements like 'whatever happens we will do our best to take care of you' are fairly non-specific but can be immensely reassuring to a sick or dying patient. Similarly telling relatives that their loved one will be made comfortable can be immeasurably important.

■ Contrary to intuition, dying patients do not need to eat. It can be cruel to force them to do so. Sometimes patients are given IV or subcutaneous fluids to help with hydration. This can be a real area of concern for relatives and requires careful explanation.

■ Never give patients a 'date or time of death'. You will probably be wrong. Also, it is awful for all concerned if the patient lingers on after they 'should have died', or if they die sooner than the date you have given.

Pain control

Pain is one of the things that dying patients are most afraid of. You can help them enormously, but you may need help:

■ Use the pain team and ask for senior advice sooner rather than later. Syringe drivers and patches can be helpful if the patient is no longer able to swallow.

■ Remember the person may not admit to being in pain (check their pulse or ask relatives and nursing staff). Physiological signs of pain include tachycardia, hypertension, sweating, lacrimation and pupillary dilation.

■ Reassure patients that severe pain can be controlled, however severe.

Symptom control

The *BNF* has a fabulous section on symptom control in terminal care (look under 'Terminal care' in the index) that we have not tried to replicate for fear of being too quickly outdated. Your hospital will often also have a local policy for prescribing for terminal care that you can use. If not you can always ask the palliative care team for advice.

Prescribing for the dying

■ Following the controversial withdrawal of the Liverpool Care Pathway (a once ubiquitous document that guided the care of dying patients) there is increased focus on the way in which the dying are cared for. The principles remain the same — maximize the patient's comfort whilst avoiding excessive medical intervention.

■ Many drugs are available as suppositories, which are useful if the patient cannot swallow or is vomiting.

■ Keep drugs as simple as possible. Only prescribe medications that the patient will actually receive a benefit from. Discontinue when close to death if not required.

■ Keep analgesia continuous. IV or SC opiate infusions are useful for this as are *pro re nata* (as required) doses to back up regular doses of analgesia. In dying patients, the ultimate aim is pain control and quality, not quantity of life. Discuss pain management with the nurses so that they do not simply stop infusions to avoid respiratory depression.

■ Consider patient-controlled analgesia. Discuss with the ward pharmacist. The pain team/anaesthetists are also experts in this and can be called upon in times of need.

■ Consider withdrawing IV fluids but discuss with seniors and relatives first. Patients' fluid requirements reduce when they are dying, so often, 12–24 hourly bags of fluid SC or IV will suffice. Excess fluids can lead to fluid overload and respiratory secretions.

■ Infusion pump troubleshooting:

1 Light not flashing – pump not plugged in and battery inserted wrongly or run out

2 Infusion running too fast or too slowly – syringe incorrectly inserted, rate wrongly set, tubing kinked or blocked and needle site tissued

Support for the dying and for you

Hospice (NHS or non-NHS), chaplain and hospital bereavement officer (if you have one).

CRUSE (widowed people caring for the newly bereaved), Cruse House, 126 Sheen Road, Richmond, Surrey TW9 1UR. Go to www.cruse.org.uk for a list of local telephone numbers.

Macmillan nurses (nurses specially trained for palliative care), part of Macmillan Cancer Relief, Anchor House, 15–19 Britten Street, London, SW3 3TZ. Tel.: 0808 808 00 00 (free phone). www.macmillan.org.uk.

Marie Curie Cancer Care, Marie Curie Memorial Foundation, Head Office, 28 Belgrave Square, London, SW1X 8QG. Tel.: 020 7599 7777 (England), 01495 740 888 (Wales), 0131 561 3900 (Scotland) and 028 9088 2060 (NI). www.mariecurie.org.uk.

Some questions to ask yourself if *you* feel excessively miserable caring for dying patients

■ Make a list of five 'significant losses' you have experienced. Write down positive outcomes that arose from those situations, and identify ways in which you developed as a result.

■ Do the same exercise for 'necessary losses' – those that you had no control over.

Death

If the patient dies, don't panic. Whilst sad, death is often merciful when people have been suffering – for them, their relatives and ward staff. You can make a big difference to relatives if you handle the paperwork efficiently, allowing them to proceed with the funeral.

What to do when a patient dies

If the patient is not for resuscitation, then:

1 View the body.

2 Confirm death:

● Fixed and dilated pupils
● No spontaneous respiratory effort
● No breath sounds for 2 minutes
● No central pulses for 2 minutes
● No heart sounds for 2 minutes

The above should be recorded for 5 minutes in total.

If you are unsure, do an ECG to look for asystole or look at the fundi. The blood in the retinal veins separates into discrete blotches after death.

3 Write in the notes: 'Called to confirm death. Write the above as per your examination'.

4 Sign your name clearly with your bleep number. It is important that coroners and bereavement officers can contact you if necessary.

5 Note date and time of confirmation of death. This is the time that you confirm the death, not the time the nurses called you.

6 If possible write down the cause(s) of death.

7 *Note whether or not the patient is fitted with a pacemaker or radioactive implant.* If the patient is to be cremated, pacemakers and radioactive implants *must* be removed or they blow up in the incinerator at considerable cost to yourself and the crematorium. It is easiest to check for these whilst you still have the patient and the notes in front of you. The body will have a pacemaker scar on their precordium (commonly on the left, but some patients do have them on the right hand side).

8 Liaise with nurses about calling next of kin. Nurses usually tell the next of kin and meet them on the ward, but relatives may want to see you. Always be available if you can.

9 Note the GP's telephone number and name. You should call him or her at the earliest opportunity to let them know.

10 Write 'GP informed' in notes once you have spoken to them.

11 Write a discharge summary to the GP so that they are aware of what happened, and they have written documentation.

12 Ask your senior early whether or not a post-mortem (PM) is desirable and what cause(s) of death should be written on the death certificate.

Telling relatives about the patient's death

1 Wherever possible, inform the relatives that their loved one is close to death so they have the chance to come in and say goodbye. Ask relatives whether they want to be contacted in the middle of the night and establish the next of kin.

2 After death, ask the nurses whether they have told the relatives about the patient's death. They will often do so – sometimes before you make it to the ward.

3 If it is up to you to inform relatives, make sure you contact the patient's designated 'next of kin'.

4 It is usually best to tell the next of kin what has happened over the phone (rather than just asking them to come in urgently). Sometimes people don't want to see the body or would rather wait until morning.

5 If you do see the relatives, take them to a private room. If they have come a long way they might be grateful for a cup of tea and some time in this private area to express their grief.

6 Try to establish the following:

● If the body is to be cremated or buried. If the former, you will need to fill out a cremation form (see the succeeding text).

● If the relatives will consent to a PM (if it is required – see the succeeding text).

Religious practices on death

Some awareness of religious or cultural customs on death is invaluable to prevent misunderstandings and often also allows the relatives to deal with their grief.

■ Buddhism: no special arrangements on death.

■ Christianity: no special arrangements on death.

■ Confucianism: no special arrangements on death.

■ Hinduism: cremation of the body.

■ Islam: burial intact by the next sunset, that is, within 24 hours.

■ Judaism: body should not be left alone. Consult with relatives for additional requirements, such as speed of burial.

■ Sikhism: do not move the body. Cremation of the body.

■ Zoroastrianism: no special arrangements on death.

PMs

■ When to perform a PM:

1 Requested by a coroner as cause of death is unknown, unexpected, violent or sudden death.

2 To learn more about a condition, or the cause of death, or for medical research purposes.

■ Preferably before the patient dies, ask your seniors if they want a PM so that you can ask the relatives when the patient dies.

■ PMs requested by the coroner are mandatory by law. Otherwise, you cannot force a next of kin to agree to a PM. Many people will oblige if you explain why you want one, what it entails (lots of people have misconceptions from films they have seen), particularly if it is a limited PM. They can receive the results of the PM if they would like. Any tissue that is taken can be returned to them at a later date or can be disposed of by the hospital. Make sure they are aware of the above, and if happy ask them to sign a consent form.

■ Send complete case notes, the next of kin's consent form and a brief synopsis of the patient's history to the PM room, together with your name and bleep number.

■ Request that the pathologist bleeps you or your senior with the results.

Death certificates

Only doctors who have seen the patient within 14 days before death are legally allowed to sign a death certificate. The next of kin then takes this to the Registrar of Births and Deaths within 5 days (8 days in Scotland). Often, the bereavement office will do all of this for you, and you simply need to fill in the death certificate.

If there is no next of kin, you must ensure that the death certificate is sent to the registrar.

Writing the death certificate

Make sure you fill in the death certificate correctly or you may be recalled by the registrar and delay the funeral. The bereavement office will help you with the details. Always check if in doubt with a senior to save yourself from hassle:

1 Part one: Fill in the sequence of conditions that caused the patient's death.

(1a) is the condition that caused death. Causes of death are recognized pathological states, such as myocardial infarction or hospital-acquired pneumonia. The more specific you are, the better. For example, organ failure is not an acceptable cause. Other unacceptable causes are tabulated in the following. Ask your senior or ring the registrar if you are unsure

about how to describe the cause of death. Do not use abbreviations or layman's terms (e.g. heart attack or MI is not good practice.)

Unacceptable 'causes' of death	
Asphyxia	Hepatic failure
Asthenia	Hepatorenal failure
Brain failure	Kidney failure
Cachexia	Renal failure
Cardiac arrest	Respiratory failure
Cardiac failure	Shock
Coma	Syncope
Debility	Uraemia
Exhaustion	Vagal inhibition
Heart failure	Vasovagal attack

(1b) and (c) are diseases underlying this condition. For example, if the cause of death was MI, the underlying disease might be ischaemic heart disease or chronic hypertension.

2 Part two: Fill in other diseases that were not directly linked with the cause of death in (1a), but which may have contributed to the patient's overall demise.

3 Sign the death certificate on the relevant part of the form.

4 Print your name, hospital and most recent medical qualification.

5 Print the name of the patient's consultant.

6 Fill in the counterfoil ('cheque-butt') part of death certificate. This retains the basic details of the death when the relatives have taken the main certificate.

7 Fill in the 'note to informant'. This is given to the next of kin:

● If you are unsure about any part of the death certificate, call the registrar's office or talk to a colleague or bereavement office. The registrar's office is in the phone book under 'Registrar of Births and Deaths'.

● If your hospital has a bereavement officer, he or she will usually discuss the request for a PM with the relatives and will help you with the death certificate.

● If your patient was a war pensioner or service-man/service woman, you can influence whether or not their spouse continues to receive war widow(er)'s pension by what you write on the death certificate. This is especially important if the person died from war-related causes.

● Doctors must record diseases that may have been due to previous employment, for example, asbestos exposure leading to mesothelioma.

Referring to the coroner (Scotland: Procurator fiscal)

1 To contact your local coroner, ask your senior, switchboard, or directory enquiries for the phone number.

2 It is the statutory obligation of the Registrar of Births and Deaths, not you, to report suspect deaths to the coroner or procurator fiscal. However, it saves time if you know what these are and can send the death certificate directly to the coroner. They are as follows:

● Unknown cause of death.
● The patient was not seen by a certifying doctor within 14 days of death.
● Death was caused by medical treatment (e.g. dying in theatre, or within 24 hours of an anaesthetic or admission to hospital).
● Death was suspicious or unexpected in any way.
● Death was caused by a road traffic accident, an industrial disease or accident, a domestic accident, violence, neglect, abortion, suicide or poisoning (including acute alcohol ingestion).
● Death occurred during legal custody.
● Where there is any claim for negligence against medical or nursing staff.
● Death may have occurred from industrial injury or employment.
● Death of a foster child, patient under Mental Health Act (1983), mentally disabled people or service pensioners.

3 The coroner can request the following:

● The issue of a normal death certificate
● A PM
● An inquest

Cremation forms and fees

You receive £78.00 for every cremation form you fill out; this is charged to the funeral director by the hospital who then passes the bill on to relatives. 'Crem forms' are legal documents to establish beyond any doubt the deceased's identity, as incinerated bodies cannot be exhumed. If you have not seen the patient since death, you must pay a visit to the morgue to confirm you are signing the form for the right person. The body cannot be released until this form is filled out.

Cremation forms are straightforward to fill out, provided you are certain that there are no radioactive or pacemaker implants in the body:

■ Ensure you fill in the same cause(s) of death on the cremation form that you did on the death certificate or you will be chased by the coroner.
■ Keep details of cremation fees you have taken as you need to declare them in your tax forms. Increasingly the Inland Revenue is checking up on doctors for non-declaration.

To check for pacemakers

■ Feel the chest.
■ Look through the notes for history of implantation of pacemaker or radioactive implant. A recent chest X-ray will show the pacemaker easily. Make sure you see it before the radiology department removes it from the inpatient file.
■ Look for ECGs that will demonstrate pacing spikes.
■ The only sure-fire way to exclude a pacemaker is to check the patient for pacemaker scars and a palpable mass from the implant itself.

Further reading

There are many excellent books and articles on death and dying. Ask your librarian. Here are some useful articles for starters:

Buckman R. (1992) *How to Break Bad News. A Guide for Health Care Professionals.* Papermac, London.

Continuing Education article series on bereavement counselling. (1994) *Nursing Standard.*

Cooke M., Cooke H., Glucksman E. (1992) Management of sudden bereavement in the accident and emergency department. *British Medical Journal* **304**:1207–1209.

Corr C. (2009) *Death and Dying, Life and Living,* 7th ed. Wadsworth Cengage Learning, Belmont.

Egan G. (1990) *The Skilled Helper. A Systematic Approach to Effective Helping,* 4th ed. Brookes-Cole, Pacific Grove, CA.

Macguire P., Faulkner L. (1988) Communicate with cancer patients: handling bad news and difficult patients. *British Medical Journal* **297**:907–909.

Hallberg I. (2004) Death and dying from old people's point of view. A literature review. *Aging Clinical and Experimental Research* **16**(2):87–103

McLauchlan C. (1990) Handling distressed relatives and breaking bad news. *British Medical Journal* **301**:1145–1149.

Raphael B. (1996) *The Anatomy of Bereavement: A Handbook for the Caring Professions.* Hutchinson, London.

Smith R. (2000) A good death. An important aim for health services and for us all. *British Medical Journal* **320**(7228):129–130.

Thayre K., Hadfield-Law L. (1993) Never going to be easy: Giving bad news. RCN Nursing Update; Continuing Education article series. *Nursing Standard* **8**:3–13.

Worden W. (2002) Grief Counselling and Grief Therapy. A Handbook for the Mental Health Practitioner, 3rd ed. Springer, London.

Wilson S.A. (1999) Family perspectives on dying in long-term care settings. *Journal of Gerontological Nursing,* **25**(11):19–25.

Chapter 10
DRUGS

Don't worry if pharmacology seems a long time ago. Prescribing and giving drugs is easier than it may seem! Although daunting at first, the more prescribing you do, the easier it becomes. In this section, we will explain how to write up drugs and infusions and walk you through prescribing controlled drugs, and at the end of the chapter, there is a table of 75 commonly used drugs with side effects and dosages.

General

■ The single most useful pharmacology tip is to always refer to the *BNF* if in any doubt about any drug. As a junior doctor, you will rarely be expected to prescribe drugs that are not in the *BNF*. Also, it's worth reading the *BNF* to improve your pharmacology knowledge; it contains lots of useful information, and time spent familiarizing yourself with the layout will seldom be wasted. For example, it contains prescribing guidelines for the elderly, the terminally ill and children.

■ Make the most of your ward pharmacist. Pharmacists have a wealth of pharmacology knowledge that they can share with you. Not only are they happy to discuss patient management and find alternatives for problematic drugs (or patients), but they are often willing to find recent articles and other information about specific drugs for you. This can be useful for clarifying unusual side effects and for academic talks. They also can tell you about drug interactions, and can help you prescribe unusual drugs as needed.

■ For easy reference, make yourself a chart of common drugs and doses used on the wards and stick it on the front of your folder. It is particularly useful to do this for antibiotics and infusion dosages, which can be painstaking to look up every time you make up an infusion. As always, check the *BNF*. We have listed the doses of the 75 most common

drugs in a table at the end of this chapter for your reference, but it is best to amend it or make your own, especially as different specialties and consultants may have favourites they like to be prescribed.

Prescribing drugs

Drug charts

Drug charts are straightforward to fill out. Basically, there are four parts to a drug chart:

1 A place for prescribing regular drugs

2 A place for 'PRN' or 'as required' drugs

3 A place for one-off drugs to be given as a 'stat' dose or immediately

4 Fluids and infusions

For each section of the chart, you need to fill in the date, the generic name of each drug, its dose, how frequently it should be prescribed and your signature and bleep number. Abbreviations for prescribing are shown in Table 10.1.

Tips for filling in drug charts

■ Write legibly. Other people have to administer drugs that you prescribe. Slips of the pens can have huge consequences. Capital letters are often best.

■ In particular, take care in writing dose amounts and units. Micrograms (abbreviated

The Hands-on Guide to the Foundation Programme, Fifth Edition. Anna Donald, Michael Stein, Ciaran Scott Hill and Selina J Chavda.
© 2015 John Wiley & Sons, Ltd. Published 2015 by John Wiley & Sons, Ltd.

Table 10.1 Abbreviations for prescribing drugs.

Abbreviation	Meaning
AC (ante cibum)	Before food
PC (post cibum)	After food
BD (bis die)	Take twice daily
mane	Take in the morning
nocte	Take in the evening
OD	Take once daily
PRN (pro re nata)	Take when required
QDS	Take four times a day
STAT	Take straight away
TDS	Take three times a day
T.	1 tablet/dose
T.T.	2 tablets/dose
T.T.T.	3 tablets/dose
x/7	x days
y/52	y weeks
z/12	z months

mcg or μg) can easily be mistaken for milligrams (mg); the *BNF* advises that 'micrograms' and 'units' be written in full. (A doctor was sued when a patient was given 125 mg of digoxin by a nurse who misread the scrawled 'mcg'. She had to open many packets of the drug to give such a dose, so also ended up in the dock for failure of common sense.) Using 'u' for 'units' is also very susceptible to be misread as an additional zero, which can have disastrous consequences. Putting a dot in the middle of the U is a common but not reliable way of attempting to make this practice safer.

■ Develop a good relationship with the ward pharmacist. They are there to help you! They review all drug charts, albeit often after the drug has been given a number of times, and will usually bleep you if you prescribe anything idiotic – this is something you should encourage! Similarly, experienced nurses, who administer many drugs, will usually let you know if you have made a prescription error.

■ Hospital pharmacists usually use green ink. To avoid confusion, use a different colour when writing on drug charts. Black pen is usually best.
■ If drug administration is complicated, write legible additional instructions on the drug chart. There is no harm in writing extra notes to nurses and doctors on the drug chart. In fact it is legally advisable to do so. For some drug administration, hospitals have drug stickers that can be stuck into the drug chart to avoid confusion, for example, with sliding scales for insulin.

Writing prescriptions

FY1 junior doctors are only permitted to write prescriptions for the hospital pharmacy, so outpatient prescriptions and FP10 forms (green general practitioner [GP] prescriptions) shouldn't be an issue. However, if you do need to write a prescription on plain paper the essential ingredients are:

■ Date
■ Name of patient
■ Patient's date of birth
■ Address of patient
■ Generic drug name and amount
■ Dose/day
■ Quantity of tablets to dispense
■ Your signature and printed name
■ Your General Medical Council registration number

Controlled drugs

Prescriptions for take-home controlled drugs have to be written in a specific way; otherwise, the pharmacy will send the prescription back. This wastes a spectacular amount of time. To write a controlled drug prescription the prescription must be in your handwriting – don't use sticky labels. Include the following:

■ Date
■ Name of patient and their date of birth
■ Address of patient
■ Generic drug name and amount (e.g. '10 mg MORPHINE SULPHATE TABS')
■ Formulation of drug, for example, tablets or patches
■ Dose/day

- *Total* number of tablets in *both* numbers and letters (e.g. '10/ten tablets')
- Your signature and printed name

> For example:
> 5/4/2014
> Mr TSD
> 2 Tatelman Street
> Wolfchester WC5
> MST continuous tablets 10 mg
> 20/twenty tablets
> 10 mg twice daily for 5 days
> (Your signature and printed name)

Verbals

It is now legally suspect to prescribe drugs for patients 'verbally' over the phone to nurses. However, in certain instances it still occurs. Typical verbal requests might be 'Mr Smith has a headache. Could he have two paracetamol please?' The nurse writes your prescription in the drug chart, with a small note saying, 'Dr X will sign this'. Verbals are fine for relatively harmless drugs, such as one-off doses of paracetamol or for doses of necessary drugs when you have been held up and coming to the ward is monumentally inconvenient such as a bag of maintenance IV fluids:

- Check your local hospital policy. Increasingly, verbals are not allowed by trusts. Some trusts only allow them if the medication is already prescribed and in use but a dose change is necessary. Verbals are NEVER acceptable for controlled drugs.
- It is important to sign verbal requests on the drug chart as soon as possible. Should any problems arise in the interim, the nurse who took the verbal is liable. Because of this, some nurses refuse to take verbals altogether and insist you come to the ward to sign the drug before it is given. This is a reasonable stance for a nurse to take, and you should think twice before you criticize it.
- Nurses will rightly usually refuse to accept verbals if they think the patient should be seen by a doctor before taking the drug. Whilst this can be frustrating, remember that nurses' scruples provide a big safety net for you. Everyone remembers times when they

were glad that nurses forced them to question what they were doing. Furthermore, blanket prescribing without thinking why that patient may be in pain or vomiting can be quite dangerous.

- Some hospitals allow a limited number of drugs (e.g. paracetamol, sublingual nitrate, lactulose, and antacids) to be prescribed by nurses after calling the duty doctor. Whilst you do not need to see the patient, it is prudent to check the reasons for the request. You may be required (depending on local policy) to sign for the drugs later.
- The bottom line is, if in doubt, quickly review the patient and make a decision on what to prescribe based on your findings. This will save you time overall, and you will be reassured that the patient is stable.

Giving drugs

Nurses usually give oral drugs, suppositories, subcutaneous and intramuscular drugs. In most hospitals nurses also give intravenous drugs. However, administration of certain drugs requires a specially trained nurse or a doctor. These vary between hospitals:

- Never rush when making up a drug or administering it. Being rushed, particularly when doing something unfamiliar, is when mistakes happen.
- Glass vials are designed to snap at the neck in the direction of the blue dot on their neck. The dot is the 'weak spot' and so the bottle is flexed 'away' from the dot to break it. Be careful when opening the vials as you can cut yourself on the glass easily. A protective wad of gauze usually helps.
- Wear gloves or use your non-dominant hand when opening multiple vials. Your dominant hand's index finger can get chaffed with minute glass splinters if you snap open many glass vials consecutively. It is common to see new doctors in areas like anaesthetics with a constant plaster around their dominant index finger!
- Avoid using normal saline as a diluent for drugs in patients with liver failure – the extra salt load can precipitate ascites; 5% dextrose is usually preferable.

■ Avoid dextrose in patients with diabetic coma. Give normal saline instead or prescribe as per DKA local hospital protocols. Refer to the *BNF* for alternative diluents for different drugs. Glucose-containing fluids are also generally avoided in brain-injured patients.

■ If making up cytotoxic drugs, always wear gloves, apron and goggles (and keep your mouth closed!). Wash your hands afterwards with water. Follow local and national protocols and do not do anything you are uncomfortable with. Chemo nurses nowadays usually give chemotherapy, so you may not have to get involved.

■ The plastic containers with prefilled syringes (e.g. adrenaline) in cardiac arrest trolleys are easily opened by holding the box with both hands and twisting it. The syringe then needs to be assembled by screwing the plunger into the syringe body. Make sure you do this at least once for practice before you attend your first arrest.

Drug infusions

Continuous infusions are easy to make up, but they are a complete pain at 4 a.m. Whilst it was traditional to make up midnight infusions like morphine, dopamine and glyceryl trinitrate (GTN) infusions before going to bed, this is now considered bad practice, and the advance preparation of medicines is frowned upon.

To make up an infusion
1 Find the vial of drug in the drug cupboard. Check the dosage and the expiry date, and ideally ask a nursing colleague to also double check.

2 Open the vial and draw up the drug into a suitably large syringe, usually 50 ml.

3 Draw into the syringe the required amount of diluent fluid. This is usually normal saline, sterile water for injection or 5% dextrose, drawn from unopened (sterile) containers.

4 Label the syringe with a large adhesive label. Specify the following on the label:
- Date and time you made infusion up
- Name of patient and DOB

- Amount of drug in amount of diluent (e.g. 50 mg GTN in 50 ml normal saline)
- Rate at which solution should run (e.g. 2 ml/hour)
- Your signature and bleep

Prescribing drug infusions

1 Prescribe infusions on the fluid section of the drug chart. In some hospitals, this is a separate sheet at the end of the patient's bed.

2 Write the following: '*a* units of *b* drug in *x* ml of *y* diluent to run at *z* ml/hour'. (e.g., '500 mg of aminophylline in 500 ml of normal saline. Run at 35 ml/hour').

3 To avoid confusion, convert the amount of drug/hour to the amount of infusion to be given every hour (i.e. ml/hour, not mg/hour). To do this, ask yourself the following questions:

- How many units of drug should the patient get per hour?
  For example, 35 mg/hour (0.5 mg/kg for a 70 kg male).
- How many units of drug are there per millilitre of infusion?
  For example, 500 mg/500 ml infusion = 1 mg/ml.
- Therefore, how many millilitres do I need to give so that the patient gets the right amount of units per hour?
  For example, 35 mg/hour ÷ 1 mg/ml = 35 ml/hour.

4 You can always write additional instructions on the drug chart regarding infusion administration.
  For example, 50 mg GTN in 50 ml saline; run at 1–10 ml/hour titrated against chest pain but maintain a systolic blood pressure >100 mmHg.

5 It is often easier to calculate by making up the drug to a concentration of 1 mg/ml as in the example in the preceding text.

6 Be mindful of the volume of drug infusions, as they are in addition to normal intravenous fluid infusions, particularly in the elderly, at risk of fluid overload.

Administering infusions

If the nurses are willing to administer infusions, all you have to do is let them know that you have made up the infusion, and where they can find it. Many nurses will make up the infusions themselves and administer them. The safest stance though is to presume that they won't until you confirm otherwise with them:

■ If you have to run the infusion yourself, then get a nurse to show you how to set up an infusion pump. It is not difficult. Essentially, insert the syringe into the pump with the drug label facing outwards, set the rate on the machine, plug it in, and turn it on. You also have to remember to connect the patient to the syringe.

■ Infusions can run through central or peripheral lines. Many infusions can run concurrently with other drugs through three-way taps or multiple-tap ('traffic light') giving sets. These are simple to set up with initial nurse supervision.

■ Some infusions cannot be mixed with others. The most problematic are those containing chelating ions, such as Ca^{2+}. Unfortunately, these require a second Venflon or need flushing with heparinized saline (Hepsal) or saline before another drug is administered through the same line. If in doubt, ask the nurses for help or check the *BNF*.

■ Place the syringe driver or infusion bag *below* the level of the patient's head to avoid the risk of siphoning.

Intravenous drugs

If you are in a hospital where nurses do not administer IV drugs, which is now thankfully rare, then you need to mix them with diluent and give them yourself. This can mean doing an IV drug round three to four times daily. In reality, you are unlikely to be asked to inject any medicines except for controlled drugs such as morphine and midazolam or if you are titrating a drug against a set value, for example, metoprolol for fast atrial fibrillation (AF):

1 Ensure the patient really needs the drug IV. Most drugs may be given PO, PR, SC or IM. It is time-consuming for you and expensive for

the NHS to give drugs through IV. It is often a fallacy that IV drugs are more effective. Many medications have only a marginally reduced oral bioavailability.

2 Read the instructions in the drug packet. Some drugs can be injected directly into the patient's vein. However, they usually need to be diluted first.

Liquid drugs not requiring dilution

If the drug can be given without dilution, draw it up with a small syringe and inject it over the recommended time. Some drugs must be given slowly to avoid anaphylaxis or pain in the patient's arm which they won't thank you for. Most drugs can be given quite quickly (over less than 30 seconds to 1 minute). Read the *BNF* and the drug's instructions – take these seriously, as complications from incorrect methods of administration (including those due to lack of knowledge) do occur and can be serious. Always check the cannula in patient first by flushing it with a small amount of normal saline. Extravasation of drugs can be serious and lead to tissue necrosis that can sometimes require plastic surgery input. Your patient will not thank you if this could have been avoided by simply recannulating them.

Liquid drugs requiring dilution

If the drug comes in liquid form that needs diluting, this is easily done by drawing the drug into a suitably large syringe (e.g. 10 or 20 ml) and then drawing in sterile saline or water for injection (available in small, sterile vials in the drug cupboard). Always use sterile fluid when diluting drugs; patients can get septic from once-sterile fluid that has been lying around unsealed.

Powdered drugs

If the drug comes in a vacuum container as a powder, you need to dissolve it with a solute, such as water for injection. Most antibiotics come this way. To avoid giving yourself and the ward a drug shower (Fig. 10.1):

1 Draw the required amount of water for injection into a suitably large syringe through a needle. Tap or push the end of the syringe to

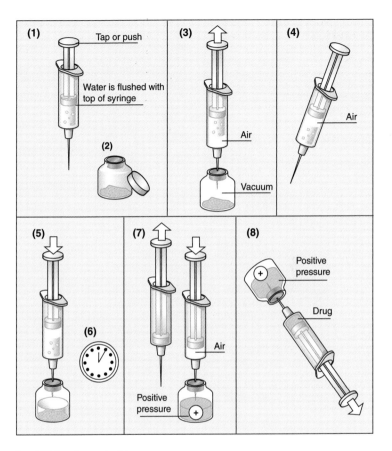

Figure 10.1 Preparing powdered drugs.

expel any air, so that the water is flushed with the top of the syringe.

2 Remove the flip-off plastic top of the drug vial, and clean with an alcohol wipe.

3 Push the needle through the rubber top of the drug vial and withdraw some air to create a vacuum inside the vial.

4 Tap or tilt the syringe upwards so that the withdrawn air moves through the water to the back of the syringe.

5 Inject the water into the vial, with the assistance of the vacuum you have just created. You may need to repeat this several times.

6 When you have injected enough water, shake the vial (or leave it to dissolve whilst you do something else).

7 Withdraw the needle. Draw some air into the syringe. Reintroduce the needle into the vial through the rubber top and inject some air to create positive pressure inside the vial.

8 Turn the vial upside down and withdraw the dissolved drug from the vial with the assistance of the positive pressure.

9 Don't worry if on first attempts you spray yourself, the desk and unwary passers-by with the drug. You will soon be able to do the whole thing perfectly in your sleep. Practice makes perfect!

Specific drug topics

Antibiotics

■ Check your hospital drug guidelines with seniors, pharmacists or ideally the consultant microbiologist. Each hospital has particular protocols that are usually published on the trust intranet. The variation in advice between hospitals is not random – the incidence of organisms is in constant flux and advice is based on regional surveillance data.

■ Always ask patients if they have known antibiotic (e.g. penicillin) allergy before prescribing any drug but in particular penicillin or cephalosporin antibiotics. Erythromycin is usually a reasonable alternative to amoxicillin and related penicillin drugs.

■ Be aware of *Clostridium difficile* in patients who have had recent broad-spectrum antibiotics (especially co-amoxiclav, cephalosporins and ciprofloxacin). Send stool for *C. difficile* toxin in any patient with abdominal pain, diarrhoea and a fever.

Also be alert to pseudomembranous colitis – a dangerous condition that is associated with *C. difficile*. Patients are at risk of toxic megacolon, and so an abdominal X-ray to look for dilated loops of bowel is essential. If your patient is diagnosed with *C. difficile*, discuss with microbiology regarding treatment (usually metronidazole orally).

■ Common antibiotic side effects include diarrhoea and vaginal (and other) candidiasis (thrush). If the patient is high risk, it may be worth prescribing an anti-candidiasis pessary or cream on the PRN side of the drug chart.

■ Warn women taking the oral contraceptive pill that antibiotics (and other drugs affecting liver metabolism) reduce its efficacy, so they should use other forms of contraception whilst on antibiotics.

■ Consider giving at least 24 hours IV treatment if the patient is very unwell.

■ Check the *BNF* and local guidelines for the most current treatment.

■ Gentamicin and vancomycin need regular peak and trough levels (see the *BNF*).

Standard treatments for common infections are listed in Table 10.2.

Anticoagulation

Foundation doctors are often required to anticoagulate patients following unstable angina, heart attacks, deep venous thromboses and pulmonary embolisms. Ask your colleagues for local protocols. These generally involve giving a low-molecular-weight heparin and warfarin together, and then stopping the heparin once the international normalized ratio (INR) (prothrombin ratio) is high enough (i.e. when the warfarin begins to work and is 'within range') (Table 10.3).

1 Check that the patient has no bleeding disorder. Check full blood count, INR and activated partial thromboplastin time (APTT).

2 If using *unfractionated* intravenous heparin (usually indicated where rapid reversal of anticoagulation may be required – now thankfully rare):

Start the patient on a heparin pump (usually 25,000 units in 50 ml of normal saline), run at 2.8 ml/hour (1400 units/hour). Check the APTT at least once a day and adjust the heparin according to a sliding scale (see the *BNF*). Ideally, the APTT should hover around 1.5–2.5 depending on the indication. The heparin should be stopped if the APTT is more than 7.

3 If using low-molecular-weight heparin:

● Prescribe daily subcutaneous low-molecular-weight heparin. Each hospital has its own preferred brand; check with your formulary and weight-adjust the dose as per *BNF* guidelines. Dosing regime will vary with brand and indication. APTT need not be checked. If a check is required then monitoring is with factor Xa activity. Note that they undergo renal

Table 10.2 Standard treatments for common infections (please refer to the protocols in your local trust for more information as regional variations exist).

Type of infection	Treatment
Community-acquired pneumonia	Oral amoxicillin (clarithromycin if penicillin allergic)
	Second choice or atypical pneumonia: clarithromycin or doxycycline. Calculate CURB score.
Severe or hospital-acquired pneumonia	IV co-amoxiclav and clarithromycin or cephalosporin, for example, cefuroxime if non-severe penicillin allergy
Aspiration pneumonia	IV amoxicillin and IV metronidazole or IV co-amoxiclav
COPD exacerbation	Oral amoxicillin or doxycycline if penicillin allergy
UTI	Oral trimethoprim or nitrofurantoin or ciprofloxacin
Tonsillitis	Penicillin V (avoid amoxicillin)
Cellulitis	Flucloxacillin and benzylpenicillin or clindamycin if with penicillin allergy
	Consider metronidazole if the wound smells strongly of anaerobes and add in teicoplanin if MRSA positive
Septicaemia of unknown source	IV cefuroxime (see hospital policy)
Clostridium difficile diarrhoea	Oral metronidazole or oral vancomycin
Meningitis	Ceftriaxone IV, add in ampicillin if pregnant, immunocompromised or over 50 to cover *Listeria*. Use chloramphenicol IV if penicillin allergic. If there is change in GCS or seizures cover for viral encephalitis with IV acyclovir
Intra-abdominal sepsis	IV cefuroxime and metronidazole
Spontaneous bacterial peritonitis	IV piperacillin/tazobactam, prophylaxis-use ciprofloxacin
Helicobacter pylori infection	Use oral PPI, clarithromycin and amoxicillin or PPI, amoxicillin and metronidazole for 7 days
Septic arthritis	Refer to surgeons for wash out and take cultures IV flucloxacillin and oral sodium fusidate, IV clindamycin in penicillin allergy
Osteomyelitis	IV flucloxacillin and oral sodium fusidate, IV clindamycin in penicillin allergy

excretion and reduced doses are often required if renal clearance is impaired. Discuss dosing with your ward pharmacist as needed.

4 Start the patient simultaneously on warfarin. Warfarin is a coumarin anticoagulant. Note that initially giving warfarin is *pro*-thrombotic due to its effects on clotting factor activity (it reduces protein C firstly); this can lead to warfarin-related skin and soft tissue necrosis. This is the reason why it is paramount that heparin cover is instituted before warfarin. The *pro*-thrombotic state obviously quickly reverses with time as the other vitamin K-dependent factors fall. The standard loading protocol is as follows:

Table 10.3 INR and warfarin dosing.

INR	Action
4.5–6	Reduce warfarin dose or omit dose. Restart warfarin when INR <5
6–8	Stop warfarin. Monitor INR and restart when INR <5
>8 and no bleeding or minor bleeding	Stop warfarin and give oral vitamin K
Major bleeding/intracranial haemorrhage	Stop warfarin. Give prothrombin complex or FFP if not available. Give vitamin K 5–10 mg IV. Discuss with haematology

- Give 10 mg of warfarin on the first day and 5 mg on the second and third, and then adjust according to the INR. This protocol may need to be modified for the elderly, frail, those with liver disease and on liver-stimulating drugs. If you dose every patient like this you will quickly encounter problems. A starting dose of 5 mg is usually more reasonable, but in those with sensitivity, this may still be too high. Be particularly cautious with postoperative patients who are at risk of bleeding, patients over the age of 60 and those with liver, renal or cardiac failure. Check with your senior if you are unsure. There may be an anticoagulation local protocol you can follow.
- You need to check the INR daily from the first dose. Reduce the warfarin dose if the INR rises too quickly or too high (e.g. above 5). Remember that the peak blood level is 36–48 hours after the dose so the INR you see will usually be 'on the way up'.

    The INR needs to be checked
    Every day for 1 week
    Every week for 3 weeks
    Every month for 3 months and
    Every 8 weeks after that

Always inform the GP in the discharge summary that the patient has been started on warfarin. Most hospitals and some GP surgeries have anticoagulation services that manage the patient's INR:

- You are usually aiming for an INR of 2–3 (but this varies depending on the condition – it may be higher in metallic valves; check with the person who has decided that the patient should be on warfarin and the *BNF*).

- Clearly explain the potential side effects of warfarin to the patient and that they must inform their GP and any other health professional that they are taking warfarin. They must be aware of the risks of bleeding and what symptoms to look out for. It is also advisable to tell the patient to keep tablets well hidden from small children. Advise patients to let their pharmacist know that they are taking warfarin before buying over-the-counter medications and to check when they are prescribed a new medication that it does not interact and cause the INR to increase or decrease.
- If the INR or APTT is too high, simply stop the warfarin and/or heparin. If the INR is greater than 10 or the patient is bleeding, give 4 units of fresh frozen plasma (FFP) and recheck the clotting. Some hospitals have access to prothrombin complex, which can be given instead of FFP, but it is very expensive. A small dose (1–2 mg) of vitamin K will reverse the clotting in a few hours. Beware of giving higher doses as this prevents further anticoagulation for weeks. Always consult with a haematologist and colleagues if a patient is bleeding or you are concerned. Beware of anaphylaxis (be prepared to treat with O_2 and adrenaline, see p. 91). FFP can also be given stat to decrease a bleeding tendency.
- The half-life of unfractionated heparin is quite short (approximately 90 minutes), so stopping the infusion is usually sufficient. Alternatively, heparin can be reversed with protamine sulphate. Use 1 mg protamine sulphate/100 IU of heparin, to a maximum of 50 mg. This should work within half an hour.

Protamine is not helpful if the patient has been given LMWH.

- Side effects of warfarin include the following:
  - Bleeding
  - Alopecia
  - Diarrhoea
  - Purple toes syndrome
  - Hepatic dysfunction with jaundice

- Side effects of LMWH and unfractionated heparin include the following:
  - Bleeding
  - Heparin-induced thrombocytopaenia
  - Osteoporosis when used long-term

Digoxin

Digoxin is commonly used to slow down the ventricular rate in atrial fibrillation. It is potentially dangerous with many side effects, such as fatigue, confusion, nausea and vomiting, anorexia, diarrhoea and arrhythmias. Digoxin also interacts with many drugs (see the BNF). In particular, beware of drugs that lower K (e.g. diuretics), as hypokalaemia predisposes to dangerous digoxin toxicity.

How to digitalize (discuss with your senior first):

1 In the non-acute situation:

- Give the patient 125–250 µg of digoxin twice daily for 1–2 days. No loading dose is required.
- Reduce dose to once daily for maintenance. Digoxin maintenance dosage varies according to age, weight and renal function. In general:

Normal dose: 125–375 µg

In the elderly: 62.5–125 µg

If in renal impairment, reduce the dose and discuss with the ward pharmacist.

Table 10.4 Therapeutic drug levels and sampling times.

Drug	Sampling time	Therapeutic range
Amiodarone	Any time when levels are stable (after 1 month)	0.6–2.5 mg/l
		Monitor LFTs and TFTs and for signs of pulmonary toxicity
Carbamazepine	Peak 3 hours after dose	Single therapy: 8–12 mg/l
		Multiple therapy: 4–8 mg/l
Digoxin	6–12 hours after dose	0.8–2 µg/l
		Check U&E and Mg Ca^{2+}, as toxicity is potentiated if Ca^{2+} is high or Mg or K^+ is low
Gentamicin and tobramicin	Peak 1 hour after dose	5–10 mg/l
	Trough (just before new dose)	<2 mg/l
Lithium	12 hours after dose	0.4–1.0 mmol/l
Phenytoin	IV peak 2–4 hours after dose	10–20 mg/l
	Oral peak 3–9 hours after dose	
Sodium valproate	Plasma levels are not a good guide to efficacy	
Vancomycin	Peak 1 hour after dose	25–40 mg/l
	Trough (just before new dose)	1–3 mg/l
		Check U&E for renal toxicity

DRUGS

- If the patient experiences side effects like blue-yellow vision (xanthopsia) or halos, nausea or delirium, then measure digoxin levels for toxicity and look for prolongation of the PR interval and an atrial tachycardia. Digoxin-specific antibodies (Digibind) are available as an antidote to digoxin poisoning.

2 In the acute situation (for more rapid control of the ventricular rate):

- Give 750–1500 μg of digoxin orally over 24 hours in divided doses until the rate is controlled (usually takes two to three doses), and then give the maintenance dose (see the preceding text) *or*
- Give 750–1000 μg IV over at least 2 hours, and then continue with maintenance doses. This method is used in the emergency setting. In the elderly, halve the above loading doses to avoid digoxin toxicity.

Therapeutic drug levels

Junior doctors are sometimes required to check the blood levels of several commonly used drugs (Table 10.4). This involves liaising with the nurse giving the drug so that you can take blood for levels at the appropriate times (e.g. at peak and trough dosage times). Ask the biochemistry technicians which tube to use (usually a yellow-top tube).

Miscellaneous tips

■ Metronidazole can be given easily and cheaply as a suppository. This is particularly useful after an appendicectomy, if the patient does not need a drip.

■ If a drug risks causing anaphylaxis (e.g. phytomenadione), ensure that you have adrenaline ready and a resuscitation trolley available. *Do not leave the ward for 5 minutes after giving these drugs.*

■ Any drug that is protein-based can cause anaphylaxis.

■ Always consider prescribing laxatives and anti-emetics prophylactically with opiate analgesia (at least on the PRN side).

■ Consider pre-emptive prescribing (i.e. prescribing certain drugs on the PRN side of the chart for all patients without contraindications) to prevent nurses bleeping you and your colleagues: paracetamol, cyclizine and laxatives (Table 10.5).

Table 10.5 75 commonly used drugs.

Drug name	Dose	Mechanism	Common side effects
Cardiovascular drugs			
Bendroflumethiazide	2.5–5 mg OD PO	Diuretic acting at DCT in kidney	Mild GI disturbances, hypokalaemia, hyponatraemia, postural hypotension
Furosemide	20 mg–1.5 g max PO/IV/infusion	Loop diuretic acting in the loop of Henle in the kidney	Mild GI disturbances, hypokalaemia, hyponatraemia, postural hypotension
Spironolactone	Dependent on reason for use: 25–400 mg daily PO	Potassium-sparing diuretic	GI disturbance, hepatotoxicity, gynaecomastia, hyperkalaemia
Atenolol	Dependent on reason for use: 25–100 mg daily PO	Beta blocker (selective β1 antagonist)	Bradycardia, peripheral vasoconstriction, bronchospasm, impotence
Doxazosin	1–16 mg max daily PO	Alpha adrenoceptor antagonist	Fatigue, cough, postural hypotension
Ramipril	1.25–10 mg max daily PO	ACE inhibitor	Care in renal impairment, hyperkalaemia, hypotension, dry cough, angioedema
Losartan	25–150 mg max daily PO (usually 50 mg daily)	Angiotensin II receptor antagonist	Hyperkalaemia, hypotension, angioedema
GTN	1–II puffs S/L, 10–200 mcg/minute and adjust according to response	Coronary vasodilator; venodilator to reduce preload	Headache, hypotension
Amlodipine	5–10 mg max daily PO	Dihydropyridine calcium channel blocker	Ankle swelling, flushing, headache
Verapamil	Dependent on reason for use: 40–120 mg, max 480 mg daily	Non-dihydropyridine calcium channel blocker	Constipation, flushing, headaches
Clopidogrel	75 mg daily (300 mg loading dose. May be higher in acute coronary syndrome)	ADP receptor inhibitor	GI bleeding, intracranial bleeding

(Continued)

Table 10.5 (*Continued*)

Drug name	Dose	Mechanism	Common side effects
Aspirin	75 mg daily	COX inhibitor	GI bleeding, bronchospasm
Simvastatin	10–80 mg max daily	HMG CoA reductase inhibitor	Myalgia, rhabdomyolysis, abnormal LFTs
Respiratory drugs			
Salbutamol	100–200 mcg inhaled QDS, or 2.5–5 mg nebulized PRN	β2 agonist	Hypokalaemia, fine tremor
Ipratropium bromide	20–40 mcg QDS inhaled, 500 mcg nebulized QDS	Muscarinic antagonist	Dry mouth, constipation, angle-closure glaucoma
Aminophylline	Loading IV 500–700 mcg/kg/hour	Phosphodiesterase inhibitor	Arrhythmias, nausea and vomiting, convulsions
Carbocisteine	2.25 g daily in divided doses PO	Mucolytic	GI disturbance
Antihistamine drugs			
Cetirizine	10 mg daily PO	H1 antagonist	Dizziness, confusion
Loratadine	10 mg daily PO	H1 antagonist	Dizziness, confusion
Chlorpheniramine	4 mg QDS, max 24 mg daily PO; 10 mg IV, max 40 mg/24 hours	H1 antagonist	Drowsiness headache
Hypnotic/anxiolytic drugs			
Zopiclone	3.75–7.5 mg max OD PO	Cyclopyrrolone	Taste disturbance, nausea, dizziness
Lorazepam	1–4 mg daily PO/IV (repeat dose sometimes given for seizures)	Benzodiazepine	Respiratory depression when given IV in seizures, drowsiness, confusion, ataxia
Chlordiazepoxide	10–30 mg QDS PO, max 240 mg in 24 hours in ETOH withdrawal	Benzodiazepine	Drowsiness, confusion, ataxia, dependence

Drug name	Dose	Mechanism	Common side effects
Antidepressant drugs			
Amitriptyline	75–200 mg max daily PO	Tricyclic–SNRI	Arrhythmias, dry eyes, urinary retention, constipation
Citalopram	10–40 mg max daily PO	SSRI	QT prolongation and arrhythmias, hepatitis
Antiemetic drugs			
Cyclizine	50 mg PO/IV/IM TDS	H1 receptor antagonist	Palpitations, drowsiness, xerostomia, dizziness/light-headed particularly on IV infusion
Metoclopramide	10 mg PO/IV/IM TDS	D2 receptor antagonist	Extrapyramidal side effects, oculogyric crisis, diarrhoea
Ondansetron	4–8 mg PO/IV/IM TDS	5-HT3 receptor antagonist	Constipation, headache, flushing
Analgesic drugs – use WHO ladder			
Paracetamol	1 g PO/IV/PR QDS	Antipyretic, analgesic	Hepatotoxic in OD
Ibuprofen	200–400 mg QDS max 2.4 g daily PO	Cyclo-oxygenase inhibitor	Renal failure, fluid overload, GI bleeding, thrombocytopaenia
Codeine	30–60 mg PO/IM QDS, 240 mg max daily	Opiate	Nausea, constipation
Tramadol	50–100 mg PO/IM QDS	Opiate	Nausea, diarrhoea, constipation
Oramorph	2.5–20 mg PO QDS	Opiate	Nausea, constipation, pruritis, respiratory depression in OD
Gabapentin	300 mg and then gradually increase up to max 3.6 g daily PO	GABA agonist	Drowsiness, nausea, vomiting, weight gain

(Continued)

DRUGS

Table 10.5 (*Continued*)

Drug name	Dose	Mechanism	Common side effects
Laxative drugs			
Senna	Two tablets OD/BD PO	Anthraquinone, stimulant	Abdominal cramps
Lactulose	10–15 ml TDS PO	Osmotic laxative	Flatulence, nausea, cramps
Movicol	One sachet OD/TDS PO	Osmotic laxative	Abdominal distension, pain, nausea, flatulence
Anti-diabetic drugs			
Metformin	500 mg–1 g TDS	Biguanide	Lactic acidosis, diarrhoea, nausea, vomiting
Gliclazide	40–80 mg daily max 320 mg daily PO	Sulphonylurea	Hypoglycaemia, weight gain, jaundice
Thyroid drugs			
Levothyroxine	25 mcg–100 mcg OD PO, max 200 mcg daily	T4 replacement	Diarrhoea, thyrotoxicosis, AF in elderly, anginal pain
Carbimazole	15–40 mg daily PO	Thyroid peroxidase inhibitor	Fever, malaise, agranulocytosis, rash
Drugs for BPH			
Tamsulosin	400 mcg PO daily	Alpha1 antagonist	Postural hypotension, dizziness
Finasteride	5 mg PO daily	5α reductase inhibitor	Gynaecomastia, hypersensitivity reactions
Antifungal drugs			
Clotrimazole	1 application top TDS	Antifungal azole	Cytochrome P450 inhibitor
Fluconazole	150 mg PO stat dose or 50 mg PO OD for 7/7	Antifungal azole	Cytochrome P450 inhibitor

Drug name	Dose	Mechanism	Common side effects
Anti-epileptic drugs			
Valproate	300 mg PO BD, increased to maintenance of 1–2 g daily	Na channel blocker; GABA transaminase inhibitor	Weight gain, abnormal LFTs, thrombocytopaenia, ataxia, tremor; teratogenic
Lamotrigine	25 mg daily, increase 100–200 mg daily maintenance PO	Na channel blocker;	Stevens–Johnson syndrome
Carbamazepine	100–200 mg OD/BD PO	Na channel blocker	Dry mouth, ataxia, dizziness
Anti-reflux drugs			
Omeprazole	20–40 mg OD PO	Proton pump inhibitor	Hyponatraemia, GI disturbance
Ranitidine	150 mg BD PO	H2 receptor antagonist	Diarrhoea, headache, dizziness
Common antibiotics			
Amoxicillin	250 mg PO TDS/500 mg–1 g IV TDS	Penicillin	Nausea, vomiting, diarrhoea, rashes
Flucloxacillin	250–500 mg PO QDS/1–2 g IV QDS	Penicillin	Nausea, vomiting, diarrhoea, rashes, hepatitis, cholestatic jaundice
Co-amoxiclav	625 mg PO TDS/1.2 g IV TDS	Penicillin	Nausea, vomiting, diarrhoea, rashes, risk of precipitating *C. difficile*
Clarithromycin	500 mg PO/IV BD	Macrolide	Tooth and tongue discoloration, stomatitis, glossitis, P450 inhibitor
Ceftriaxone	1 g IM/1–2 g IV BD	Cephalosporin	Diarrhoea, precipitates in urine and gall bladder, pancreatitis, risk of precipitating *C. difficile*
Cefuroxime	750 mg IV TDS	Cephalosporin	Diarrhoea, jaundice, eosinophilia, risk of precipitating *C. difficile*

(Continued)

DRUGS

Table 10.5 (Continued)

Drug name	Dose	Mechanism	Common side effects
Ciprofloxacin	500 mg PO BD, only give IV if NBM (400 mg IV BD)	Quinolone	Diarrhoea, risk of precipitating *C. difficile*, and erythema nodosum; avoid in G6PD deficiency and myasthenia gravis
Gentamicin	5–7 mg/kg initially and then dose adjusted according to serum concentration	Aminoglycoside	Nephrotoxicity, ototoxicity, hypomagnesaemia; contraindicated in myasthenia gravis
Nitrofurantoin	50 mg PO QDS	Damages bacterial DNA, mechanism unknown	Pulmonary fibrosis, peripheral neuropathy, lupus erythematosus-like reaction
Trimethoprim	200 mg PO BD	Dihydrofolate reductase inhibitors	Raised creatinine, rashes, erythema multiforme
Vancomycin	125–250 mg PO QDS, 1–1.5 g IV BD	Glycopeptide	Nephrotoxicity, ototoxicity, neutropenia, agranulocytosis
Teicoplanin	400 mg IV BD for first three doses, then OD thereafter	Glycopeptide	Rash, fever, angiodema, eosinophilia
Piperacillin/ tazobactam	4.5 g IV TDS	Penicillin	Diarrhoea, vomiting, stomatitis, risk of precipitating *C. difficile*
Meropenem	1 g IV TDS	Carbapenem	Nausea, vomiting, diarrhoea, thrombocythaemia, positive Coombs test
Doxycycline	200 mg PO stat on first day and then 100 mg PO thereafter	Tetracycline	Photosensitivity rash, anorexia, tinnitus, headache and visual disturbance if pt has BIH
Clindamycin	450 mg PO QDS; only give IV if NBM (450–600 mg IVQDS)	Lincosamide	Diarrhoea, risk of precipitating *C. difficile*, oesophageal ulceration
Metronidazole	400 mg PO TDS; only give IV if NBM (500 mg IV TDS)	Nitroimidazole	Taste disturbances, mucositis, anorexia
Co-trimoxazole	960 mg PO/IV BD	(Trimethoprim + sulphamethoxazole)	Stephen–Johnson syndrome, toxic epidermal necrolysis, photosensitivity, hyperkalaemia

Drug name	Dose	Mechanism	Common side effects
Antivirals			
Acyclovir	200 mg PO five times a day/10 mg/kg IV TDS	Nucleoside analogue	Nausea, vomiting, abdominal pain, diarrhoea, photosensitivity
Lamivudine	150 mg PO BD	Nucleoside reverse transcriptase inhibitor	Peripheral neuropathy, rhabdomyolysis, alopecia
Emergency drugs			
Adrenaline	0.5 mg (0.5 ml of 1:1000) IM for anaphylaxis 1 mg (10 ml of 1:10,000) IV for cardiac arrest	α- and β-adrenoceptor agonist	VT, arrhythmias, peripheral vasoconstriction, hypertension
Amiodarone	900 mg IV loading dose and then 300 mg IV maintenance 200 mg PO TDS for 1 week and then 200 mg PO BD for 1 week, then 200 mg OD maintenance	Prolongs cardiac action potential	P450 inhibitor, hypo-/hyperthyroidism, slate-grey skin, phototoxicity, hepatitis, pulmonary fibrosis, peripheral neuropathy, corneal microdeposits
Adenosine	6 mg, then 12 mg and then 12 mg IV as bolus doses via a large peripheral cannula	Transient AV node blockade	Transient facial flushing, bronchospasm, chest pain, dyspnoea
Atropine	300–600 mcg IV	Muscarinic antagonist	Constipation, urinary retention, dry eyes and mouth, angle-closure glaucoma
Local anaesthetics			
Lignocaine	Comes in 2% or 1% vial. Max dose is 3 mg/kg	Na channel blocker	Respiratory depression, convulsions, hypotension, bradycardia – can lead to cardiac arrest

If in doubt, consult *BNF*.

DRUGS

Chapter 11
HANDLE WITH CARE

Some patients need special attention as they are especially vulnerable from physical or mental frailty and stigma. This chapter covers the above patients and some specialist scenarios you may have to deal with including oncological and haematological emergencies. There is also a section on issues relating to capacity.

Alcoholism

Many more of your patients will be dependent on alcohol than you may first appreciate. This is something that you should routinely assess when taking a history. Never make assumptions. There have been many times when I have routinely asked elderly ladies how much they drink and have been told matter-of-factly: 'only a bottle of sherry a day, and two if my friends come round!'. This can be an issue when these patients come into hospital, as they do not have access to alcohol and so are at risk of withdrawal (see the following text).

To assess alcoholism, do the CAGE questionnaire,[1] which is remarkably reliable for picking up alcoholism:

1 Have you ever felt you should **C**UT down on drinking?

2 Have people made you **A**NGRY by asking about your alcohol intake?

3 Have you ever felt **G**UILTY about your drinking?

4 Do you ever drink first thing in the morning (or take an **E**YE-OPENER)?

[1] Mayfield D., McLeod G., Hall P. (1974) The CAGE questionnaire: validation of a new alcoholism screening instrument. *American Journal of Psychiatry* **131:**1121–1123.

Answering 'yes' to two or more of the above questions gives the patient an 80% chance of having an alcohol problem.

When taking an alcohol history, try to incorporate the following questions:

● Ask the patient for a typical day, with the amount and type of alcohol taken at each time.
● Have they always drunk those quantities or has it increased?
● Have they ever given up alcohol before? Do they want to now?
● Do they feel they have a dependence on alcohol?
● Do they drink for a specific reason? (Are they depressed or have financial/social issues?)
● Do they have any other substance misuse problems?
● Is there any history of mental health problems?
● How is this affecting their lives?
● Tactfully ask relatives or friends about the patient if you suspect denial of alcoholism.
● Request a full blood count (FBC) with mean cell volume to look for macrocytosis. Also check liver function tests and gamma-glutamyl transferase (GGT). Both rise with prolonged use of alcohol, and the former can take approximately 2–3 months to return to normal following abstention (the latter usually reduces in days to weeks depending on the degree of liver damage). Note that there are other

The Hands-on Guide to the Foundation Programme, Fifth Edition. Anna Donald, Michael Stein, Ciaran Scott Hill and Selina J Chavda.
© 2015 John Wiley & Sons, Ltd. Published 2015 by John Wiley & Sons, Ltd.

causes of a raised GGT like benzodiazepines, phenytoin, obesity, gall bladder and pancreatic disease. Patients with alcoholic liver disease also have a relative thrombocytopaenia.

• Consider a nutritional screen and vitamin supplementation (especially B, D and K groups). If the patient is being admitted, prescribe 48 hours of Pabrinex (a multi-B vitamin complex) IV BD, and then prescribe both thiamine 100 mg BD and vitamin B compound strong tablets, 1 tablet TDS.

• Offer the patient local alcoholic support services, as an inpatient and an outpatient also. The general practitioner (GP) can be very helpful in providing these services. Some practices also have links to counsellors or psychologists if the patient needs them. In some hospitals, all patients admitted with an alcohol-related complications need referral to alcohol support services. This even includes drunk teenagers who hurt themselves or require a period of observation until they sober up. This is an opportunity to educate and change behaviour before more serious problems develop.

• Try not to be judgemental; as alcohol dependence is a complex multifactorial disorder and you should approach it as such.

Alcohol withdrawal

Some patients will be admitted specifically to withdraw from alcohol, either as an inpatient in hospital if they have other medical problems requiring admission or as part of inpatient rehabilitation. Others will have their alcohol dependence unmasked in hospital. Always consider alcohol (and nicotine) withdrawal if your patient suddenly becomes unexpectedly agitated. If you reassure patients with addictions at an early stage that they will be supported, then this reduces their anxiety and makes them more likely to be cooperative and not self-discharge:

■ Ask your senior for local protocols.

■ Always prescribe more chlordiazepoxide on the as-required side of the drug chart, to a maximum daily dose of 240 mg including the regular dosing.

■ Watch for hypotension, dehydration, hypoglycaemia and electrolyte imbalance. Patients with alcohol excess often do not eat and so are at risk of re-feeding syndrome. Monitor their phosphate and magnesium levels. Ensure 4-hourly observation and regular urea and electrolytes, glucose and FBC.

■ Benzodiazepines such as chlordiazepoxide, clomethiazole and lorazepam are all used; chlordiazepoxide is the most commonly used nowadays.

See Table 11.1 for dosing regimen of chlordiazepoxide.

■ Consider IV clomethiazole if the patient is vomiting. A 0.8% infusion of clomethiazole at 3–7.5 ml (24–60 mg)/minute, reducing to 0.5–1 ml (4–8 mg)/minute, should keep the patient lightly sedated. Consult with your senior before administering IV clomethiazole, as this is quite extreme. A resuscitation trolley must be available at all times and frequent observations performed, as the patient may become too deeply sedated and at risk of respiratory arrest. Similarly as it impairs the rate of alcohol

Table 11.1 Prescribing chlordiazepoxide.

Day	Dose of chlordiazepoxide (mg)	Tablet timing
Days 1–2	10–20	Four times daily
Days 3–4	10	Thrice daily
Days 5–6	10	Twice daily
Day 7	10	Once daily

Do not treat with chlordiazepoxide for more than 9 days.

breakdown if the patient drinks whilst receiving the medication, the results can easily be fatal.

■ Be careful with any benzodiazepines. Patients should not drive for 48 hours after taking the last dose. Sedation may mask hepatic coma. Avoid prolonged use and abrupt withdrawal. Dependence becomes a problem after about 9 days.

■ Nowadays, patients are rarely admitted into hospital as an inpatient solely for detoxification. The reasons for this are multifactorial but include service reorganization with a focus on community care and a perception that patients who may succeed in detoxification must actively engage in their own care.

Capacity

The issue of capacity can often be tricky to deal with as a junior. A general rule of thumb is to involve seniors early on if you suspect there is an issue with a patient's capacity. Similarly, it is also prudent to recheck the patient's capacity if you are unsure as to whether they lack capacity. This is often an issue in the elderly population, especially those with dementia.

Remember, all adults are deemed to have capacity to make decisions as they are mentally competent. If you suspect someone does not have capacity, you need to test it in accordance with the Mental Capacity Act 2005.

In order for a patient to have capacity, they must be able to:

■ Understand the information given.
■ Retain the information.
■ Weigh up the information.
■ Communicate their decision, by whatever means possible to you.

Importantly, a bad or irrational decision does not mean the patient does not have capacity. You also cannot presume someone lacks capacity simply because they have mental health problems or have communication problems (blind/deaf) or because they make decisions that you disagree with.

Capacity can also be fluctuant, so a patient may have capacity to make a decision on one day and not another. Similarly, capacity is not an 'all or nothing' phenomenon. Just because a patient lacks the capacity to make a decision on their discharge destination does not mean they automatically lack the capacity to decide what to have for breakfast.

Assessing capacity is a skill, and the best people I have seen performing the assessment are geriatricians. Often the best way to learn is to sit in during an assessment.

Involving other members of the multidisciplinary team can be helpful to assess whether someone has capacity to make specific decisions such as psychiatrists, neurologists and senior team members. Social workers are also able to perform capacity assessments.

If a patient is deemed to lack capacity, then the doctors must act in the patients' best interests. Ideally, if the patient is likely to lack capacity only for a temporary time period, the doctors should act in the least restrictive manner possible, so that when the patient does regain capacity, they can make their own decision.

The doctor should find out if the patient:

1 Has an advanced decision

This is a legal document signed by the patient and a third party stating what treatments the patient would not want to have. The patient will have written this when they had capacity.

2 Had any advanced statements

These are similar to advanced decisions but are not a legal document. They are essentially a group of beliefs or wishes the patient would have wanted.

3 Has a lasting power of attorney

This is someone the patient has legally appointed to act on their behalf and make decisions regarding their care/finances when they lack the capacity to do so.

Relatives views and those close to the patient should also be sought, but ultimately, unless the patient has a valid advanced directive, the management plan is determined by the doctor. Usually these decisions are made by the consultant in charge, so you do not need to worry too much. If you have any concerns, you should contact your defence union for advice.

Ultimately, if there are major disagreements between relatives and the medical team, legal action is sought and a court decision may be required.

If the patient has no relatives or next of kin, then an Independent Mental Capacity Advocate (IMCA) may be required. They will review the case and then offer an opinion on the treatment plan. They cannot refuse life-saving treatment on the patient's behalf.

Children

You may work with children as a surgical junior doctor or in A & E, although you are not expected to provide full paediatric care. The following tips may help:

■ If you normally power dress you may wish to consider outfits that are more casual; it helps to avoid doctor phobia and unnecessary formality. This does not mean that you should be scruffy or unclean but you may want to consider less formal wear.

■ For children under 16, get consent from parents/guardians whilst they are on the ward, or you will have to call them in from home.

■ Minors can legally sign for themselves if they are deemed to have Gillick competence and they are consenting for treatment, but it is usually a good idea to get parental or guardian consent unless there is an emergency.

■ NO minor can refuse treatment that is deemed medically in their best interests, even if they are deemed Gillick competent if someone with parental responsibility has given consent.

■ Ask the anaesthetist to insert cannulae when the child is asleep for theatre, to minimize needle trauma and phobia. Young children usually undergo an anaesthetic induction with volatile inhalation agents and so do not require IV access as a prerequisite.

■ Paediatric blood bottles minimize the amount of blood needed.

■ Use local anaesthetic cream before inserting cannulae and taking blood in young children.

■ Be cautious when prescribing IV fluids and drugs – different-sized children have very different fluid and drug needs. Consult the *BNF for Children* if in doubt, and this is preferable to asking colleagues. If you do ask a colleague, the paediatric registrar or a senior paediatric nurse is probably the best person, as they can check your calculation and give you advice on where to find the information you require. However, remember you are ultimately responsible for any prescriptions you write.

■ In emergencies, intraosseous access is preferable to a delay in finding intravenous access. You ideally need to practice this on a model before doing it for the first time. Although scalp veins may be easy to access in those under 10 months (and can even be used to site central cannulae), you are advised to seek a senior opinion before you attempt to access them. If doing so, an elastic band can act as a useful tourniquet. Be strict with your aseptic non-touch technique infections of the scalp can lead to meningitis.

Depression

People in hospital often suffer with depression. Hospitals can be frightening, intimidating places, full of the unknown, with an endless array of tests and painful procedures in between interminable waiting. Patients may not be forthcoming about their depression, and it may take some skilful rapport building on your part to acquire this information.

Be alert to sudden mood changes and negative conversation. Ask patients about their fears. You may be able to help immediately with reassurance or liaison with social workers, nurses, psychiatrists and medical colleagues.

■ Interestingly, many elderly patients suffering from acute conditions such as ACS or strokes have been recently bereaved. Your patient may be grieving. In addition, a lot of elderly patients suffer from loneliness, which can lead to depression. The most saddening thing I had ever heard from a patient when she came to clinic was that I was the first person she had spoken to in over 2 weeks.

■ If your patient seems low in mood, they may be suffering from undiagnosed pain, hypoxia, alcohol or drug withdrawal, electrolyte and thyroid imbalances, as well as concerns about employment, finances and home care.

■ Alert psychiatrists and colleagues if you think a patient is in danger of attempting suicide (see Chapter 4, Overdose).

● Be aware of the physical and psychological signs of depression.

Physical signs (constipation, early morning wakening, reduced appetite)

Psychological signs (anhedonia, tearful, anxious, visual or auditory hallucinations in psychotic depression)

Elderly patients

Like children, elderly patients can present with non-specific, understated symptoms. Elderly patients are often stoical and may hide quite severe pain. They come to hospital either because they have been brought by carers, or because something has caused them to reduce their ability to function in their current state. They can often be confused or unable to give you a history. A collateral from a carer, GP or relative that knows the patient well is invaluable in these circumstances. When taking a history, it is important to take a detailed social history. The following are some useful questions to ask:

■ Where do they live? In a house or flat?
■ Who do they live with?
■ Does their accommodation have stairs (both indoors and out)?
■ Do they have a lift/stair lift?
■ Do they have carers? If so, how often do they come in? What do they help the patient with?
■ Are they able to dress/wash/feed themselves?
■ Are they continent of urine and faeces?
■ How do they walk about? Do they have a stick or a frame? What is their mobility like?
■ Do they have family nearby?
■ Who does the shopping/cooking/cleaning?
■ Do they feel they are coping at home, or do they need some extra help?

These questions are helpful to get an understanding of their baseline status and will greatly aid discharge planning.

Investigations to do:

1 Monitor vital signs. Consider checking core temperature. Beware, the elderly may not spike a temperature even if they are septic, as they may not mount an inflammatory response like younger patients do. Cold sepsis is also particularly dangerous, as it is often missed.

2 Go through a checklist of systems to make sure you're not missing something serious. In particular, watch for:

● Fractures: old people often don't complain of pain. Be particularly wary if they have had a fall recently. Look at the limbs (especially the hips, legs and wrists) and feel for crepitus.

● Hypoxia: people may present with euphoria. Measure the respiratory rate and do pulse oximetry or blood gases if concerned. Remember that lots of elderly patients may have undiagnosed chronic obstructive pulmonary disease and may be at risk of CO_2 narcosis.

■ Fluid overload and electrolyte imbalance: prescribe IV fluids cautiously at a slow rate in the elderly and slow down or stop fluids if necessary. Monitor electrolytes daily and regularly reconsider whether the patient needs IV fluids.

■ A basic IV fluid regime for a small elderly person who is not septic would look something like this:

---

500 ml of normal saline with 20 mmol KCl over 6 hours

500 ml of normal saline with 20 mmol KCl over 6 hours

500 ml of 5% dextrose with 20 mmol KCl over 6 hours

500 ml of 5% dextrose with 20 mmol KCl over 6 hours

■ Hypothermia: consider checking rectal temperature – a patient's 'peripheral' temperature as measured with a tympanic or oral probe may not reflect their true core temperature. Put a bair hugger on the patient, and consider giving warmed IV fluids if temperature not improving.

■ Malnutrition: look for flaky skin, poor gums, unhealed bruises or scratches. The elderly classically have a 'tea and toast diet'. Vitamin deficiencies are common and can have serious consequences if not treated. Consider a nutritional screen and a vitamin D level in those with all over body pain. Vitamin K deficiency is particularly common and can lead to abnormal clotting with a raised international normalized ratio (prothrombin ratio) (INR).

■ K⁺-wasting with diuretics. Check K⁺ and supplement orally if necessary. Be careful not to produce hyperkalaemia. If you send the patient home with K supplements, be sure to notify both the patient and the GP, so K⁺ can be monitored – it is usual to only prescribe 3 days worth to avoid hyperkalaemia. There are lots of other ways to orally supplement K naturally such as with bananas, tomatoes and chocolate.

■ Infantilization of elderly patients. Remember that 80% of elderly patients live at home. Only 14% of people over 75 have any form of dementia. Junior doctors often get a skewed perspective of the elderly, as most interactions in hospital are with those who are very sick or with complex care needs. Be careful not to treat elderly people like children, and always be respectful towards them like any other patient.

Haemophilia patients

Haemophilia is a rare X-linked disorder affecting clotting factors. Adult UK haemophiliacs are not uncommonly hepatitis B/C and/or HIV positive, from previous blood product transfusions. This is no longer an issue as recombinant products are used, and testing of blood products is much more stringent, so the risks are much lower.

Haemophilia can be crippling, and haemophilia patients often have many bad hospital experiences. More than most, this group needs open and honest communication. Because of the high rate of infectivity, you need to take the following precautions.

Taking blood

■ Minimize taking blood unless clinically indicated. Question your colleagues if they have requested frequent routine blood tests.
■ Phone a haematologist or ideally the nearest haemophiliac service; usually, they will advise on management from the haemophilia point of view.

■ Paediatric bottles from the paediatrics ward can be used to minimize the amount of blood needed.
■ Don't use a vacutainer; its 18-gauge needle is too big. Use the smallest possible needle or blue butterfly on small veins. Knuckle veins can be useful, as these patients may have poor venous access due to repeated blood tests/cannulae in the past.
■ Never use a tourniquet. It causes excessive bruising and occasionally major bleeds from pressure trauma to blood vessels. If you need pressure to find a vein, very gently inflate a blood pressure cuff, but release the pressure as soon as you are in the vein, or you will cause major bruising. A good alternative is to get a nurse to gently squeeze the arm.
■ Never give or prescribe drugs IM, and avoid non-steroidal anti-inflammatory drugs as they can precipitate bleeding.
■ Always use standard precautions for taking blood samples.
■ Always alert the lab to the haemophiliac status of a patient and their hepatitis/HIV status if known.

For theatre

■ Do a full clotting screen (INR, bleeding time, activated partial thromboplastin time, fibrinogen) preoperatively and a screen for antibodies. A group and screen is essential. Liaise with the haematologist. Any deficiency of factors VIII or IX must be corrected before theatre. If the deficiency is corrected, the patient can be treated like other patients post-operatively, except:
■ Factor VIII levels should be tested post-operatively twice per day (factor IX levels once per day). Make sure the first level is taken before the patient is bathed and the wound dressed.
■ Delay suture removal beyond the usual 10 days, as haemophiliacs are prone to bleeding about this time. Get senior advice.
■ For patients with haemophilia A, desmopressin can be given for minor surgery and mild bleeding (desmopressin is not useful in haemophilia B patients). The antifibronolytic agent tranexamic acid is useful for cuts and dental procedures.

HIV/AIDS

It goes without saying that these patients need special care. They face both death and stigma. You face potentially dangerous needlestick injuries. Time, care and an honest, open approach are essential.

Taking blood

■ It is completely fine to touch HIV/AIDS patients without gloves just about anywhere – just not in a major artery! It is really awful for such patients if health professionals are scared to treat them normally.

■ However, do always wear gloves when taking blood. Always have plenty of space for your tray and sharps. Dispose of sharps immediately after using them. Ideally use sharps with a safety device that clicks shut immediately after use to reduce the risk of needlesticks.

■ Use universal precautions if doing more invasive procedures. Although not necessary for simple venepuncture if the procedure you are undertaking has a risk of body fluids splashing into your eyes then goggles or a full face mask should be worn.

■ Don't do things in a hurry. Leave plenty of time for procedures and explanations.

■ Label blood samples with high-risk stickies (not in front of the patient). These are available from the labs if they are not already on your ward. It is your responsibility if a lab worker contracts HIV from an unlabelled sample. Alternatively call the lab in advance to warn them.

■ Use two specimen bags for high-risk samples.

■ Always warn theatre staff if a patient has HIV or AIDS.

■ Treat oral *Candida* with nystatin lozenges (mild) or fluconazole (see the *BNF*). When prescribing new medications, make sure they do not interact with the patient's antiretrovirals (ARVs). Check the *BNF* or use the following website: www.hiv-druginteractions.org/.

■ Be aware that HIV/AIDS patients may suffer from depression and may consider suicide. Consider referring to the psychiatrists or social workers. Discuss concerns with the nursing staff – and the patient, of course!

■ AIDS patients may suffer from multiple serious medical problems that may require urgent or aggressive therapy. Common problems include fever, atypical pneumonia, diarrhoea, skin sores, atypical malignancies and drug reactions. For reasons that are as yet poorly understood, allergies are much more common in patients with HIV/AIDS. If you find yourself looking after an HIV patient in a general ward, get expert advice from infectious disease staff.

■ Always check with a patient whether they are happy for you to disclose the diagnosis with their GP or family. Some patients keep their diagnosis a secret from everyone, and it is not your place to break confidentiality.

■ If you get a needlestick injury, don't panic. Only a tiny minority of needlestick injuries (even from HIV patients) transmit an infection (1 in 250), and even fewer do so after prophylaxis. Wash out the injury and get rid of the sharp; bleeding the wound is controversial and not currently recommended by the Centre for Communicable Disease. Call occupational health to arrange for prophylaxis or testing. If it is out of hours, get hold of the on-call microbiologist or go to accident and emergency. They will give you post-exposure prophylaxis and arrange the necessary bloods to be taken from you and the donor. It may be difficult after a needlestick to focus on patient care so you may need to hand over the continuation of the patients' management until you have settled your nerves.

HIV testing

Patients need counselling and preparation for HIV tests. Discuss doing HIV tests with seniors; they can advise you on hospital policy. The genitourinary specialist nurse may be able to help you with this. The important thing is to be professional and not make a big deal out of it. HIV is common, and a large proportion of people are not diagnosed. The antiretroviral treatments now available mean that HIV is now more like a chronic illness like diabetes or ischaemic heart disease (IHD) rather than the death sentence many patients think it might be. In fact, an appropriately treated HIV-positive patient may now have a normal life expectancy.

■ Explain HIV/AIDS. Being HIV positive is not the same thing as having AIDS. At present, 50% of asymptomatic HIV-positive patients get AIDS after 10 years.

■ Explain the benefits of the test. If the patient is HIV positive, there are drugs available to help treat it. They do not cure the patient but can help keep the levels of the virus down. You can monitor their T-cell function and treat infection better, and they can practise safe sex in order to protect their partner; 24 hour support is available for people with HIV.

■ Explain the problems of the test particularly the window period (the time between an initial infection/exposure and the test becoming positive). Some life insurance companies may discriminate against the HIV-positive person (this is being phased out). A way around this is to get tested anonymously at a genitourinary medicine clinic.

■ Tell the patient at what time the result will be back. If there is any delay, let the patient know and reassure him or her that it is not due to the sample being infected.

■ Always discuss the results in person, not over the phone.

Jehovah's Witnesses/ Christian Scientists

■ As with any person, you cannot force a Jehovah's Witness or Christian Scientist to accept treatment (e.g. a blood transfusion). Make sure they sign a statement acknowledging refusal of treatment. Most hospitals have policy documents and suitable consent or exemption forms. Discuss with the patient what blood products, if any, they are willing to accept. Discuss the case with your seniors. Plan operations very carefully in these patients, and ask how they feel about autologous blood transfusions. IV iron can also be a good way to boost the haemoglobin (Hb).

■ Some of the larger hospitals will have access to a Jehovah's Witness liaison who can talk to the patient and provide them with information and advocacy. Not all Jehovah's witnesses will refuse all blood products. Depending on interpretation, some may accept products that circulate in the blood but are not technically part of it, that is, clotting factors.

■ In an emergency, you can legally instigate treatment to save someone's life unless it is clear that the patient has given an informed refusal of that treatment that remains in force. Again, get senior advice and, if necessary, advice from your defence organization. The General Medical Council has issued guidance on this subject – 'Personal Beliefs and Medical Practice'.

Pregnant women

■ Get senior advice about X-rays in pregnancy. Make sure you notify the radiologist and radiographer that the patient is pregnant – write it clearly on the form and preferably speak to the team yourself.

■ Always ask women of childbearing age the date of their last menstrual period and whether or not they are likely to be pregnant. Most will agree to a urinary pregnancy test if asked.

■ Pregnant women have hyperdynamic, volume-expanded circulations. Their jugular venous pressures (JVPs) are usually slightly raised. This is okay, but it also means that they can lose a lot of blood before they exhibit signs of hypovolaemia.

■ Most drugs are potentially toxic. Check the BNF for guidance. Make sure you know the trimester and always get senior or pharmacist advice before prescribing. The obstetrics team can be helpful in these situations.

■ Foetuses consume folate, iron, Ca and other vitamins that would normally go to the mother. Ensure that pregnant women have adequate nutrition and supplement if necessary. Monitor Hb.

● Always monitor BP in pregnancy. Women over 40 and under 20, nulliparous females, women with diabetes mellitus and twin pregnancies are all at increased risk of pre-eclampsia. Always do a urine dip to look for protein and get early advice from both medical and obstetrics teams.

■ Be wary of pregnant women with abdominal pain. Organs such as the appendix get displaced, and inflammation can present in bizarre ways. For example, appendicitis may present as chest pain if it irritates the diaphragm. Always seek specialist advice and consider consulting with an obstetrician.

Sickle cell anaemia

Be alert to sickle cell anaemia in any black, Arabic, Indian or Mediterranean patient within the United Kingdom with acute pain in the spine, joints, chest or abdomen. Within the United Kingdom, all patients of African descent need a sickling test before surgery, and females can be tested with their partners when they become pregnant.

Heterozygous patients are only likely to suffer severe symptoms when hypoxic, as may occur during anaesthesia or at high altitudes. However, in homozygous patients, sickling crises are precipitated by hypoxia, dehydration, infection and cold weather. Sickling crises can develop with alarming rapidity and can be fatal without prompt treatment. The patient will often know when they are going into crisis:

1 Symptoms of a sickle crisis include severe bone pain, acute abdominal pain, shortness of breath (SOB) and neurological symptoms such as fits and cranial nerve palsies.

2 Basic management includes prompt analgesia. Some patients have a key record that states exactly what analgesia they will require in a crisis to help you. This will be available in their medical records or they may bring it with them.

● Perform a brief, initial assessment using airway, breathing and circulation (ABC).

● O_2 therapy, rehydration (ensure fluid intake of at least 3 l/day) and antibiotics if pyrexial or evidence of infection are essential.

● Make sure the patient is warm as cold can worsen sickling.

● Seek urgent, expert help from intensive therapy unit (ITU) and haematology especially if they do not improve quickly – these patients can deteriorate within hours!

● Lung involvement is particularly worrying as it may signify acute chest syndrome. Continuous positive airways pressure can help, or in severe cases, they may need intubation. Treat for atypical bacteria such as *Mycoplasma* or *Haemophilus*.

3 Investigations: the patient will need urgent IV access and baseline bloods, crossmatch, FBC, reticulocyte count and film, lactate dehydrogenase, blood cultures, midstream urine and chest X-ray (CXR). Include arterial blood gases if there is any CXR shadowing, respiratory symptoms or infection. Measure Hb daily.

4 If the patient needs surgery, make sure a suitable experienced anaesthetist is involved; this may require seeking specialist advice. If you know a patient will need surgery on an elective basis make sure the sickle testing is done in advance. If it is positive then involve the anaesthetist early so they have adequate time to plan their anaesthetic. If it is discovered on the morning of the surgery then they may be reluctant to proceed.

5 Patients will require lifelong penicillin prophylaxis, folate supplementation and pneumococcal vaccinations.

The patient on steroids

Patients on long-term steroids are vulnerable to infection and other multitude of side effects that steroids cause. They may require additional steroid cover whilst ill. Anti-inflammatory steroid equivalent doses are shown in Table 11.2.

Side effects of steroids

Mineralocorticoid effects:

■ Na and water retention and hypertension
■ Hypokalaemia

Glucocorticoid effects:

■ Hyperglycaemia/diabetes
■ Changes in fat distribution – centripetal adiposity

Table 11.2 Anti-inflammatory steroid equivalent doses.

Steroid	Dose (mg)
Dexamethasone and betamethasone	0.75
Methylprednisolone and triamcinolone	4
Prednisolone	5
Hydrocortisone	20

■ Changes in protein mobilization: osteoporosis, skin atrophy, striae, muscle wasting and delayed wound healing

■ Psychiatric problems. These occur in most patients. They vary from subtle changes to frank paranoid psychosis. Warn the patient (and relatives and friends!) that they may become easily irritable or 'difficult' and that they should inform the doctor if this causes problems. Initial euphoria, sleep disturbance and increased appetite are common.

■ Infection

– *Candida* infection: oral (visible plaques coating tongue and mouth), oesophageal (dysphagia) or vaginal (itching or discharge)

– Disseminated viral infection: measles, varicella zoster and herpes zoster

– Bacterial infection. The inflammatory response is suppressed hence late presentation and rapid systemic spread of infection. Be alert to the 'silent' abdomen, septicaemia and tuberculosis.

Other effects

■ Peptic ulceration: severe dyspepsia is common and peptic ulceration can occur. GI bleeding can result from severe peptic or oesophageal ulcers.

■ Acne is common.

■ Withdrawal reactions (see the following).

■ Ophthalmological – cataracts, glaucoma and papilloedema.

■ Musculoskeletal – myopathy, fractures and osteonecrosis.

Managing ill patients on steroids

Illness (acute stress, especially surgery or infection) increases steroid requirements. Decide if your patient needs additional steroids or not, or ask the endocrinologists for advice. Prescribe hydrocortisone 25–100 mg QDS (or equivalent) in addition to existing steroid dose if required. Always be aware of 'silent' infections in a patient on high-dose steroids (see side effects). Never stop steroids suddenly in those taking them long-term as you risk precipitating an Addisonian crisis. Patients should carry a steroid card with them at all times to alert health care professionals to the reason for taking them and the dosage. During times of illness or physiological stress, a patient on long-term steroids will not be able to produce the appropriate response of generating more steroids, and therefore, you may need to administer an extra exogenous dose.

Treating common side effects

1 *Candida* infection. Prescribe nystatin lozenges/oral solution for oral/oesophageal infection. If severe, give 50 mg daily for 7 days. Clotrimazole (Canesten) cream/vaginal pessaries is usually given for vaginal infection. A stat dose of 150 mg fluconazole can also be given to help clear the infection. Fluconazole 50 mg PO daily is useful as prophylaxis for high-dose steroids.

2 If the patient is known to suffer from cold sores or shingles, tell the patient to start high-dose acyclovir at the earliest sign of recurrence.

3 Reflux symptoms. Prescribe ranitidine 150 mg BD. Avoid PPIs unless specific indication due to risk of *C. difficile*.

Withdrawing steroid therapy

The longer the patient has been on steroids, the more gradual the reduction of steroids needs to be. Therapy for longer than 2 weeks can lead to adrenal suppression.

You can reduce steroids from high doses by 5 mg of prednisolone (or equivalent)/week until you reach the equivalent of 10 mg prednisolone/

day. Thereafter, reduce by 2.5 mg/week until you reach 5 mg/day. After this, the rate of reduction depends on the preceding length of therapy. If this was greater than 3 months, reduce slowly, for example, by 1–2 mg/week.

Withdrawal reactions include Addisonian crisis (hypotension, dehydration, hyperkalaemia, hyponatraemia), arthralgia, conjunctivitis, mood change, rhinitis, skin rashes (itchy nodules or acne) and weight loss. Morning irritability can be prevented by taking the daily dose BD; note, however, that taking steroids on a BD basis is less physiological and more likely to cause Cushingoid symptoms.

Haematological and oncological emergencies

These patients are a special subset and should be treated warily. They tend to be on complicated chemotherapy regimens, which can cause multiple side effects. If in doubt, speak to a senior from the medical team urgently, and get specialist advice from the haematologist/oncologist early. These patients can become very sick very quickly, so you need to initiate treatment in a timely fashion.

We have summarized the treatment of some common haematology/oncological emergencies.

Spinal cord compression

Spinal cord compression requires a high index of suspicion on the clinician's part and requires fast treatment to preserve neurological function. Cord compression commonly occurs from extradural metastases, but can occur due to a crush fracture, or less commonly from direct extension of the tumour.

Patients can present with the following symptoms:

■ Back pain – particularly thoracic that is radicular in nature and worse on sneezing, coughing and laughing
■ Reduced mobility
■ Bowel/bladder dysfunction (this often presents late)
■ Sensory impairment

Perform a full neurological examination. Check for spinal tenderness, perianal sensation (to both light touch and pinprick) and anal tone. If the patient is catheterized, see if they can feel a gentle catheter tug. A thorough assessment requires completion of an American Spinal Injuries Association (ASIA) score chart otherwise known as an 'International Standards for Neurological Classification of SCI (ISNCSCI) Exam Worksheet'. This is extremely useful as it guides you through the whole examination. If your hospital does not hold the proforma on the ward, you can download them for free along with learning materials (www.asia-spinalinjury.org/elearning/ISNCSCI.php).

Management

Get an urgent magnetic resonance imaging (MRI) of the whole spine, not just the area where there is pain, as patients can have multiple metastases at multiple sites.

Give dexamethasone 8–16 mg PO as a stat dose and then continue on a regular regimen (4 mg QDS or similar).

Check their clotting.

If the MRI shows an acute cord compression, then refer as an emergency to clinical oncologists as they may be able to give radiotherapy to the affected area. You will also need to discuss the case with neurosurgery as although uncommon, there is sometimes an indication for decompression or stabilization. They will want to know the patient's prognosis, so try and have this ready before your referral if possible.

If in any doubt about spinal stability then put the patient on flat bed rest with log rolling until you have discussed with the specialist teams.

Superior vena cava obstruction and airway compromise

Superior vena cava obstruction (SVCO) is an emergency if the patient has concomitant tracheal compression and airway compromise. Lung cancer with mediastinal metastases or a central lung Ca (SCLC) is the usual culprit, but lymphomas and germ cell tumours can also cause SVCO as well as thrombotic disorders such as Behcet's syndrome.

Symptoms include the following:

- SOB and orthopnoea
- Facial, neck and arm swelling
- Facial plethora and cyanosis
- Engorged neck veins

Check the JVP as this will be raised and non-pulsatile, and listen for stridor.

Management

Get an urgent CXR and CT of the chest to assess the severity of disease. Give dexamethasone 4 mg QDS, and get urgent senior help. Inform the oncology team, who may be able to give radiotherapy or chemotherapy to shrink the tumour, and also contact the interventional radiologists who can try and perform superior vena cava stenting.

Raised intracranial pressure

Raised intracranial pressure can be due to either metastatic disease to the brain (commonly from the breast and lung) or due to a primary central nervous system tumour. If a primary, the tumour can be malignant or a benign lesion like a meningioma causing mass effect. Patients often get early morning headaches that get better through the day, which are worse on coughing/sneezing/bending over. They can present with seizures, weakness, cranial nerve palsies, and nausea and vomiting. Always perform a full neurological exam and assess the fundi to look for papilloedema but remember that absence of papilloedema, whilst reassuring, is no guarantee of normal intracranial pressure.

Request an urgent CT with contrast/MRI head to assess the disease, and give a stat dose of dexamethasone 8–16 mg. Treat any seizures as per usual emergency management of seizures with a benzodiazepine and consider a loading dose of phenytoin. If the scan shows solitary metastases, a posterior fossa lesion, herniation, haemorrhage or hydrocephalus, discuss the patient with the neurosurgeons. Inform the oncologists who can then plan for discussion in a multidisciplinary meeting to make decisions regarding biopsy/resection or whole-brain radiotherapy +/− chemotherapy.

Tumour lysis syndrome

This condition is more likely to occur in patients with a high tumour burden (i.e. widespread disease) or those with a rapidly proliferating cancer. It is more common in patients with leukaemia, lymphoma, myeloma and germ cell tumours. It occurs when chemotherapy is first given to the patient, causing all the cancer cells to die and release their intracellular contents. This causes a rise in serum urate, K and PO_4, which can precipitate renal failure.

As always prevention is better than cure. Give hydration IV and orally prior to starting chemotherapy and start allopurinol the day before. Rasburicase is an expensive alternative for patients with an intolerance to allopurinol.

If the patient develops renal failure, they may require haemodialysis whilst having the chemotherapy.

Hyperviscosity

This is common in haematological malignancies where there are blast cells in the peripheral circulation such as acute myeloid leukaemia/acute lymphoblastic leukaemia or in the presence of large monoclonal immunoglobulins such as Waldenströms macroglobulinaemia. It can also occur when there is an increase in the number of circulating red blood cells, as occurs in polycythaemia rubra vera.

Patients classically present with headache, visual disturbances and lethargy. In severe cases, they can become confused and drop their conscious level.

IF you suspect this, you need to get senior specialist help as an emergency.

Treatment includes leucophoresis if the cause of the hyperviscosity is due to blasts, venesection of 500 ml of blood and replacement with N saline or packed red blood cells if Hb < 7 if due to polycythaemia and plasma exchange if due to monoclonal immunoglobulins.

Treating the underlying cause will also help to prevent the hyperviscosity from recurring.

Febrile neutropenia (see Chapter 8 – The immunocompromised patient with fever – for detailed management)

Essentially management includes the following:

■ Brief initial assessment – ABC.

■ Take cultures – blood, urine, sputum, stool if diarrhoea, line cultures and respiratory swab for viral polymerase chain reaction.

■ Initiate broad-spectrum antibiotics: most hospitals have a local policy, but usually, patients are given tazocin and a stat dose of gentamicin. Ciprofloxacin is given instead of gentamicin in patients with myeloma or sarcoma due to the risk of nephrotoxicity. Contact microbiology if there are concerns.

■ Treat for sepsis with aggressive IV fluids.

■ If needed, contact ITU early, and get advice from the specialist team urgently.

Hypercalcaemia: (see Chapter 8 – Hypercalcaemia – for more detailed management)

Hypercalcaemia is commonly caused by myeloma, cancers secreting parathyroid hormone-related peptide (squamous cell lung Ca) or osteoclast-activating factors and bony deposits.

Patients present with non-specific symptoms – the classical 'moans, stones and abdominal groans'.

Take blood urgently to measure albumin and calcium levels, as well as renal function and routine bloods. Calculate the corrected calcium if your lab does not automatically do this.

The first, key step in management is to rehydrate the patient with IV fluids (normal saline), and give pamidronate IV (bisphosphonate). Monitor calcium levels, and watch for fluid overload in small elderly frail patients.

Chapter 12
APPROACH TO THE MEDICAL PATIENT

With contributions from Dr Magda Sbai
This section provides a practical approach to the history and examination of a medical patient and outlines how to optimize your time in getting to know them and developing a feel for their problems. This chapter also gives a brief outline of common procedures or investigations that you may be expected to explain to patients during your medical post and looks at situations when referral to a speciality is indicated and the necessary investigations you should consider for patients presenting with certain pathologies.

History and examination

With the introduction of shift work, it is inevitable that you will find yourself looking after patients you did not admit and may have never met. It is well worth the effort to re-clerk these patients, albeit briefly. If this is not possible due to time constraints then an alternative is constructing a patient summary or problem list. It takes less time than you may think.

Before seeing a patient, review their medical records, so that you have some idea what their presenting problem might be due to; for example, if they have known inflammatory bowel disease and present with diarrhoea, you should consider if this is a flare of their disease. Information gathering is a key part of medical detective work and developing a thorough approach when tackling problems will protect you from errors in the longer term.

An approach to history taking comprises two essential parts, which enable management to be tailored to the individual patient and their condition:

1 Getting to know the patient (the person and their medical background)

2 Getting to know the condition (the presenting problem)

Getting to know the patient as a person

- Patient identification – age/sex
- Occupation
- Social support – family, friends, finances
- Mobility
- Home help and other services accessed in the community
- Problems as perceived by the patient – expectations, worries and fears

The medical background

- Past medical history (MJ THREADS acronym is helpful – i.e. in addition to any volunteered medical conditions, you should specifically ask about myocardial infarction/heart disease, jaundice, thyroid disorders/

tuberculosis (TB), hypertension, rheumatoid arthritis/rheumatic fever, epilepsy, asthma/respiratory disease, diabetes or stroke)
- Past surgical history
- Allergies and drug history
- Family history
- Social history

Getting to know the disease

Presenting complaint

Identify as clearly as possible the reason for the patient presenting now to the hospital. What was the trigger? Think of the possible causes for the symptoms, so that you establish an early differential diagnosis. Do not take a history blindly without this kind of forethought, as it is likely to be inefficient and will not lead you to a diagnosis quickly.

The present history

This is what the patient tells you about their present illness. Listen carefully and ask clarifying questions. Attempt to live the patient's life from the onset of the symptoms so that you become aware of important details that will refine your differential diagnosis. This will also help you form a detailed social history.

Next, try to rank your differential diagnosis and identify those features of the most likely diseases that have emerged thus far. Ask about these features now – the specific directed enquiry – and write down your differential diagnosis and problem list before the examination.

The systematic (or functional) enquiry

This is usually the least useful part of the history. Whilst it provides a convenient list of symptoms, it encourages thoughtless history taking that overworked junior doctors do not need! It should therefore be left until last and although it can sometimes be shortened it is inadvisable to omit in its entirety. On an odd occasion it may identify important information that the patient may not have

thought was relevant. If you have taken a thorough history of presenting complaint you will find that you have asked many of the questions for the relevant systems already and the systems enquiry should then consist of a short run through of the remaining systems. For the detailed list of symptoms, see Figure 12.1.

The examination

The same general examination for all patients should be followed by a directed systemic examination, based on the diagnostic possibilities elicited in your history. For example, you would make a careful check for signs of infective endocarditis in a patient with a history of valvular heart disease and a recent decrease in exercise tolerance with fevers. Note the important negative findings, for example, no splinter haemorrhages, no vasculitic skin lesions, no splenomegaly. Fully document your findings in the medical notes.

We have provided an outline of the general and systematic examination of the medical patient in Figure 12.2. Whilst it is structured in the order for 'routine' examination, few patients are 'routine', and you should examine some systems in more detail according to your differential diagnosis. Equally, examination may not be possible to a detailed level if your patient is confused or drowsy.

Once you have examined a few patients, you will develop your own style doing this.

Summing up

At the end of your history and examination, it is a good idea to summarize your findings for presenting on ward rounds, to seniors or to other specialist teams:

1 Patient ID and salient medical background. Mention what is pertinent to the present problem such as any cardiac risk factors if the patient presented with chest pain.

2 Presenting complaint.

3 Current problems – medical, pharmacological and social.

History — Getting to know the patient as a person

Patient ID – age, sex, etc. ....

Work .... Mobility ....

Lives with .... Home help ....

Social support – Problems as perceived by the patient,

family, friends .... worries, fears ....

Finances ....

The medical background

Past medical history

1 CVS – IHD, CHF, rheumatic fever, hypertension, other ....

2 RS – asthma, smoker, COPD, TB, exposure to irritants ....

3 Diabetes, thyroid disease, CVA/TIA, Epilepsy, other medical illnesses ....

Past surgical history

What operations ....

Any anaesthetic complications ....

Drug history and allergies

Current medication ....

Relevant past medication ....

Allergies ....

Family history ....

Hobbies and pets ....

Getting to know the disease

Presenting complaint/s ....

....

(STOP–THINK–CONSTRUCT A RANKED DIFFERENTIAL DIAGNOSIS)

The present history and the specific directed enquiry

(What the patient tells you about their illness and directed questions to define the differential.)

Systematic (or functional) enquiry

1 General – loss of appetite, loss of weight, fever, night sweats, any lumps, itch and rashes
2 CVS/RS – chest pain, dyspnoea, orthopnoea, PND, cough, wheeze, haemoptysis, sputum, ankle oedema, intermittent claudication
3 GIT – dyspepsia, nausea, vomiting, abdominal pain, diarrhoea, change in bowel habit, blood or mucus PR
4 GU – dysuria, frequency, urgency, nocturia, haematuria, polyuria, incontinence, terminal dribbling, hesitancy
5 Gynaecology – vaginal discharge, menses, first day of last period (LMP), menarche, menopause, pregnancy, previous births, miscarriages
6 CNS – fits, blackouts, headaches, visual disturbances, sensory disturbances, weakness/paralysis, falls, loss of hearing. Higher mental function
7 MSK/skin – joint pain/swelling, stiffness

Refined differential diagnosis

....

....

Figure 12.1 Approach to history taking.

Examination

In order of examination

1. Appearance. Does the patient look ill? General nutrition
2. Temperature

Working up the arm:

3. Hands, nails
4. Pulse
5. Respiratory rate
6. While doing the above, consider evidence of endocrine disease (pituitary, thyroid, Addison's), Paget's; body hair, skin pigmentation, skin lesions.
7. BP
8. Eyes – pallor, jaundice, corneal arcus, xanthelasma
9. Mouth and tongue – cyanosis, smooth or furred tongue, any lesions, mouth ulcers, xerostomia, cheilitis, angular stomatitis?
10. Examine the neck – nodes, goitre

CVS examination with patient at 45°:

11. JVP and carotid pulses
12. Praecordium – inspect, palpate, auscultate
13. Sacral oedema? Ankle oedema?

RS examination with patient at 90°:

14. Chest – inspect, palpate (trachea, expansion), percuss, auscultate
15. Breasts and axillary nodes

GIT examination with patient lying flat:

16. Abdomen – inspect, palpate (tenderness, visceromegaly), percuss (organomegaly and ascites) auscultate (bowel sounds)

Legs:

17. Swelling, pulses

CNS examination:

The detail of this examination depends on the differential diagnosis. The essentials include the following:

18. Cranial nerves – pupil responses; visual acuity; fundi; corneal reflexes; 'Open your mouth; stick out your tongue; show me your teeth; shut your eyes tightly; raise your eyebrows; shrug your shoulders'.
19. Peripheral nerves and motor function – wasting; sensation (vibration, light touch); tone; power; gait
20. Speech and higher mental functions
21. Do PR and FOB test. Consider PV.
22. Dipstick urine and consider microscopy.
23. Summarize findings and list your plan for solving the patient's problems:
    - Patient ID and salient medical background
    - Presenting complaint/s ....
    ....
    - Current problem/s ....
    ....
    - Investigations ....
    ....
    - Plan for discharge ....
    ....

Figure 12.2 Approach to examination.

4 Results of relevant investigations.

5 Plan for discharge – any anticipated obstacles and the estimated date of discharge from hospital.

Another way of doing this is by summarizing the main problems, starting with medical issues and then any social issues that are likely to prevent discharge.

History and examination

Figures 12.1 and 12.2 provide an outline of the above approach to history and examination. Retype and photocopy if you want.

Clinical stalemate

Your patient sits in bed day after day, and no progress is made. What do you do?

1 Decide if the patient is improving or deteriorating.

2 If the patient is ill or deteriorating, then identify the main problems and make a management plan. Ask seniors early on if unsure.

3 Having addressed any obvious problems, review the case:

• Main complaint
• History of main complaint
• PMH
• Drugs, allergies, habits, foreign travel, etc.

4 Repeat a complete examination. Examine test results critically – Are they reliable or spurious? If spurious, do they need repeating? Are they up to date? Is a more in-depth investigation needed?

5 Formulate a list of problems, differential diagnoses and investigations to be requested.

6 Now write a summary in the notes of your findings at this stage. If appropriate, use tables for important serial data.

7 Discuss the patient with your seniors, escalate appropriately, and identify if any other specialists need to be involved, for example, intensive care or other medical specialties.

Preparing patients for medical procedures

During your placement, you will prepare patients for many different procedures. It is important to realize that whilst most procedures are routine for you, they are usually frightening for patients and can cause a lot of anxiety. Probably the scariest thing is not knowing what will happen next, so appropriate information and communication can make a big difference. A list of patients' common concerns about procedures includes:

1 What does the procedure entail?

2 Why are they having this done?

3 How long will the procedure take?

4 Do they need a general anaesthetic?

5 Will the procedure be painful?

6 What should they do if they have pain or other symptoms after the procedure?

7 When can they eat/drink/drive/have sex?

8 Will they have any scars/permanent after-effects?

9 Who is doing the procedure?

The General Medical Council guidance on consent now states that it should only be undertaken by someone who fully understands the procedure and its alternatives/complications and ideally be taken by one who is capable of doing the procedure themselves but as a minimum has training in taking consent. This is usually the consultant in charge of the patients or a nominated deputy. If you are unsure whether you should be taking consent for a particular procedure always clarify with your seniors before proceeding. In medicine the boundaries of where your job begins and where it ends are often blurred. However, consent taking is definitely one area where you should not be acting outside out of your sphere of competence, regardless of how unwell the patient is or urgent the task appears.

Cardiac catheterization

Preparation

1 Consent (if angioplasty or stenting is planned in addition to diagnostic catheterization, this should be explained). There are variants of the procedure, for example, left and right heart catheters, coronary angiography, electrophysiological studies, depending on the indication. Ask the cardiologists what they intend to do.

2 Make sure the patient has stopped oral anticoagulants at least 3 days prior to the procedure. In cases where stopping anticoagulants carries a clinical risk, for instance, when a patient has a metal valve replacement and is taking warfarin, the patient should be switched to low molecular weight heparin. If required, they may need to be admitted for heparinization. Low molecular weight heparin is shorter acting and can be omitted prior to the procedure. Always anticipate this issue in advance, and discuss the case with your local anticoagulation team or haematologists to formulate a bridging plan for around the time of the procedure.

3 Request full blood count (FBC), clotting studies, group and save (G&S), urea and electrolytes (U&E) and creatinine to check renal function.

4 Secure peripheral venous access.

5 Check all peripheral pulses (this acts as a baseline, since rarely, cardiac catheterization can cause peripheral arterial thromboembolism).

6 If the patient has renal impairment or diabetes, seek senior advice regarding delaying procedure and the possibility of a sliding scale.

Tell the patient

1 Why they require cardiac catheterization.

2 The procedure will be done under local anaesthetic and sometimes mild sedation, via the blood vessels in the groin, arm or wrist.

3 The procedure takes place in a special unit (the 'cath lab'), under X-ray guidance.

4 The process may be diagnostic (coronary arteriogram) or therapeutic (angioplasty or stent). Explain each of these procedures in further detail as needed, using diagrams if necessary.

5 Afterwards, the patient will need to lie flat for about 4–6 hours.

6 Afterwards, there may be some bruising, and sometimes an ache in the groin, but this should subside.

Complications

1 Bleeding/bruising at groin puncture site

2 Pseudoaneurysm in the groin

3 Stroke/death/myocardial infarction (MI)/contrast nephropathy/anaphylaxis to contrast (risk is <1/1000 but varies with procedure and baseline characteristics of the patient – ask the cardiologists what risk should be quoted or defer the question to when consent is being obtained)

Following the procedure

1 Patients must lie flat for several hours.

2 Check groin wound is clean, and there is no evidence of pseudoaneurysm/infection before discharge.

3 Driving – this is something that must be heeded carefully. Different rules apply for different procedures and for group two vehicle licence holders, for example, lorry drivers or bus drivers. Generally post-angioplasty patients must not drive for 1 week. Patients who have had MIs treated by angioplasty should not drive for 1 week; otherwise, the rule is cessation of driving for 1 month. Refer to the DVLA guidance for more information

(https://www.gov.uk/government/publications/at-a-glance).

Elective DC cardioversion

Preparation

1 Electrocardiogram (ECG) (check if there is still an indication for cardioversion).

2 International normalized ratio (prothrombin ratio) (INR) (check that INR is between 2 and 3 and has been for the last month).

3 U&E (check that serum potassium >3.5 mmol/l and that other electrolytes are in the normal range, in particular magnesium).

4 Patient has been nil by mouth (NBM) for 4 hours prior to attempted cardioversion.

5 If patient is taking digoxin, exclude symptoms of digoxin toxicity, that is, nausea, diarrhoea, visual disturbance and confusion, and consider sending a digoxin level.

6 Gain peripheral venous access.

7 If the patient has renal impairment, seek senior advice.

8 Inform the anaesthetist and the staff who are required for the procedure. In some centres, the procedure is carried out in theatre recovery or in the induction room, in which case the theatre manager needs to be informed and the patient added to the emergency list. In other places, it is done on the cardiac day ward, in which case the ward staff should be informed.

9 Obtain informed consent.

10 Ensure that the skin overlying the right sternal border and the cardiac apex is shaved.

Tell the patient

1 Why they require DC cardioversion.

2 It is done under a brief general anaesthetic.

3 What the procedure involves – a pulse of electricity is delivered to the heart via electrodes/pads on the skin to stimulate the heart back into a normal rhythm.

4 There is no guarantee that it will cause reversion to sinus rhythm, but that successful cardioversion should bring symptomatic benefit. The probability of success is variable. In young people with no structural heart disease and fairly recent onset, the chances of success are high; in older people with structural abnormalities and chronic disease, the chances are slim. If the procedure is successful, there is still a chance that they will revert back to the abnormal rhythm.

5 Procedure is usually a day case. The patient can go home once the anaesthetic has worn off, but should be taken home by somebody else,

and should not drive or operate machinery for the rest of the day.

Complications

1 Small risk of major complications such as thromboembolism, life-threatening arrhythmia and aspiration

2 Skin burns where pads were applied

Following the procedure

1 Repeat ECG, and put in medical notes.

2 Inform patient whether the procedure was successful or unsuccessful. If successful, warn patient that effects may not be sustained indefinitely and that arrhythmia may reoccur.

3 Continue medications and arrange outpatient clinic appointment.

4 Wait for 2–3 hours before discharging. Ensure that patients do not go home on their own and that there is somebody at home to supervise them for the rest of the day.

5 They should be kept nil by mouth until fully alert and awake. If unsure, ask for help from a senior or the anaesthetist supervising the procedure.

Upper gastrointestinal endoscopy

Preparation

1 Obtain consent.

2 NBM for 4 hours beforehand. If you suspect gastric outlet obstruction, allow only water for 8 hours and then NBM for 4 hours. Make sure NBM decision communicated to nursing staff and patient as procedure will be cancelled if patient has been given something to eat.

3 FBC and INR (in case of biopsy).

4 Insert cannula in the arm that will make endoscopic manoeuvring easiest (usually the right arm).

5 Barium can block the suction channel of the endoscope, so delay for 24 hours following upper GI barium studies.

Tell the patient

1 What endoscopy is and why they are having it.

2 That the procedure usually takes about 5–10 minutes.

3 During the procedure, they may be given IV sedation to make them drowsy. However, they will not be given a general anaesthetic and their throat will be sprayed with local anaesthetic so that they won't feel the endoscope.

4 An endoscope (tube with a camera inside) that is the thickness of a little finger is passed into the food pipe and into the stomach. It may be uncomfortable but should not be painful.

5 The doctor might take a tiny sample of the inside of the gullet or stomach to examine under a microscope. This is painless.

6 The patient should be able to eat and drink after the local anaesthetic and sedation has worn off, which should take about half an hour. However, they may be restricted to sips for a while if treatment such as clipping has been given. They might have a sore throat, which should get better within a few days.

7 They should not drive for the rest of the day.

Complications

1 Transient sore throat and possible numbness

2 Rarely oesophageal perforation (about 1 in 1000)

3 Mild bleeding (and rarely haemorrhage) following a biopsy

Colonoscopy

Preparation

1 Obtain consent.

2 Low residue diet for 36 hours and fluids only for 12 hours before the procedure. If sedation is being used, patient will need to be NBM for the last 4 hours.

3 Give bowel prep 24 hours before the procedure. Check local hospital guidelines for prescribing protocols. Do not give to patients with inflamed colonic mucosa (ulcerative colitis, Crohn's, etc.).

4 If maintaining oral fluid intake may be problematic, consider whether patient needs maintenance IV fluids or admission the night before the procedure for IV hydration.

Tell the patient

1 What a colonoscopy entails (a way of looking directly at the bowel) and why they are having it.

2 Warn that bowel prep causes explosive diarrhoea. They need to drink plenty of clear fluids to maintain hydration (2–3 l/day: three to four jugs of squash).

3 IV sedation is given that will make them drowsy, but it is not a general anaesthetic.

4 A flexible tube with a camera is passed into their back passage.

5 The whole procedure takes about 20–30 minutes, and the patient can go home accompanied as soon as the sedation has worn off – usually in about 2 hours. They should not drive until the following day.

Complications

1 Mild abdominal discomfort during and after the procedure is common due to a small amount of gas that is pumped in to aid vision through the colonoscope during the procedure.

2 Incomplete examination, requiring a second examination or barium enema, occurs in up to 10% of cases.

3 Perforation occurs about 1 in 500, more commonly in acute colitis or extensive diverticulosis. If this unlikely event happens, the person usually will need to have their bowel repaired surgically under a general anaesthetic.

4 Serious haemorrhage post-biopsy or polypectomy is rare.

Flexible sigmoidoscopy

Preparation

1 Phosphate enema usually 6 hours before procedure may need repeat enema if results are unsatisfactory.

2 Explanation as for colonoscopy except sedation is not usually needed, and so patient does not have to be NBM.

Liver biopsy

Preparation

1 Consent.

2 Bloods: FBC, clotting, liver biochemistry and G&S.

3 Abdominal USS/CT beforehand to check anatomy.

4 Mild premedications, such as pethidine (50 mg) and prochlorperazine (12.5 mg), are usually given (but check local protocols).

5 IV access with at least a green cannula.

Tell the patient

1 What a liver biopsy is and indications.

2 The procedure is performed on the ward or in an operating theatre. The biopsy itself is very quick (a few seconds) but the whole procedure might take up to 30 minutes. They will have to stay in hospital overnight for regular observations.

3 The procedure does not usually involve heavy sedation or a general anaesthetic.

4 The site of the biopsy is on the patient's right side, between the 8th and 10th ribs. The patient will need to help by holding their breath during the biopsy.

Complications

1 Shoulder tip or local abdominal pain from a few hours – up to 2 days is common but usually relieved by paracetamol 1 g 6 hourly.

2 Bleeding possibly requiring transfusion (about 1 in 50).

3 Infection, abscess, pneumothorax (rarely requiring drainage) and biliary peritonitis are uncommon (<1:1000).

Following the procedure

1 The patient should lie on their right side for at least 2 hours and remain in bed (absolute bed rest) overnight.

2 Observations: BP and pulse every 15 minutes for 1 hour, then every 30 minutes for 2 hours, then hourly for 6 hours. Ask to be informed if the BP falls (>15 mmHg) or if the pulse rises (>15 bpm).

3 Ensure that an IV line is secure and that analgesia is written up.

4 Review patient at 4 and 8 hours following the biopsy for pain and vital signs.

Pacemaker insertion

Preparation

1 Informed consent

2 FBC and INR

3 *Methicillin-resistant Staphylococcus aureus* screening swab

Tell the patient

1 What a pacemaker is and why he or she needs one.

2 A very small wire is threaded via a large vein (internal jugular/subclavian) into one of the chambers of the heart under X-ray screening. The wire is gently inserted into the wall of the heart. The other end of the wire is connected to a machine called a pacemaker that generates heart beats, which is placed into a small pocket, fashioned in the fatty tissues of the chest. Its battery will not run out! The pacemaker causes a small lump under the skin on the upper thorax, but nowadays, the generators are so small that these are hardly noticeable. The patient will have a small scar on their chest wall.

3 The procedure is performed under local anaesthetic, sometimes with mild sedation.

4 The procedure is mostly painless. It takes 30–60 minutes.

5 In future, the patient will need to carry a card that says they are fitted with a permanent pacemaker, in case they ever need emergency treatment. A Medic alert bracelet is recommended. Most pacemakers nowadays are MRI safe.

6 They will also need to attend pacemaker checks to ensure the device is working properly.

7 Caution in pregnancy, as X-ray screening is used during the procedure.

Complications

1 As for central line placement – pneumothorax, bleeding, risk of infection.

2 Dislodgement of the wire leading to pacing failure. Electrical faults are uncommon.

Following the procedure

1 The patient will need a chest X-ray (CXR) post-procedure to check lead placement and to exclude pneumothorax.

2 A pacemaker check ECG to make sure the pacemaker is capturing correctly.

Renal biopsy

Preparation

1 Consent.

2 Bloods: FBC, INR and G&S.

Abdominal USS is essential to check that two kidneys are present and the anatomy of the patient.

3 Mild premedication as per local policy.

4 IV access with at least a green cannula.

Tell the patient

1 What a renal biopsy is and why they need one.

2 The procedure is usually done in theatre or on the renal unit and takes a few minutes. Sedation but not always a general anaesthetic is given.

3 The biopsy is taken through the left or right flank. The patient will need to hold their breath briefly during the biopsy.

4 The patient should drink a lot of fluids after the biopsy, to flush the kidneys and avoid renal colic.

Complications

1 Local pain (prescribe analgesia) and mild haematuria are common.

2 Haemorrhage requiring transfusion is less common (about 1 in 30–60). Surgical intervention for massive haemorrhage is rare (can result in nephrectomy if unable to control bleeding).

3 Renal colic from clots may occur.

Following the procedure

1 Patient should lie on the side of the biopsy for at least 2 hours and remain in bed (absolute bed rest) overnight.

2 Observation: as per liver biopsy.

3 Check for gross haematuria.

4 Ensure IV access and that adequate analgesia is prescribed.

5 Review patient at 4 and 8 hours following biopsy for pain, vital signs and gross haematuria or bleeding.

Specialist referrals and investigating the medical case

Most consultants have their own preferred investigations. Be guided by ward protocols, but ask a senior if you do not understand the rationale for a particular investigation. Protocols often become outdated, and frequently, the team forgets to inform the new junior doctors.

If a patient is unwell enough to be admitted, you should have the following results as a minimum:

1 Weight

2 Temperature, blood pressure, pulse, respiratory rate and oxygen saturations

3 Urine dipstick

4 FBC/urea/electrolytes/creatinine/C-reactive protein (CRP)+/−liver function tests (LFTs)/clotting

When indicated (for most medical patients):

5 CXR

6 ECG

A list of further investigations to anticipate is provided, listed under system headings for commonly encountered pathologies.

Cardiology

Essential investigations before referral to a cardiologist include ECG and CXR.

Suspected acute MI

1 Serial ECGs to look for dynamic changes (at least every hour if equivocal and then for three consecutive days).

2 Serial serum cardiac enzymes including troponin assay which, when taken after 12 hours, offers a more specific and sensitive marker of MI. Some trusts are now adopting 6 hour troponins or even immediate 'triple panel' assays (troponin, creatine kinase cardiac isoenzyme and myoglobin) so check local protocol.

3 If within 6 hours of onset of chest pain, you can check lipid profile (levels are unreliable after this).

Ischaemic heart disease

1 ECG (preferably both during an episode of chest pain and when pain-free).

2 Serum cholesterol and triglycerides, ideally fasted sample.

3 Formal blood sugar, again ideally a fasted sample. The finger prick capillary blood glucose is not accurate enough. Also an HbA1c/ glycosylated haemoglobin.

Heart failure (recent onset)

1 Echocardiography (ECHO): this is urgent if there are murmurs or you suspect infective endocarditis (consider transoesophageal ECHO if suspicion is high) or pericardial disease.

2 A plasma B natriuretic peptide is also helpful to confirm or exclude the diagnosis. This is an expensive test, so check with your local hospital if it is performed, and if a junior is allowed to request it. In some trusts only a cardiologist can request the test.

Hypertension

1 Cholesterol and triglycerides.

2 Midstream urine (MSU) for microscopy, culture and sensitivity (MC&S) if blood or protein on urinary dipstick. Microscopy of the urine to look for casts or red cells.

3 If the urine dip is positive for protein, send a urine protein–creatinine ratio or 24 hour urinary protein.

4 Ensure there is a recent ECG, CXR and serum biochemistry.

5 USS of the kidneys if symptoms are suggestive of clinical renal disease (history of nephritis, renal problems in childhood, family history of renal disease) or sudden onset of poorly controlled BP (renal artery stenosis).

6 Fundoscopic examination for hypertensive changes.

Infective endocarditis

1 Blood cultures, at least three sets – ideally from different sites.

2 FBC, CRP, U&E and LFT.

3 Urine dipstick and microscopy (microscopic haematuria).

4 Blood film, serum haptoglobins and urinary haemosiderin to look for evidence of haemolysis.

5 Consider transoesophageal ECHO if transthoracic ECHO normal and suspicion high.

6 Document peripheral stigmata of infective endocarditis.

Endocrinology

Except for diabetes mellitus, endocrine disorders are relatively rare. Special tests are required according to the differential diagnosis before referral.

Diabetes mellitus

1 Flow chart of the patient's blood glucose readings and glycosylated Hb (HbA1c) if available.

2 Renal function:

• Flow chart of creatinine and urea levels

- 24 hour urine collection for creatinine clearance and protein

3 Careful fundoscopy and ophthalmology referral for retinal screening.

4 Peripheral nerve examination – sensory neuropathy and for signs of diabetic foot disease.

5 Cholesterol and triglycerides.

6 ECG – have old ECGs to compare.

7 Arrange follow-up in diabetic clinic, arrange diabetic dietary advice by dietician, and involve diabetic specialist nurse.

Cushing's disease/syndrome

Consult a specialized lab for advice. Different labs prefer different tests.

Standard tests done in most labs include those listed in the following:

1 Midnight (or at least after 10 p.m.) and 9 a.m. cortisol levels. The night level is usually lower than the morning level, but this diurnal cycle is lost in Cushing's. The midnight level is often called a 'sleeping level' – this can be done soon after waking the patient, not whilst they are actually asleep!

2 Shortened low-dose dexamethasone suppression test: 1 mg dexamethasone PO at 11 p.m. and measure the cortisol level in the morning at around 9 a.m. In Cushing's, the cortisol levels are not suppressed, whereas in pseudo-Cushing's (e.g. depression, severe obesity and alcoholism), the cortisol level is suppressed.

3 High-dose dexamethasone suppression test: 0.5 mg dexamethasone 6-hourly for 48 hours. Next, measure the morning cortisol level at 24 and 48 hours. This suppresses cortisol levels in pituitary-dependent Cushing's disease, whilst it does not suppress cortisol levels in adrenal adenomas and ectopic adrenocorticotropic hormone (Cushing's syndrome).

4 Measure urinary-free cortisol (24 hour urine collections).

Phaeochromocytoma

Consult a specialized lab for advice. Different labs prefer different tests. Standard tests done in most labs include those listed in the following:

1 Three 24 hour urine collections for catecholamines (adrenaline, noradrenaline metabolites (HMMA/VMA) or total metadrenalines). This requires a special urine collection bottle. Tell the patient to avoid vanilla, bananas and aspirin.

2 CT or MRI scan of the chest and abdomen (phaeochromocytomas can arise anywhere along the sympathetic chain), and/or special isotope (MIBG) scan, if the urine test is positive to localize lesion.

Thyroid disease

1 Hypothyroidism: raised thyroid-stimulating hormone (TSH) and low T_4. Request thyroid auto antibodies to exclude Hashimoto's.

2 Secondary hypothyroidism (rare): low T_4 and T_3 but TSH is not raised; look for pituitary failure.

3 Hyperthyroidism: suppressed TSH and raised T_4 or T_3. In 10% of patients with hyperthyroidism, only the T_3 is raised.

4 If Graves' disease is suspected, send thyroid antibodies and refer to ophthalmology.

Gastroenterology

Always do a **per rectum** (PR) before referring to a gastroenterologist. Gastroenterologists often request some unusual tests so investigate according to the differential diagnosis.

Upper GI symptoms

1 Barium meal or gastroscopy

2 FBC and haematinics for iron deficiency anaemia

GI bleeds

1 Crossmatch at least 4 units.

2 Hb, platelets and clotting studies.

3 Check LFTs and U&E.

4 Endoscopy.

5 Consider surgical consultation.

6 If severe bleeding, may need to activate major haemorrhage protocol.

Chronic diarrhoea

1 Foreign travel history (giardiasis).

2 Hot stool for MC&S including ova, cysts and parasites (×3), **Clostridium difficile** toxin and culture.

3 FBC (including mean cell volume [MCV]).

4 LFTs (albumin).

5 Ca^{2+} and phosphate.

6 Thyroid function tests (TFTs).

7 Amylase will be low/normal in chronic pancreatitis, and faecal lipase/elastase may be more useful.

8 24 hour 5-hydroxyindoleacetic acid or chromogranin A (carcinoid syndrome).

9 Coeliac antibodies.

10 Colonoscopy.

Chronic lower GIT symptoms

1 Faecal occult bloods – used as a screening tool for colorectal malignancies.

2 FBC and MCV.

3 Flexible sigmoidoscopy.

4 Consider barium enema or colonoscopy and small bowel meal.

5 Consider other sources (e.g. GU tract) for symptoms.

Ascites of unknown origin

1 History of alcohol consumption.

2 Bloods for LFTs, viral hepatitis serology. Consider checking anti-mitochondrial antibodies (for primary biliary cirrhosis) and anti-smooth muscle cell antibodies (for chronic autoimmune hepatitis). Consider alpha-fetoprotein and Ca-125 if malignancy is suspected.

3 Tap the ascites (paracentesis). Re-examine following aspiration, especially for female pelvic organs. A vaginal examination is essential if the cause of ascites is unclear particularly in older females as ovarian cancer is an often overlooked culprit.

4 USS abdomen and pelvis (consider aspiration under US guidance if there is a small or loculated collection). USS is most useful after aspiration. Specific points on US: Is the portal vein patent or is there a thrombosis? Look at size and texture of liver and spleen. Look for portal hypertension and a cirrhotic liver. Are there porta hepatis nodes raising suspicion of malignancy?

5 Consider a CT scan.

6 Consider endoscopy for varices.

7 Consider peritoneoscopy or laparotomy after discussion with seniors and surgical colleagues.

Liver disease

1 INR, platelets, bleeding time (full clotting studies)

2 Liver function tests and general biochemistry

3 Urine for bilirubin and urobilinogen

4 Liver screen to include hepatitis screen – B and C (A if acute) – iron/total iron binding capacity, caeruloplasmin, alpha-fetoprotein and auto antibodies

5 USS abdomen

6 Stool chart

Haematology

Essential investigations before referral include FBC, differential, film, haematinics and erythrocyte sedimentation rate (ESR).

Suspected DIC

1 Fibrin degradation products (FDPs)

2 INR and activated partial thromboplastin time

3 LFTs

4 Urine dipstick and microscopy

5 Blood cultures

(DIC [disseminated intravascular coagulation] is not an end diagnosis – you must find the cause.)

Anaemia

1 Reticulocyte count and sickle cell status.

2 Serum bilirubin, lactate dehydrogenase (LDH) and serum haptoglobins (markers of haemolysis).

3 Haematinics (iron studies/vitamin B$_{12}$/serum and red cell folate).

4 CRP and ESR.

5 Consider Hb electrophoresis.

6 Consider bone marrow biopsy.

7 Upper GI endoscopy and colonoscopy if unexplained iron deficiency anaemia.

Suspected paraprotein/myeloma

1 FBC/ESR.

2 Serum and urine electrophoresis, urine collection for light chains (15% of patients have urinary light chains only).

3 Serum calcium levels/creatinine.

4 Skeletal survey.

5 Consider bone marrow biopsy.

Neurology

A thorough history and detailed examination are by far the most important things before you consider any referral.

Meningism

1 Initiate emergency treatment early. Start antibiotics immediately unless you can get a cerebrospinal fluid (CSF) sample without any significant delay. Culture of CSF may be negative if antibiotics have been given before taking the sample. However, the risk of delaying treatment is not justifiable unless the lumbar puncture (LP) can be done quickly. You are generally safe in performing an LP if there are no signs of raised intracranial pressure (rising BP and falling HR, papilloedema or depressed loss of consciousness) or contraindications like bleeding disorders. If possible, perform a CT prior to performing LP, to rule out hydrocephalus or compression of intracranial structures like the basal cisterns. CT *must* be performed before LP in patients with focal neurology or altered conscious level or who are immune-compromised; otherwise, you expose the patient to the risk of herniation due to CSF drainage in the presence of a space-occupying lesion:

● Opening pressure with a manometer.

● Note appearance of CSF fluid.

● MC&S, cell count and xanthochromia.

● Consider Indian ink stains for *Cryptococcus*, Ziehl–Neelsen stain for acid-fast bacillus (AFBs) and viral polymerase chain reaction.

● Glucose (ensure you take a matched serum glucose sample at time of LP for comparison).

● Protein.

2 Consider serology for *Cryptococcus*, syphilis and viral causes of meningitis.

Unexplained coma

Before referral, you should:

1 Ensure that the patient's airway, breathing and circulation are not compromised, and involve anaesthetist immediately if airway not being safely maintained.

2 Obtain a history from relatives, friends and GP, especially regarding epilepsy, possible drug overdose/recreational drugs or recent travel abroad.

3 Do a secondary neurological examination for clues. The neurological exam would initially have been restricted to the Glasgow Coma Scale and hard localizing signs.

4 Have the following results clearly documented (if available):

● Blood glucose that was done immediately on admission

● FBC, U&E, Ca, phosphate and blood glucose

● Liver biochemistry

● Urine dipstick and MC&S

● Arterial blood gases and toxicology screen

5 Arrange an urgent CT scan head followed by LP.

6 Send a CSF sample for storage 'CSF save'.

Unexplained weakness

Before referral, you should:

1 Send off the following initial tests:

● FBC, U&E, creatinine kinase and LFT

● ESR, Ca^{2+} and protein electrophoresis

● Vitamin B$_{12}$, folate, blood glucose and TFTs

2 Consider electromyography or nerve conduction studies and paraneoplastic screen in elderly.

Renal medicine

Renal physicians rely heavily on biochemistry to manage their patients, so have a flow chart of the patient's U&E and creatinine results. Get their help early if a patient's renal function is deteriorating.

Renal failure/nephrotics/nephritics

1 BP.

2 Fresh urine for microscopy and send sample for MC&S.

3 Daily weights.

4 Fluid input/output chart.

5 Serology.

• Virology: cytomegalovirus, Epstein–Barr virus, hepatitis B and C and HIV if candidate for haemodialysis/transplant (counsel the patient)
• Bacteriology: VDRL (syphilis) and atypical serology
• Immunology: CRP, immunoglobulins and serum electrophoresis, complement and auto-antibodies, antinuclear antigen (ANA), anti-neutrophil cytoplasmic antigen, anti-glomerular basement membrane and cryoglobulins

6 Biochemistry: in addition to renal and hepatic indices, request: Ca, total protein, albumin and phosphate.

7 Urine protein:creatinine ratio and 24 hour urine collection for protein and creatinine clearance.

8 Renal USS – do early to exclude obstruction, especially if the renal function is deteriorating.

9 Consider renal biopsy.

Recurrent UTIs

1 BP and MSU.

2 Creatinine clearance.

3 Abdominal X-ray and/or non-contrast CT of the kidneys, ureter and bladder to look for calculi.

4 USS kidneys (document the size).

5 Consider a micturating cystogram (reflux) – this is mainly used in children and is only usually requested in a specialist setting.

6 PR and proctoscopy.

7 *Per vaginum* and speculum examination.

8 Consider urology referral.

Respiratory medicine

Essential investigations before referral to a respiratory physician are CXRs, ECGs, results of lung function tests and arterial blood gases.

Pneumonia

1 CXR.

2 Sputum for MC&S, cytology and AFB.

3 Physiotherapy if bronchopneumonia or exacerbation of chronic obstructive pulmonary disease – arrange as soon as possible. Physiotherapy is not indicated for lobar pneumonia.

4 Arterial blood gases (ABGs) are mandatory for any severe respiratory illness. Always document how much O_2 the patient was receiving when the ABG is taken.

5 Serology for atypical pneumonia, for example, mycoplasma.

6 Urinary antigens for legionella and pneumococcus.

7 Consider HIV test in young patients.

If you suspect TB

1 Sputum for AFB (hypertonic 5% saline nebulizer will encourage productive coughing if sputum is difficult to obtain).

2 3+ early morning specimens of urine or sputum for AFB.

3 Mantoux test or interferon gamma testing (Quantiferon test).

4 Consider bronchoscopy and broncho-alveolar lavage or Endoscopic bronchial Ultrasound (EBUS) for lymph node biopsy.

(If TB is suspected, remember that patient will need to have respiratory isolation precautions.)

Obstructive lung disease

Lung function tests: pre- and post-bronchodilators

Respiratory failure

ABGs and acid–base balance (raised bicarbonate or base excess is a useful indicator of chronic CO_2 retention)

Pleural effusion

1 Send aspirate for:

- Protein, LDH, amylase and pH
- MC&S, Gram stain, AFBs and TB culture
- Cytology and cell count
- Glucose
- Immunology if indicated (rheumatoid factor, ANA, complement)

2 Consider pleural biopsy if pleural fluid results are inconclusive.

Rheumatology

'Look, feel and move' all salient joints; FBC, ESR and CRP; X-rays of relevant joints

Monoarthritis

1 FBC and CRP

2 Urate

3 Blood cultures

4 INR if on warfarin

5 X-ray of affected joint

6 Joint aspiration for gram stain, MC&S and crystals (do not aspirate if joint is replaced)

(Remember septic arthritis requires prompt antibiotics and urgent orthopaedic input.)

Polyarthritis

1 Urate.

2 Fresh urine for microscopy.

3 X-ray affected joints.

4 CRP.

5 Antistreptolysin O titre, serum sample for storage.

6 Rheumatoid factor.

7 Autoantibodies screen – ANAs and anti-cyclic citrullinated peptide antibody.

8 Consider joint aspiration ± synovial biopsy.

Chapter 13
PRACTICAL PROCEDURES

As a junior doctor, you will be expected to perform procedures on your patients safely. As you become more senior, the complexity of the procedures will increase and the supervision will decrease. Just remember that practice makes perfect and the more procedures you do the more confident you will become.

This section is aimed to guide you through most procedures you will encounter as a foundation doctor. Becoming competent, safe and skilful in undertaking interventions to help patients is one of the great joys of medicine.

General hints

■ Obtain consent from the patient – often, verbal consent will suffice, but if in doubt, be sure to at least document that you have discussed the procedure and risks and that the patient agreed.

■ Never perform a procedure on your own unless you have been supervised at least once.

■ Never undertake a procedure where you cannot deal with all potential complications unless there is someone available who can. If you think there is a realistic potential for needing support it is better to prewarn them before embarking on the procedure.

■ Being methodical and having space and a spare pair of hands make procedures much easier. Before starting, get everything you need ready on a trolley. Mentally run through the procedure and check you have the necessary equipment at each stage. Take a sharps bin to where you are working or have a kidney dish ready. Make sure you have enough local anaesthetic, needles and gloves. If possible take extra equipment in case you fail first time round.

■ Consider taking the patient to a side room for the procedure, rather than performing it at the bedside which can be embarrassing for the patient and others on the ward. Always draw the curtains round.

■ A warm, confident approach is useful even if you are nervous. Try to avoid negative comments before a procedure: 'you look like you have difficult veins, this may be a struggle'; this will simply heighten the patient's anxiety and will diminish their confidence in you. It is, however, acceptable (and – in the case of a 'difficult' patient – advisable) to warn them that there is no guarantee that you will be successful the first time. Never promise you will get it first time – even the best miss sometimes!

■ Never be afraid to ask for help.

■ Wear gloves for all procedures. Remember that the most unlikely people have hepatitis B.

■ Nurses can help in positioning and reassuring the patient. They can also be those useful extra pair of hands when you are doing fiddly procedures.

■ Use local anaesthetic for all but the smallest procedures – it is a good habit to have.

■ Remember that you always have more time than you think, even during emergencies. If necessary, hand your bleep to a nursing or medical colleague.

■ Use every single opportunity to be assessed. Bring a supervisor and have them complete the assessment documentation immediately if at all possible.

The Hands-on Guide to the Foundation Programme, Fifth Edition. Anna Donald, Michael Stein, Ciaran Scott Hill and Selina J Chavda.
© 2015 John Wiley & Sons, Ltd. Published 2015 by John Wiley & Sons, Ltd.

> **Arterial blood gases**
> Bleeding tendency or anticoagulation is a relative contraindication for taking arterial blood gases (ABGs). Always apply pressure for at least 5 minutes after taking ABGs from patients on warfarin or heparin or those with low platelets.

Arteries in order of preference

1 Radial – check collateral blood supply from the ulnar artery by asking the patient to make a tight fist and applying pressure over the radial artery. Ask the patient to relax the hand. If it remains white after 10 seconds, try the other arm (this is Allen's test).

2 Femoral – however, it is easy to hit the vein. You need to apply strong pressure to the puncture site for at least 5 minutes after taking blood.

3 Brachial – use this as a last resort. Use a 20–22G needle. The problem with this artery is that it is an end artery and collaterals may be insufficient if it occludes.

Have ready

1 Lidocaine 1% *without* adrenaline

2 One 3 ml syringe

3 One 23G (blue) and 25G (orange) needle (alternatively a 1 ml insulin needle with pre-attached syringe can work excellently and is even less painful than a 25G)

4 Heparinized ABG syringe

5 Alcohol swabs

6 Sterile swabs/cotton wool balls

7 Plastic bag or carton with a few ice cubes at the bottom

In lots of hospitals, two to four come made up in an ABG packet.

The procedure
(See Figs. 13.1 and 13.2.)

1 Ask your colleagues where the blood gas machine is before taking an ABG sample (it is often in intensive therapy unit, accident and emergency (A&E) or the respiratory ward).

2 Most ABG syringes come with heparin already in them. Expel the heparin completely – classical teaching states that excess heparin will cause an erroneous acidosis; however, in reality this is minimal and most effects are dilutional with a rise in $PaCO_2$ and a fall in PaO_2. You only need a few molecules of heparin to prevent the blood from clotting.

3 Clean the skin and infiltrate superficially with a small bleb of local anaesthetic if there is no emergency.

4 Hold the syringe at a 60–90° angle to the skin and slowly advance the needle. Keep very still and the syringe will usually fill due to arterial pressure with 1–2 ml of bright red blood. If this is not forthcoming, you can gently aspirate 1–2 ml; however, this often indicates a venous puncture that will be confirmed by the results.

5 Withdraw and apply pressure for at least 3 minutes (5 minutes if the patient is anticoagulated).

6 Expel all air from the syringe. Cap the syringe, gently roll between your hands and either take to the ABG machine immediately (within a maximum of 15 minutes) or place on ice and read as soon as possible (1 hour).

7 Note the oxygen concentration that the patient is on. This is important for interpretation. Take the blood gas from the patient at least 10 minutes after a change in oxygen concentration. It is not acceptable to take a hypoxic patient off oxygen for a 'baseline' blood gas.

If you fail

■ Withdraw the needle to a point near the skin, redirect the needle, and try again. The artery is usually only a few millimetres under the skin; it is not unusual to transect the artery. Try aiming the needle at a shallower angle. This allows a steadier approach. Try not to remove the needle completely, as the two most painful parts are piercing the skin and then the artery. The artery is often more medial than you may think so re-angle the needle in this direction and you will be likely to be successful.

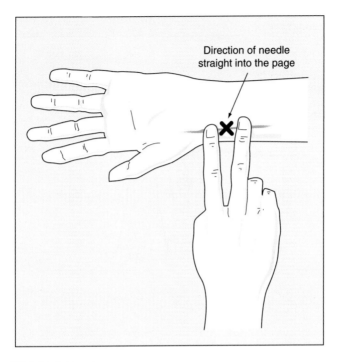

Direction of needle straight into the page

Figure 13.1 Radial arterial puncture.

■ Try to avoid bones and tendons. If you hit a bone, withdraw whilst gently aspirating.

Hints

■ It is important to expel all the air from the sample to prevent erroneous readings of false oxygenation. Once this is done, ice only serves to slow cellular use of O_2 which is negligible over 60 minutes.

■ Do not expect immediate ABG changes after adjusting someone's O_2 supply. It takes up to 20 minutes for the ABGs to equilibrate to a change in inspired O_2 concentration, although 10 minutes is usually enough. If a reading looks suspiciously high or low, repeat it.

■ You can tell the difference between arterial and venous blood by its percentage saturation: 50% or less suggests venous blood, whilst 80% or above is certainly arterial – unless they have an arteriovenous shunt!

Interpreting ABGs

Normal ABG values are shown in Table 13.1.

Points to consider when interpreting ABGs

PO_2 and $PaCO_2$

First ask yourself: does the patient have abnormally low O_2 for them? What is their baseline PaO_2 value? Many patients with chronic respiratory disease live quite happily with a PaO_2 of 7.5 kPa. Check the results of previous ABGs when the patient was well to see how much they have decompensated.

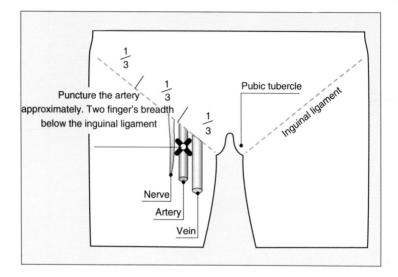

Figure 13.2 Femoral arterial puncture: inguinal canal anatomy may be remembered using the mnemonic 'NAVY' – nerve, artery, vein and Y-fronts (!).

Table 13.1 Normal ABG values.

pH	7.35–7.45
PCO_2	4.3–6.0 kPa
Base excess	±2 mmol/l
PO_2	10.5–14.0 kPa
Serum HCO_3^-	22–26 mmol/l
O_2 saturation	95–100%

Next check if the patient is retaining CO_2. This will determine the amount of O_2 therapy you can give and will guide you to the degree that a respiratory component is determining their blood gas. The body never overcompensates; so if the $PaCO_2$ is high, the patient is not ventilating adequately. The pH will tell you if the acidosis is of respiratory origin or if it is compensatory (if there is a metabolic alkalosis and the patient is hypoventilating to try and compensate for this).

Remember that the O_2 saturation curve for haemoglobin (Hb) is a steep sigmoid curve that starts to plateau around a PaO_2 of 9.1 kPa (70 mmHg). This means a patient may have a PaO_2 of 8.5 kPa and still have better than 90% O_2 saturation. However, in the steep part of the curve (PaO_2 of 6–8 kPa), small changes in PaO_2 dramatically affect O_2 saturation and are clinically significant.

pH
Check to see if the pH is normal or if there is an acidosis (pH <7.35) or an alkalosis (pH >7.45). If either exists, decide if it is metabolic or respiratory and whether or not it is compensated (see Table 13.2).

A compensated acid–base disorder suggests chronic disease, over days to weeks, whilst an uncompensated acidosis or alkalosis suggests a more acute problem. In general, the body compensates for changes in pH by altering the respiratory rate (e.g. in metabolic acidosis, CO_2 is 'blown off') and regulating renal excretion of HCO_3. Respiratory compensation occurs much quicker (minutes) than renal compensation (hours to days).

Table 13.2 Interpreting acid–base disorders.

	pH	PCO$_2$	HCO$_3^-$	K$^+$
Acidosis				
Metabolic – early	↓	Normal	↓	Usually ↑
Metabolic – compensated	Normal	↓	↓	Normal or ↓
Respiratory – early	↓	↑	Normal or ↑	↑
Respiratory – compensated	Normal	↑	↑↑	
Alkalosis				
Metabolic – early	↑	Normal	↑	↓
Metabolic – compensated	↑	Normal	↑↑	↑
Respiratory – early	↑	↓	Normal or ↓	↓
Respiratory – compensated	Normal	↓	↓↓	Normal or ↑

Reproduced from Zilva J.F., Pannall P.R., Mayne P. (1989) *Clinical Chemistry in Diagnosis and Treatment.* Lloyd-Luke (Medical Books) Ltd, London.

Serum electrolytes (Na$^+$, Cl$^-$ and HCO$_3$)

If the patient is acidotic, you will need to calculate the anion gap ([Na + K] − [Cl + HCO$_3$]) in order to refine the differential diagnosis. A raised anion gap is due to the addition of unmeasured acid to the system, for example, methanol, urea, diabetes (ketones), paraldehyde, isoniazid, lactic acid (in anaerobic metabolism), ethanol and salicylic acid. A good mnemonic for this is 'MUD PILES'.

A normal anion gap acidosis is usually due to loss of base, for example, from use of acetazolamide or other carbonic anhydrase inhibitors, diarrhoea and renal tubular acidosis.

Hints

■ A patient with a mixed picture or who is well compensated may have a normal pH. Check all the parameters of the ABG analysis, not just the pH and PO$_2$.

● If the results of the ABG analysis are very poor, you may have sampled venous blood.
● ABGs will also give you results of several electrolytes such as K, Na, Ca, Cl as well as Hb. These are relatively accurate if the machine has been calibrated, so if they are grossly abnormal you should act to correct them. Always remember to send a formal set of bloods to the lab at the same time.

■ Patients with decompensated organ failure (e.g. cirrhosis, congestive cardiac failure, respiratory or renal insufficiency) may have developed acid–base and electrolyte disturbances over weeks. Do not be tempted to correct them in a day.

Respiratory disease and ABGs interpretation

Type 1 respiratory failure:

■ PaO$_2$ less than 8.0 kPa (60 mmHg)
■ PaCO$_2$ less than 6.0 kPa (45 mmHg)

If stable, their ABGs will reveal a compensated respiratory alkalosis.

Type 2 respiratory failure:

■ PaO$_2$ less than 8.0 kPa (60 mmHg)
■ PaCO$_2$ greater than 6.0 kPa (45 mmHg)

If stable, their ABGs will reveal a compensated respiratory acidosis. They will often have a very high bicarbonate.

Patients with type 1 failure progress to type 2 as they tire.

Bladder catheterization

Female nurses usually (but not always) catheterize women; you will certainly end up catheterizing men (whether you are a man or a woman).

Men

Have ready

1 Catheterization pack – kidney bowl, gauze swabs, sterile towels, etc.

2 Sterile gloves – two sets.

3 Cleaning solution, either normal saline or sterile water.

4 Sterile tube of lidocaine jelly.

5 10 ml syringe and 10 ml sterile water (this often comes with the catheter).

6 Several Foley catheters. For the first attempt, 14F is the usual size. If you cannot pass a 14F due to a large prostate, try a bigger size to circumnavigate benign prostatic hypertrophy.

7 Urine bag and stand.

The procedure

1 Get a clean trolley that has been swabbed with an alcohol wipe and place the catheter pack on it.

2 Wash your hands thoroughly.

3 Fully expose the patient's penis. Make sure there are no bedclothes in the way that might dirty the working area. Urinary tract infections are easy to induce with catheterization.

4 Tell the patient what you are about to do and why you are doing it.

5 Open the catheter pack, and put sterile gloves, tube of lidocaine jelly, syringe, water and catheter onto the trolley in a sterile fashion. Pour the cleaning solution into a receptacle.

6 Put on gloves.

7 Drape the sterile towels to leave only the patient's penis exposed.

8 Gently retract the foreskin and clean the urethral opening with cleaning solution.

9 Gently squeeze the contents of the tube of lidocaine jelly into the urethra. Give this 5 minutes to work and use the time to change your gloves to ensure you are as sterile as possible.

10 Open the catheter wrapping at the tip end only and insert the catheter into the urethra, withdrawing the plastic covering in stages as you go. This is the trickiest part of the procedure. Make sure the end is in the kidney bowl to collect urine. You should get some urine back when you reach the bladder from all but the most dehydrated patients.

11 If you feel resistance, gently pull the shaft of the penis upwards. *Never* use force.

12 Once fully inserted, inflate the catheter balloon with 5–10 ml of sterile water by placing the syringe directly over the proximal opening (no needle) and pushing hard. Stop immediately if the patient experiences pain, as the balloon may be in the urethra. Once inflated, gently pull the catheter until you feel resistance of the balloon, indicating it is stable in the bladder.

13 Always remember to gently replace the foreskin over the penis tip and document this in the notes. If you cannot, gently try again. If the foreskin genuinely gets stuck and starts to swell, get senior help immediately. Paraphimosis is a surgical emergency.

14 Connect the end of the catheter to the bag and mount on a catheter stand.

15 Document in the notes and record the residual volume.

16 Send a sample of urine for microscopy, culture and sensitivity (MC&S).

17 If the patient is septic, consider giving a stat dose of gentamicin IV/IM. Consult your local microbiology policy or discuss with your microbiologist if this is appropriate.

If you fail

■ The catheter may be blocked with jelly. Aspirate the catheter with the syringe or gently massage the bladder above the pubic bone to encourage urine flow.

■ The patient may have a large prostate or penile stricture. For strictures, a smaller size catheter should be used – proceed with care and be ready to abandon the procedure! For large prostates, *larger* catheters are useful, particularly stiff, silastic ones.

■ If after several attempts with different size catheters you cannot access the bladder, call for help. Even the most senior urologists have trouble sometimes and can show you tricks for really difficult urethras.

Suprapubic catheterization is a useful last resort. It is useful to perform a bladder scan to get an idea of the bladder volume before such a procedure.

Women

Have ready
Same equipment as for the men

The procedure

1 Position the patient as for a vaginal examination. Ask her to lie flat on her back, knees bent, feet together and to allow her knees to fall down in full abduction.

2 Part the labia minora and clean the area with cleaning solution.

3 Locate the urethral opening just posterior to the clitoris and introduce a well-lubricated catheter tip. Female catheterization is usually much less problematic because they have no prostate and a short urethra.

Be aware of underlying causes for problems in catheterization such as tumours. If concerned, do a PV and call for help.

Blood cultures

If you are going to the trouble of doing blood cultures, it is better to do two sets from different sites, particularly if accurate diagnosis is important. Three sets for infective endocarditis are the gold standard.

Have ready

1 One or two sets of culture bottles

2 Two 20 ml syringes and needles or a vacutainer system

3 Lots of alcohol swabs

The procedure

1 Select a vein.

2 Clean the skin with alcohol, from the centre out. Allow to dry for at least 30 seconds.

3 Without relocating the vein, cannulate and withdraw at least 10 ml of blood for each set of cultures.

4 Inject at least 5 ml into each bottle.

5 Place in incubator as soon as possible.

Hints

■ It is not necessary to change needles between taking blood and inserting it into the culture bottles. There is increased risk of needlestick injury and little increase in contamination.

■ It is also unnecessary to clean flip-cap culture bottle tops. Try to avoid getting air in the anaerobic bottle.

■ The above technique is fine for easy veins. If not, keep your gloves sterile, as this will allow you to palpate for veins.

Venepuncture

Have ready

1 Tourniquet

2 Needles (green or blue)

3 Syringe(s) of adequate size for the bloods you need to take

4 Alcohol swab(s)

5 Cotton wool ball or small plaster

6 Blood tubes

7 A sharps container

Vacutainers are much quicker to use than needles and syringes but have no 'flashback' to let you know when you have entered the vein.

The procedure

1 Put on gloves.

2 Tell the patient what you are doing and why.

3 Choose the preferred arm – not a drip arm; tighten the tourniquet above the elbow and find a vein.

4 Alcohol swab the insertion area.

5 Put the needle on the syringe. Holding the patient's skin taut around the vein (tether it

distally), gently advance the needle into the vein. After breaching the skin with the bevel up, make sure the needle is very shallow. With practice you feel the vein give way when you are through. You should get a small 'flashback' in the base of the syringe.

6 Draw back the plunger until you have enough blood.

7 Undo the tourniquet *before* withdrawing the needle.

8 Apply pressure to the puncture site with cotton wool.

9 Taking care not to needlestick yourself, insert the needle into the blood tubes and allow the vacuum to withdraw the blood. Some labs recommend that you remove the needle from the syringe, uncap the tube and gently squirt the blood directly into the tube. This prevents needlestick injuries. Never squirt blood into the tube through small needles as this risks haemolysis and false readings. The main benefit of vacutainer systems is avoiding this high-risk transfer of blood.

10 Tidy up, especially sharps.

11 Send blood to the lab.

Choosing a vein

Ask the patient for their preferred arm. Obvious forearm or cubital fossa veins are good. In dialysis patients, never use their arteriovenous (AV) fistula arm. Likewise, never use an arm with lymphoedema or one that has had its lymph nodes removed or irradiated.

If you can't find a vein

1 Hang the arm over the edge of the bed, 'milking' it or tapping the back of the hand. Hitting the skin releases histamine and brings up the veins.

2 Use a sphygmomanometer; it is better than a tourniquet. Pump it up to diastolic pressure; you are aiming for the artery to fill the limb in systole but prevent venous drainage. Also, ask the patient to pump their hand. An experienced assistant who squeezes the arm may be equally effective.

3 Immerse the arm or hand in a bowl of warm water for 2 minutes; pump the sphygmomanometer up with the arm in the water; dry the arm and quickly look for veins.

4 If all else fails, a femoral stab can be much less painful than repeated failed venepuncture attempts. It is a useful skill to have and in peri-arrest or arrest situations is often the only way you will get blood.

Hints

■ Don't overfill heparinized tubes – they will clot.

■ Paediatric tubes, which only require a few drops of blood, can be used for patients with very difficult veins (though your lab-based colleagues may disagree and question you when they note the date of birth!).

■ Find out from the labs how much blood is really necessary for standard tests at your hospital. Often you need very little, particularly for biochemistry. Clotting is usually the exception and requires a full bottle.

Cannulation (Venflon/line insertion)

(See Fig. 13.3)

Cannulation often worries junior doctors as it is something that they are routinely required to do and is initially a difficult skill to acquire. Anyone who tells you that they never had trouble cannulating is lying! That said, it is a skill that anyone can acquire but practice really is the only way to be good at this. Here we outline the basic procedure but the best way to learn is to get someone with good technique to show you.

Have ready

1 Tourniquet

2 Appropriate size cannula (see Table 13.3)

3 Cannula dressing (wing shaped)

4 5–10 ml syringe

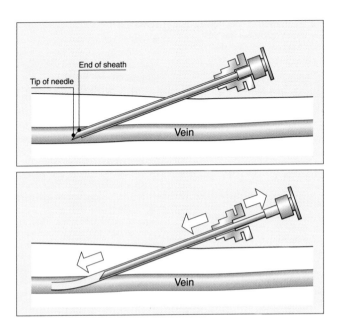

Figure 13.3 Cannulating a vein.

Table 13.3 Cannula sizes.

Colour	Size	Use
Yellow	24G	Paediatric or oncology patients and intravenous (IV) drug users
Blue	22G	Small, fragile veins
Pink	20G	Regular IV drugs and fluid administration
Green	18G	Blood transfusions and fluids
White	17G	As above – rarely available
Grey	16G	Rapid fluid administration, GI bleeds
Brown/orange	14G	Major bleeds, usually placed prophylactically in theatre

5 Saline flush

6 Alcohol swab(s)

7 Cotton wool ball/small plaster

8 Bandage and tape

The basic procedure

1 Put on gloves. Take lots of gauze to mop up any blood or spillages.

2 Tell the patient what you are doing and why.

3 Choose your preferred arm. Tighten the tourniquet above the elbow and find a vein. Vein choice is key.

4 Swab the insertion area and allow to dry (or it will sting).

5 Advance the needle into the vein. You should get a small 'flashback' of blood in the base of the cannula. The flashback is an indication that the *tip* of the cannula has entered the vein (but not necessarily the plastic of the cannula); with the cannula flat, advance the needle a millimetre or two more. The gap between needle tip and plastic sheath is longer in larger cannula.

6 Advance the plastic cannula into the vein – ideally with one hand – in effect covering the tip of the needle; *only then* when the plastic is in the vein withdraw the metal stylet. Quickly attach a vacutainer system or syringe to take blood or a bung.

7 Undo the tourniquet and secure the cannula with a dressing. It is a good idea to secure the cannula with a covering bandage to prevent it catching on bedclothes.

8 Tidy up, especially sharps. Beware that although many cannulae have a safety sheath that deploys once the needle is fully withdrawn, these are typically absent on the smallest needles.

Choosing a vein

1 Ask the patient for his or her preferred arm. Remember that the dorsum of the hand is more convenient for you but less so for the patient. Obvious forearm veins are good (in dialysis patients, never use their AV fistula arm).

2 Avoid sites where two vein joins are tethered. Whilst these can be easier to cannulate, the drip is more likely to tissue as a result of poor flexibility.

3 Avoid foot veins except as a last resort. They thrombose more readily and are prone to infection.

4 Avoid crossing joints.

5 Shave hairy arms for ease of cannulation and to reduce pain when removing the drip.

Hints

■ Emla anaesthetic cream is extremely useful for squeamish patients. Keep a tube handy. Apply over selected veins and cover with an occlusive dressing. Simply wipe off in 30 minutes to 1 hour and site the drip as usual. Injection of local anaesthetic is less useful as it often obscures the vein.

■ It is helpful to take blood at the same time as putting in the cannula. This must not be done with 'precious' veins. Once the cannula is secured, elevate the arm above the level of the left atrium. Remove the cap and place a syringe into the back of the cannula. Lower the arm (sometimes you need to reinflate the cuff gently) and *very gently* aspirate the required amount of blood (rapid aspiration causes the vein to collapse down into the cannula). You may need to withdraw the cannula slightly or lift the wings of the Venflon away from the skin a little way to initiate the flow of blood into the syringe (it is not unusual for blood to fail to flow because the tip of the cannula sits against a valve).

■ Pink, rather than green, cannulae are adequate for most routine purposes, such as saline infusions, IV drugs and CT scans with contrast.

Saving a dying drip or cannula

When asked to resite a cannula because it has tissued:

1 Ask whether or not it is still really necessary and check the cannula yourself; it is not unusual for an inexperienced nurse to mistake a fully functioning cannula for one that has 'tissued' because of a loose connection, three-way tap in an off position or infusion pump problem. Many cannulae are also 'positional' and work perfectly well provided the limb is kept in a certain, usually neutral, position.

2 Many lines can be flushed gently with 5 ml of heparinized saline (HepSal) that clears any minor blockage. Small syringes (2 ml) are most effective at clearing minor blocks.

3 Always remove the cannula if the site is inflamed. Phlebitis is not to be ignored!

Times when a cannula **MUST** be in place, even at night

■ In the acutely ill or unstable patient, it is often essential to secure peripheral access before removing central lines in post-operative patients. The day you don't do this is the day you'll regret.
■ Hypovolaemia or poor oral intake.
■ Danger of blood or fluid loss.
■ IV drug infusions.

Problems with temporary and tunnelled central lines

You will often be called to sort out line problems. The most common are

■ *Sepsis.* If a patient with a central line develops a fever, take peripheral and central blood cultures. If the patient is clearly septic, discuss removing the line with your senior. Tunnelled lines can sometimes be treated with antibiotic line locks if the patient is otherwise well, but this cannot be done for short-term lines when the track is much shorter. After removal of any central line, always cut the tip off with a sterile pair of scissors and send it for culture.
■ *Blocked lumen.* This is prevented by daily flushing with HepSal. If the line is blocked, flush using a 1–2 ml syringe with HepSal, applying moderate pressure. Remember to put in a heparin–saline lock after flushing. If still no luck, a dilute solution of urokinase can be instilled by repeated aspiration and injection. Leave it for 30 minutes, and then try flushing again.

Hints

■ Taking blood from central lines should only be performed as a last resort. Phlebotomists should be counselled about refusing to bleed patients with central lines. There is a high risk of infection. You need to discard the first 15 ml of blood and use a good aseptic technique. Do not take samples for aminoglycoside levels from a central line as these drugs are absorbed by the line.

Using central lines

Hickman and Groshong lines are tunnelled lines intended for long-term use such as for chemotherapy or total parenteral nutrition. Groshong lines have a special three-way valve system at the tip of each lumen that prevents blockage after flushing and facilitates taking of blood samples. It is extremely useful to know how to handle these lines. Infection is the major problem and most patients are trained in looking after their own line. Therefore, before handling a line, ask a nurse or medical colleague to give you a tutorial. The basic technique outlined in the succeeding text is a guide only. For setting up an IV, giving drugs or taking blood via a tunnelled line, you will need to

1 Open up:

● Dressing pack
● Sterile gloves
● One 5-ml syringe and heparin–saline or saline
● One sterile bung (end plug for cannula)
● Four alcohol swabs
● Cleaning solution, for example, Betadine solution, and container

2 Get an assistant.

3 Scrub up.

4 Keep one hand absolutely sterile.

5 Handle the line with dry sterile gauze.

6 Remove the bung from the end of the line using a swab and discard.

7 Always open and shut the gate or clamp between procedures.

8 Attach drip or take bloods as appropriate.

Chest drains

Whilst you may be forgiven for being unfamiliar with inserting chest drains, you will be expected to manage and remove them. The following paragraphs give general guidelines for maintaining and removing drains (see Fig. 13.4).

Indications

Pneumothorax (A = air = apical drain), haemothorax, effusions or empyema (B = blood = basal drain)

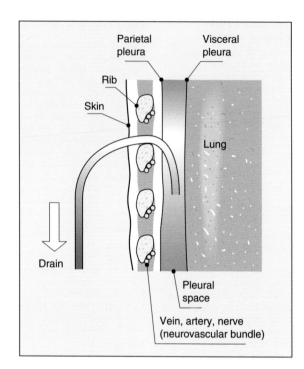

Parietal pleura
Visceral pleura
Rib
Skin
Lung
Drain
Pleural space
Vein, artery, nerve (neurovascular bundle)

Figure 13.4 Cross section through chest cage to illustrate chest drain.

Managing a chest drain

Pneumothorax

1 Check for an air leak by asking the patient to cough. A bubbling drain implies an air leak from an unsealed hole, fistula or a leak in the tubing. You may need to apply suction to the drain if you suspect a hole or fistula. Consult a respiratory or cardiothoracic specialist, and note that suction is not a panacea and can in fact hold open a pneumothorax. Exercise is difficult whilst on suction, but a bedside exercise bike can help with lung inflation and has been used effectively in some centres.

2 After the lung has re-expanded and the drain is no longer bubbling, remove the drain, and re-X-ray. Never clamp a drain inserted for pneumothorax – this can rapidly convert an open pneumothorax into a fatal tension pneumothorax.

3 If the pneumothorax is present after a surgical procedure like a pleurodesis, then avoid non-steroidal anti-inflammatory drugs as they will inhibit inflammatory response and adhesion to the chest wall.

Effusion/haemothorax

1 Large effusions can drain over several days, up to a maximum of 1 l/hour and not more than 4 l/day (otherwise, there is a risk of 'reflex' pulmonary oedema). Remove the drain when the chest X-ray (CXR) reveals no further fluid.

2 For recurrent effusions you may consider talc/chemical pleurodesis; discuss with your team.

3 Empyema drains require special consideration. Get a specialist opinion.

How to remove a drain

Have ready

1 Gloves

2 Clamping forceps

3 Pair of scissors

4 One occlusive dressing

The procedure

1 Clamp the tube with the forceps.

2 The entry point of the tube should have been secured with a purse-string suture that must be untied (not cut) and the ends firmly pulled to seal the hole as the tube slides out. Take your time the first few times you do this. It is easy to lose the stitching. Some of the newer drains do not require suturing in, and so all you need to do is cut the strings and pull the drain out.

3 Withdraw the tube with positive intrathoracic pressure by asking the patient to blow hard against a closed nose and mouth ('make your ears pop'). Alternatively, ask the patient to take a deep breath and hold. Withdraw quickly and smoothly. You should hear the hiss of the expulsion of the last bit of air as the end comes out. Quickly pull the purse string to seal the hole. Apply an occlusive dressing.

4 Do a CXR to assess the success of the drain and as a comparison for future X-rays.

Hint

Have a 4 × 4 cm gauze swab to hand to place over the hole in the event of a failed purse-string closure. Later, replace this with a large clear occlusive dressing over the hole.

DC cardioversion

As a junior doctor rotating through cardiology, you may be asked to do the elective cardioversion list. This may seem daunting, but in reality is a straightforward procedure.

Similarly, you may be required to undertake this procedure in the emergency department if the patient is haemodynamically compromised:

1 Position the gel pads before the patient is anaesthetized. Anteroposterior position may be more effective, but the anterolateral position is most commonly used for convenience.

2 Once the patient has been anaesthetized, ask the anaesthetist whether he or she is happy for you to continue.

3 Ensure that the defibrillator is set to 'synchronized'. Check that the defibrillator is sensing QRS complexes rather than T or P waves. You may need to adjust the gain to achieve this. If you do not sync the defibrillator, you run the risk of precipitating ventricular fibrillation (VF) and cardiac arrest.

4 Set defibrillator to 100 J.

5 Warn all present that you are about to charge the defibrillator, and make sure everyone is standing clear as well as stating that the oxygen should be removed.

6 Deploy the shock by pressing the button. From the time you press the button to administer the shock, there may be some delay before the shock is deployed. This is because the defibrillator is waiting for the next QRS complex. During this delay, do not be tempted to think the paddles have not worked. It is sometimes the case that the machine cannot synchronize properly and so doesn't deliver a shock.

7 Check the electrocardiogram (ECG) or rhythm monitor. (Once the shock has been delivered, the anaesthetist will continue ventilation.)

8 If the procedure has not worked, repeat at 200 J. If this too does not work, repeat at 360 J. Check the gel pads between each shock to make sure that they have not dried out, as this will lead to skin burns.

9 If, at 360 J, the procedure has not caused reversion to sinus rhythm, consider repositioning the paddles, with one at the left sternal border and one to the left of the spine at the same level, and administering another 360 J shock.

10 At the end of the procedure, do a formal 12-lead ECG, and ensure the patient is in the recovery position and is self-ventilating well, with good oxygen saturation.

Hints

Do not be too hasty in judging whether a treatment cycle has been successful or unsuccessful on the basis of the rhythm monitor. It may take a few seconds for the rhythm to settle into sinus after a shock, and likewise, the initial appearance of sinus rhythm may give way to atrial fibrillation within a minute or so.

Electrocardiogram

There are many indications to performing an ECG. They are harmless; if in doubt, just do one. It is always useful to have a routine ECG on admission for comparison.

The procedure

1 Have the patient lie with their chest exposed. Explain to them what you are doing and reassure them that there they will not get an electric shock.

2 Attach limb leads to the inner aspect of the forearm just below the wrist and the outer aspects of the leg above the ankle. The wires are usually labelled, but if not the colour code is most often as follows:

> Red = right arm
> Yellow = left arm
> Green = left leg
> Black = right leg

The lead placement is often remembered as 'ride your green bike' in a clockwise direction.

3 Ensure good contact with the skin.

4 For chest leads, see Figure 13.5.

Hints
Preventing spurious results

■ The patient should be completely relaxed.
■ Make sure the chest lead electrodes do not overlap.

■ Lightly shave hairy areas for proper contact.
■ If the patient has a hand tremor (e.g. Parkinson's), attach the leads higher up the arm.
■ The black (right leg) lead is an earth lead and can be attached to any part of the body.
■ For leg amputees, the green (left leg) lead can be placed on either leg. However, the arm leads must not be crossed. For an arm amputee, ensure that the arm electrodes are equidistant from the heart (they may be placed on the shoulders).

Exercise stress test

Exercise (ECG) stress tests take approximately 20 minutes to perform. Your job is to encourage the patient to attain their peak heart rate if possible (=220 − patient age) and to watch their ECG closely. Your aim is to detect and measure the severity of coronary artery disease and uncover arrhythmias.

Relative contraindications (discuss with senior)

Aortic stenosis
Hypertrophic obstructive cardiomyopathy
Left bundle branch block on ECG
Systolic BP >200 mmHg and diastolic BP >100 mmHg
Unstable angina
Uncontrolled arrhythmias
Note: Beta blockers should be stopped 2 days before the test.

The procedure

1 Make sure that there is resuscitation equipment immediately available. Approximately 1 per 4000 patients arrests during stress tests. Also have glyceryl trinitrate (GTN) ready.

2 Assess peak heart rate (about 220 − patient age).

3 Follow the instructions of the ECG technician.

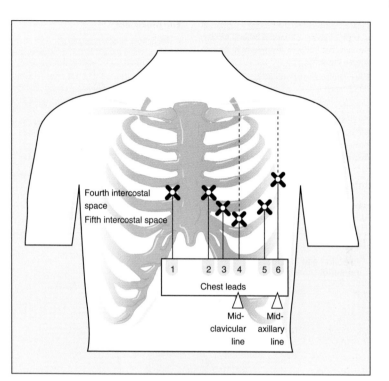

Figure 13.5 ECG chest lead placement.

4 *Stop the test* if the patient complains of:

- Increasingly severe chest pain or faintness/dyspnoea. Consider administering GTN.
- A fall in systolic BP of more than 20 mmHg.
- A fall in heart rate.
- Ventricular tachycardia (VT) or VF.
- Progressive ST elevation.
- ST depression greater than or equal to 2 mm.
- Three or more consecutive ventricular ectopics.
- Peak heart rate is attained.

5 You must remain present at all times and monitor BP and pulse at regular intervals. This includes the recovery period when the test may become positive or the patient may go into VT.

Injections

Subcutaneous

Have ready

1 23–25G needle

2 Alcohol swab

The procedure

1 Choose a fatty site and use the smallest possible needle.

2 Clean site with an alcohol swab and allow to dry.

3 Gently pinch skin between your thumb and index finger.

4 Place the needle on the skin for 3 seconds at an angle of about 60° before pushing through the skin. This reduces the sensation of pain. Release the skin.

5 Aspirate to ensure you do not inject into a blood vessel.

6 Slowly depress the plunger. Rapid injection will cause pain.

7 If you aspirate blood, remove and replace the needle and explain the need to repeat the injection.

Intramuscular

Have ready
As for SC

The procedure

1 The deltoid muscle is usually good for small injections. If the patient is thin or wasted, use the gluteal muscles – choose the upper and outer quadrant below the iliac crest to avoid the sciatic nerve by drawing an imaginary line between the anterior superior iliac spine and the greater trochanter of the femur and injecting posteriorly to and above this line (see Fig. 13.6).

2 Pull the skin taut and inject at 90° to the skin (pulling the skin ensures that the injection doesn't leak after you pull the needle out).

3 Aspirate to ensure that you do not inject into a blood vessel. Inject slowly.

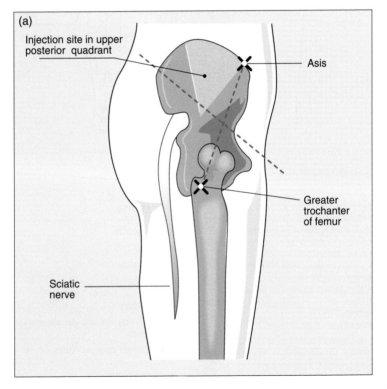

Figure 13.6 Site for intramuscular injections: (a) lateral view.

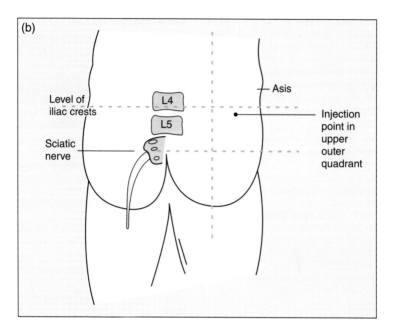

Figure 13.6 (continued)(b) Posterior view.

Joint aspiration/ injection

This is a useful procedure to learn from an expert, especially if you are an aspiring general practitioner (GP) (or GP with special interest). Superb aseptic technique is vital as is a sound knowledge of the anatomy. Each joint requires a slightly different approach, but the basic technique is the same.

Aspiration

Indications

Diagnostic:
■ Recent onset arthritis
■ To rule out infection (acute and chronic)
■ Joint effusion – particularly a traumatic haemarthroses with pain

Therapeutic:
■ Steroid injections
■ Drainage of septic arthritis

Have ready

1 Three syringes (5, 10 and 50 ml)

2 Two needles (25G and 21G)

3 Lidocaine 2%

4 Sterile gloves

5 Sterile dressing pack

6 Betadine/chlorhexidine

7 Three specimen containers, blood culture bottles and a fluoride tube (grey top)

The procedure

1 Obtain written consent.

2 Find the site of maximal effusion and mark this point with indelible ink.

3 Scrub up and clean the area with Betadine. Allow it to dry and wipe over the site of aspiration with an alcohol swab. Allow it to dry completely. Even small amounts of Betadine will ruin your culture results.

4 Anaesthetize the area, being careful to avoid injecting local anaesthetic into the joint – lidocaine is also bactericidal so it will affect cultures.

5 Insert the aspiration needle and advance it slowly. When you hit the effusion, drain it completely.

6 Never inject steroids if infection is a possibility. To inject steroids after tapping an effusion, disconnect the syringe, leaving the needle in place. Attach the syringe containing the steroid. Aspirate to ensure you are not in a vessel, then inject. There should be minimal resistance. Stop if you feel you are in the tissues and try again.

7 Remove the needle and apply pressure for a minute. Dress the wound.

Hints

■ Phone microbiology to request urgent microscopy and gram stain on the joint fluid. Some labs insist on special transport media when certain infections are suspected – get advice from the microbiologist.

Injecting joints

Many rheumatology departments teach a simple no-touch technique. The risk of infection following this method is no worse than that outlined in the preceding text.

Have ready

1 Two 5 ml syringes – one for lidocaine (to anaesthetize the skin) if deemed necessary, and one for the steroid, ± lidocaine.

2 Two alcohol swabs.

3 A small plaster.

4 Triamcinolone 5–20 mg or methylprednisolone 10–40 mg for steroid injections. The dose will depend on the size of the joint.

The procedure

1 Inform the patient of the small risk of infection (see the preceding text).

2 Draw up the lidocaine and the steroid for injection. The latter is now available with lidocaine added. This limits the potentially painful response to the injection and lasts for about 2–3 hours. Note that lidocaine for skin anaesthesia is still advisable for squeamish patients.

3 Locate the site for injection; clean with an alcohol swab and allow to dry. Without touching the site again, push through the skin and anaesthetize the skin down to the joint. Remember to aspirate to ensure you are not in a vessel. Remove and allow a minute for the local anaesthetic to work.

4 Repeat (3) except this time inject the joint with steroid. There should be minimal resistance to the injection.

5 Remove the needle and apply pressure for a minute. Dress the wound.

Hints

■ Tell the patient that mild pain and redness can occur after steroid injections and may persist for up to 24 hours. They are due to a reaction to the crystalline suspension used in long-acting steroids, but be wary of iatrogenic infection.

Local anaesthesia (for any procedure)

Have ready

1 21G and 23G needle

2 5–10 ml syringe

3 Alcohol swabs

4 1–2% lidocaine ampoules

The procedure

1 Start with a 23–25G needle. Infiltrate the skin and SC tissues raising a small bleb. If deeper anaesthesia is required, switch to a larger needle (21G), wait 1 minute, and then pass through the same puncture site.

2 Aspirate for blood before injecting anything. If you hit blood, withdraw a little and try again.

3 Wait at least 2 minutes for effect.

Hints

■ Lidocaine lasts approximately 2 hours. Marcaine and bupivacaine are longer acting (8 hours) and useful for intercostal blocks.

■ Use lidocaine with adrenaline for very vascular sites where you need to incise skin, as adrenaline causes vasoconstriction, for example, the scalp. Never use adrenaline for a nerve block of an extremity, for example, a finger ring block or nose, or you will cause disastrous ischaemia.

■ To work out the dose of lidocaine in mg/ml, multiply the percentage concentration by 10. The maximum doses of lidocaine within 24 hours are:

○ Without adrenaline: 3 mg/kg (i.e. 20 ml of 1% lidocaine for a 70 kg adult)
○ With adrenaline: 7 mg/kg

Lumbar puncture

Lumbar punctures (LPs)/spinal taps are easy once you get the hang of them. The thing to do is to reassure the patient that it is an uncomfortable but relatively painless procedure and that it might take up to 30 minutes – so you don't feel rushed.

Indications

Diagnostic:
■ Meningitis, subarachnoid haemorrhage, multiple sclerosis (MS) diagnosis and neurological rarities

Therapeutic:
■ Intrathecal drugs (never to be given by junior doctors)

● Benign intracranial hypertension – removal of cerebrospinal fluid (CSF) to alleviate symptoms

Contraindications (get help)

1 Local sepsis.

2 A space occupying lesion or an obstructive hydrocephalus. The symptoms and signs of raised intracranial pressure (ICP) (vomiting, bradycardia, drowsiness, papilloedema) are generally a warning that an LP may be dangerous. Please note however that in rare circumstances such as a communicating hydrocephalus, the treatment may actually be an LP. In these cases, expert guidance should always be taken.

3 Suspicion of a cord or posterior fossa mass.

4 Coagulopathy, anticoagulation or platelet count <50.

If patient is drowsy, is unconscious or has evidence of raised ICP, request an urgent CT scan before doing an LP.

Have ready

1 LP pack, or if none available:
2 Two sterile drapes
3 One gallipot
4 One pack of gauze swabs
5 One pack of cotton wool balls
6 Two LP needles (an 18G (yellow) or a 20G (black); open one)
7 One sterile, disposable manometer
8 Three sterile, 20 ml specimen containers
9 Antiseptic (povidone/Betadine/chlorhexidine solution)
10 5–10 ml lidocaine 2%
11 10 ml syringe
12 23G and 21G needles
13 Sterile gloves

The procedure
(See Fig. 13.7.)

1 Obtain consent. Explain to the patient what you are doing and that the procedure may take some time but that it is not very painful – just uncomfortable.

2 Ask the patient to lie as indicated in Figure 13.7a – with the knees tucked up under the chin as much as possible (to draw the spinal cord out of the way). Ensure the vertebral column is parallel to the bed (the hips are perpendicular to the edge of the bed).

3 Get an LP pack ready on a trolley with plenty of room to manoeuvre. Make room for sharps and dirty items.

4 Scrub up as for a sterile technique.

5 Prepare skin with Betadine and cover with a sterile drape.

6 Unscrew the tops of the three sterile sample containers and label.

7 Locate the puncture site L3–L4 or L4–L5 by drawing two imaginary lines, one joining

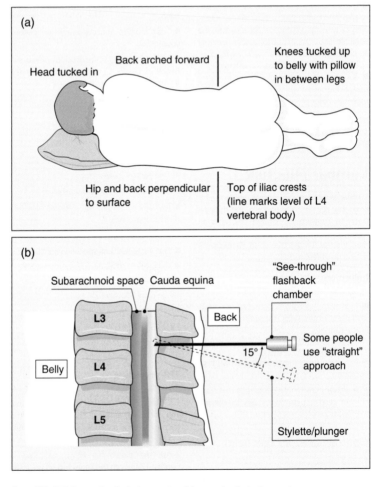

Figure 13.7 (a) Patient position for lumbar puncture, (b) approaches for lumbar puncture.

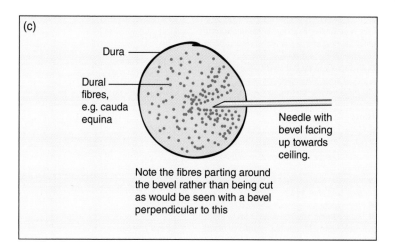

Figure 13.7 (continued) (c) Close-up of lumbar puncture.

the top of the iliac crests and the other running down the spine. These intersect at L3–L4. The spinal cord ends at L1–L2, so the L2–L3 interspace is safe if you cannot use the lower interspaces for some reason, but ensure the patient is properly curled up.

8 Anaesthetize using a 23G needle for superficial skin and SC infiltration. Switch to a 21G needle for deeper infiltration into the interspinous ligament. Inject slowly, waiting at least 2 minutes for effect.

9 Assemble the LP equipment, check that the stylet moves freely within the needle, and check how to use the manometer taps.

10 Insert the needle in the midline between the two spinous processes. Advance towards the patient's umbilicus. Resistance increases as the needle passes through the interspinous ligament. A small 'give' is felt as the needle punctures and passes through the ligamentum flavum. Withdraw the stylet to check for a flashback of CSF. If there is no CSF, advance the needle a few millimetres and check again.

11 Attach the manometer and measure the opening pressure (recorded in cmH_2O, normal range 10–20 cmH_2O).

12 Disconnect the manometer. From the open end of the needle, collect

- 2–5 drops for biochemistry
- 5–10 drops for bacteriology (MC&S)
- Up to 5–10 drops for cytology

If performing the procedure for benign intracranial hypertension, attain a closing pressure so that you know your treatment has been of therapeutic benefit.

13 Replace the stylet and withdraw the needle. Dress the wound.

14 The patient should lie flat for 4 hours; this is usually done on the basis of convention as the evidence base does not actually support this. They may have a moderate headache afterwards. If they experience a severe headache they should inform the nurses or doctors. Severe low pressure headaches sometimes require an epidural blood patch. Advise them to have a caffeinated drink also to stimulate CSF production.

If you fail

■ Correct positioning is the key to success. If you fail, recheck the patient's position. Try another interspace if necessary.

■ If the patient is anatomically 'difficult' (e.g. very large or has an abnormal spinal column), enlist the help of a radiologist who can do the LP under X-ray screening.

■ If you feel you are in the right place but there is no CSF, then lightly rotate the needle through 90°; the bevel may be lying against a nerve root.

Hints

■ Sedate the patient if required: 2.5–5 mg diazepam or 1 mg of lorazepam orally 30 minutes before the procedure should do the trick.

■ Warn the patient that headaches can occur up to 3 days after an LP.

■ *Never* apply suction to a CSF needle.

■ Subarachnoid haemorrhage is easily distinguishable from a bloody tap by uniform blood staining of the three consecutive samples and xanthochromia in the supernatant (12 hours after the headache onset). The samples from a bloody tap gradually clear. Send samples for a cell count.

Normal values

- Opening pressure: 10–20 cmH$_2$O
- Red cells: <5/mm^3
- Lymphocytes (WBC): <5/mm^3
- Neutrophils: nil
- Protein: <0.4 g/l
- Glucose: >50% of plasma level
- Colour: clear (if no vessels are hit, you may obtain a 'champagne tap'; if this clear-coloured CSF is obtained on your first ever attempt, then custom dictates that your senior should buy you a bottle of champagne to celebrate!)

Mantoux test

Indication

A Mantoux tests for a delayed-type hypersensitivity reaction to a partially purified protein derivative (PPD) from *Mycobacterium tuberculosis*. For routine pre-'bacillus Calmette–Guérin' (BCG) skin testing, the 10-unit dose of tuberculin PPD is used.

Have ready

1 PPD

2 1 ml diabetic syringe (26G 1 cm needle)

3 Alcohol swab

The procedure

1 Dilute PPD to a concentration of 100 TU/ml.

2 Draw up 0.1 ml (10 TU) into a diabetic syringe.

3 Clean a small area on the left forearm (convention).

4 Indicate the area to be injected with a marker pen.

5 Keeping the needle almost horizontal to the skin, carefully insert the needle intra dermally and inject 0.1 ml so that a small bleb is raised.

6 A negative reaction at 48 hours indicates a negative response (either no infection/immunization *or* overwhelming infection).

7 Read at 72 hours. Measure the diameter of induration, not the erythema:

- >10 mm = positive, suggestive of previous or current infection, not necessarily disease
- >20 mm = strongly positive, highly suggestive of active disease

Nasogastric tubes

Nurses are usually experienced at inserting nasogastric (NG) tubes; you are usually called only if they fail. They are straightforward.

Have ready

1 An apron and non-sterile gloves

2 Fresh NG tube – size 10 (small)–16 (large)

3 Kidney bowl and catheter drainage bag

4 KY jelly

5 Glass of water

The procedure

1 Sit the patient upright with chin on chest.

2 Tell the patient what you are doing and ask for their help in swallowing the tube.

3 Lubricate the tube with jelly and insert into a nostril. Gently advance the tube

towards the occiput (not upwards). Ask the patient to swallow when they feel the tube at the back of their throat and advance the tube as they swallow. They may find swallowing the water simultaneously to be helpful.

4 To assess position, aspirate some contents using a small syringe and test with pH paper to check that the contents are gastric (pH <5.5). If in doubt, get a CXR to confirm placement. The NPSA has issued a safety alert in 2005 and 2008, giving guidance on how to confirm placement. They specifically state that you should not use signs of respiratory distress or the 'whoosh' test (blowing air down the tube and listening for gurgling) to assess where the NG tube is.

Never use an NG tube for feeding unless you are confident of its placement.
5 Attach the drainage bag.

If you fail

- Try the other nostril.
- Sometimes keeping tubes in the fridge stiffens them and can help.
- Consider endoscopic/X-ray placement under mild sedation.

Hints

- NG tubes are uncomfortable and predispose to sinusitis and mucosal ulceration. Remove as soon as possible.
- Use fine-bore tubes for enteral feeding and large-bore ones (Ryles) for drainage.

Peritoneal tap (paracentesis)

Like pleural aspiration, paracentesis is straightforward.

The procedure

1 Ask the patient to empty their bladder. Explain what you are doing and why. Stress that the procedure is painless except for initial anaesthesia.

2 Lie the patient as flat as possible.

3 Percuss out the ascites.

4 Scrub up, prepare the skin, and drape. Give local anaesthetic in the sites indicated in Figure 13.8.

5 Follow the same procedure as for pleural aspiration (see the succeeding text).

6 For therapeutic taps, use a suprapubic or peritoneal dialysis catheter and attach a drainage bags.

7 Send samples for biochemistry (protein, albumin, glucose, lactate dehydrogenase [LDH]), bacteriology (MC&S, Ziehl–Neelsen stain [ZN] stain and tuberculosis [TB] culture) and cytology. Send for culture in blood culture bottles.

Hints

- Do not remove more than 500 ml in the first 10 minutes and no more than 1200 ml in 24 hours.
- Avoid going too close to old surgical scars as bowel may be attached to the abdominal wall.
- You may need to reposition the catheter or ask the patient to mobilize to maintain the flow.
- Bizarre cells on cytology often represent reactive mesothelial cells, not malignancy. Always get a formal report. If it is unclear, call the pathologist for clarification.
- Complications are rare but include perforated bowel, peritonitis, intra-abdominal haemorrhage and perforated bladder.
- Paracentesis is essential to rule out peritonitis in patients with cirrhosis and decompensated ascites.

Pleural aspiration

Like many invasive procedures it is now common to have this undertaken by radiologists or the puncture site marked by USS.

Indications

Diagnostic:
- Infection

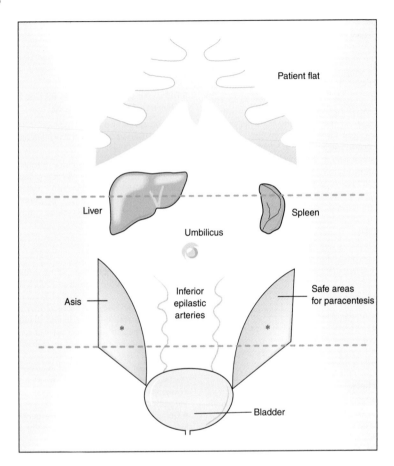

Figure 13.8 Site for tapping ascites.

- Malignancy

Therapeutic:
- Large effusions for relief of dyspnoea

Have ready

1 Dressing pack

2 Sterile gloves

3 One 10 ml syringe

4 One blue needle

5 One orange needle

6 One green needle

7 10 ml 1% lidocaine

8 Three specimen jars (sterile) For therapeutic taps, add:

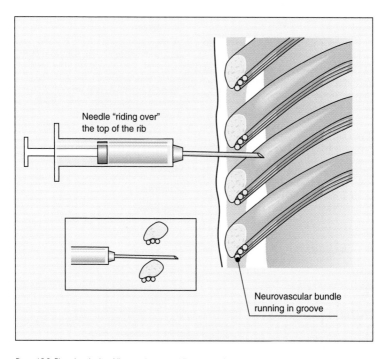

9 One large-bore IV cannula (brown or grey Venflon)

10 One three-way tap

11 IV giving set and an empty, sterile bowl or saline bag

The procedure

1 Confirm the size and extent of the effusion on the most recent CXR. Scrub up. Tell the patient what you are doing.

2 Sit the patient upright in bed leaning forwards over the side of the bed or on a bedside table, resting their elbows on a pillow.

3 Select the insertion site by tapping out the effusion. The best sites are usually two to three spaces below the lowest point

(angle) of the scapula or at the same level in the posterior axillary line. Avoid the mid-clavicular line on the left (and so the heart!).

4 Scrub up and drape the patient.

5 Anaesthetize the skin with an orange needle for superficial infiltration and then with a green needle for deeper infiltration. The track of the needle should hug the upper border of the rib to avoid the neurovascular bundle (Figure 13.9).

6 Attach a 20 ml syringe to the end of a green needle and insert the needle through the area already anaesthetized. Aspirate as you push forwards. The flashback of fluid indicates that you have reached the effusion.

Needle "riding over" the top of the rib

Neurovascular bundle running in groove

Figure 13.9 Pleural aspiration (diagram shows an oblique section).

7 Gently aspirate 20 ml of fluid for analysis. Send for:

- Bacteriology: MC&S, ZN stains and TB culture
- Chemistry: protein, glucose, LDH and amylase
- Cytology: the more fluid, the better (up to 10 ml) as the sample is spun down to concentrate the cells

8 For therapeutic taps, attach a large (green/grey) cannula to a 50 ml syringe; after the flashback of fluid, advance the Venflon and withdraw the needle, leaving the flexible cannula in place. Secure the cannula with tape if you are aspirating a large effusion.

9 Aspirate 50 ml at a time, emptying the syringe contents into the bowl or saline bag. Do not remove more than 1000 ml at one sitting.

10 Withdraw the cannula, asking the patient to breathe out as you do so. Apply an occlusive dressing.

11 Perform a CXR after the procedure to exclude a pneumothorax.

12 Document the procedure, including the macroscopic appearance of the fluid (straw coloured/blood stained/containing pus), the volume aspirated and what the CXR shows.

If you fail

A dry tap indicates a possible loculated effusion or empyema. Try redirecting the needle. Otherwise, ask for help from a colleague or radiologist. In many hospitals, it is now routine to ask a radiologist to perform the aspirate under ultrasound guidance.

Hints

■ Ask the patient to cough as you reach the end; this aids in expelling fluid.
■ Have a vial of atropine to hand for vasovagals (1 ampoule (0.6 mg) IV stat).

Pulsus paradoxus

This is not a procedure per se but complex enough to make it into this section and certainly worth knowing about! During inspiration, intrathoracic pressure falls, which reduces the systolic ejection volume and therefore systolic pressure. Normally, the difference in systolic pressure during inspiration and expiration is less than 10 mmHg. This pressure difference is exaggerated by a large drop in intrathoracic pressure that occurs during inhalation in serious conditions, including severe asthma and cardiac tamponade. Pulsus paradoxus is defined by a difference in systolic BP between inspiration and expiration of more than 10 mmHg.

Have ready

A stethoscope and a sphygmomanometer

The procedure

1 Inflate the cuff above systolic pressure, and then slowly deflate until the first, intermittent sounds are heard (during expiration). Note the pressure.

2 Continue to deflate the cuff slowly until the sounds are continuous (i.e. heard during inspiration and expiration). The drop in mmHg between when the first sound is heard (intermittent) and when it becomes continuous represents the degree of paradox.

Respiratory function tests

Spirometry

Have ready

A spirometer, a vitalograph paper and a disposable mouthpiece

The procedure

1 Explain the procedure to the patient.

2 Plug the machine in. Place the vitalograph paper in position on the spirometer. Make sure the spirometer's needle is set to zero. Place the disposable mouthpiece in the end of the spirometer's hosepipe.

3 Ask the patient to take a couple of deep breaths. When they are ready, ask them to breathe in and then breathe all the way out into the mouthpiece until the needle reaches the end of the graph paper.

4 Depending on how automated the machine is, you may need to push the record button whilst the patient is exhaling.

5 Repeat several times.

6 Record the best forced expiratory volume in first second (FEV_1) and forced vital capacity (FVC) in the notes, with expected values for the patient (see Tables 13.4 and 13.5).

The patient has a restrictive picture if FVC is reduced and FEV_1/FVC >75%.

The patient has an obstructive picture if FEV_1/FVC <75%.

Peak expiratory flow rate

This measures the maximum expiratory flow rate in the first 2 ms of expiration and is useful for assessing the respiratory status

of patients with asthma, chronic obstructive pulmonary disease and other respiratory conditions.

Have ready

A peak flow meter and disposable mouthpiece

The procedure

1 Put the disposable mouthpiece into the peak flow meter.

2 Ask the patient to breathe in as deeply as possible.

3 With their lips tightly sealed around the mouthpiece, ask them to blow out forcefully and quickly.

4 Have them repeat it at least three times.

5 Record the best value in the notes, with the expected value (Table 13.6).

Table 13.4 Expected values for FEV_1 (litre).

Age (years)	Height (m)				
	1.5	1.6	1.7	1.8	1.9
Males					
15–20	2.80	3.30	3.55	3.90	4.30
20–25	3.25	3.60	3.95	4.35	4.70
25–35	3.10	3.45	3.80	4.20	4.55
35–45	2.80	3.15	3.50	3.90	4.25
45–55	2.50	2.85	3.20	3.60	3.90
55–65	2.15	2.50	2.90	3.25	3.60
65–75	1.85	2.20	2.60	2.95	3.30
75–85	1.55	1.90	2.25	2.65	3.00
85+	1.40	1.75	2.10	2.50	2.85
Females					
15–25	2.45	2.80	3.15	3.45	3.75
25–35	2.35	2.65	2.95	3.30	3.65
35–45	2.05	2.35	2.65	3.05	3.35
45–55	1.75	2.05	2.35	2.75	3.05
55–65	1.45	1.75	2.10	2.45	2.75
65–75	1.15	1.45	1.85	2.15	2.45
75–85	0.85	1.20	1.55	1.85	2.15
85+	0.75	1.05	1.35	1.70	2.05

Table 13.5 Expected normal values for FVC (litre).

Age (years)	Height (m)				
	1.5	1.6	1.7	1.8	1.9
Males					
15–20	3.45	4.00	4.50	5.05	5.55
20–25	3.65	4.15	4.70	5.20	5.75
25–35	3.55	4.05	4.60	5.10	5.60
35–45	3.30	3.85	4.35	4.90	5.40
45–55	3.10	3.60	4.15	4.65	5.20
55–65	2.85	3.40	3.95	4.45	4.95
65–75	2.65	3.15	3.70	4.20	4.75
75–85	2.45	2.95	3.45	4.00	4.50
85+	2.35	2.85	3.35	3.90	4.40
Females					
15–25	2.90	3.40	3.85	4.35	4.75
25–35	2.75	3.25	3.70	4.15	4.65
35–45	2.45	2.95	3.45	3.90	4.35
45–55	2.20	2.65	3.15	3.60	4.05
55–65	1.90	2.35	2.85	3.30	3.75
65–75	1.60	2.10	2.55	3.00	3.45
75–85	1.30	1.80	2.25	2.70	3.20
85+	1.20	1.65	2.10	2.60	3.05

Table 13.6 Predicted values for PEFR (l/minute).

Age (years)	Height (m)			
	1.5	1.6	1.7	1.8
Males				
15–20	440	475	510	545
20–25	535	570	610	645
25–35	525	560	595	630
35–45	500	535	570	605
45–55	480	510	545	575
55–65	455	490	520	550
65–75	435	465	495	525
75–85	410	440	465	495
85+	410	430	455	480
Females				
15–25	360	395	435	470
25–35	350	385	420	460
35–45	325	365	400	440
45–55	305	345	380	420
55–65	285	320	360	395
65–75	265	300	340	375
75–85	245	280	315	355
85+	235	270	305	345

Table 13.7 When to remove sutures.

Area sutured	When to remove sutures
Face and neck	3–5 days
Scalp	5–7 days
Abdomen and chest	5–10 days
If impaired wound healing (e.g. steroids, cachexia, severe infection)	14 or more days

Sutures

Suturing is best learnt with a model in the skills lab before being applied initially in A&E or in theatre. Table 13.7 discusses times for suture removal.

Materials

1 Non-absorbable: Nylon (Ethilon)/Ethibond/Prolene*/Silk*

2 Absorbable: Plain catgut (5–10 days)/chromic gut (10–20 days)/Vicryl (60–90 days)*/Dexon (60–90 days)*

3 Sizes:

● Very coarse, 2, 1, 0, 1/0, 2/0, etc.; very fine, 6/0, 5/0, etc. (think of 2/0 as two zeros after the point, i.e. 0.001).

● 3/0 and 4/0 are suitable for the skin on the arms and legs.

● 5/0 and 6/0 for the face and back of the hand.

● 2/0 is most often used for securing lines and 1/0 for chest drains.

Hints

■ Nylon is less comfortable for patients. Use softer, non-absorbable material (silk or Prolene) for securing lines and chest drains.

■ Some synthetic sutures are made as mono- or polyfilament. Monofilament sutures are more slippery but are better if there is a high risk of infection. Polyfilament sutures tie well and hold securely, but they can theoretically facilitate tracking of fluid down the suture, leading to infection.

*Most commonly used for normal ward procedures.

Chapter 14
RADIOLOGY

With contributions from Dr Rahul Mukherjee

Radiology is central to the clinical practice of medicine. Information gained from different imaging modalities can be used for diagnosis, monitoring treatment, assessing progression and detecting relapses of a wide variety of medical conditions in a minimally invasive and anatomically precise manner. As a junior doctor, you will spend much of your time requesting radiological investigations and explaining the results to patients. Many of the following guidelines come from the Royal College of Radiologists. Your hospital may also have its own which you should follow.

Requesting investigations

Radiology registrars are notorious for grilling you on exactly why a scan is required and how it is going to change your management plan. Radiologists have a duty not to expose a patient to unnecessary radiation. Scanners and radiographers are often overstretched resulting in some reluctance on the part of radiology staff to perform unjustified investigations. Take this as a learning exercise and a challenging opportunity to practice your communication skills. The ability to convince a reluctant radiologist to agree to a scan is a rite of passage! It saves a lot of time if you can supply logical and clinically coherent answers, so don't be shy to ask your seniors why the investigation is needed and what you expect to find. If it isn't clear to you then it probably won't be clear to radiology either. By asking your seniors, you will also reinforce your understanding of the indications for certain investigations.

1 Always book procedures as early as possible. Most radiological departments are overbooked. This is particularly true for contrast studies, CTs and particularly magnetic resonance imagings (MRIs). For urgent studies needed on the same day, it is usually best to go down to the department and speak to a radiologist face-to-face early on in the day. In some hospitals, approvals for specialized scans such as MRIs can only come from a registrar or even a consultant. It is best to prepare yourself beforehand with the patient's details, brief history, results of investigations so far, differential diagnoses and why you think the scan will help to either make the diagnosis or change the management plan.

2 The following information must be included on the radiology request form.

- Patient ID.
- Whether pregnant or not. Any reactions to contrast media.
- Whether the patient has any infective issues, for example, *Clostridium difficile* or *methicillin-resistant Staphylococcus aureus* (MRSA) positive.
- A specific question to be answered. Imagine being the radiologist reporting these scans without the benefit of patient history, examination or indeed notes. This is why writing a misleading request card to get a scan done more urgently is dangerous and completely unacceptable.

The Hands-on Guide to the Foundation Programme, Fifth Edition. Anna Donald, Michael Stein,
Ciaran Scott Hill and Selina J Chavda.
© 2015 John Wiley & Sons, Ltd. Published 2015 by John Wiley & Sons, Ltd.

• Clinical features (not just suspected diagnosis).
• How the results will affect the management plan.
• Any factors which may complicate the procedure (e.g. diabetes, epilepsy).

3 Ask the radiographers about how to prepare patients for investigations if you are unsure, such as barium enemas. Often, the radiographer will liaise directly with the ward nurse, in which case you don't have to do anything except prescribe preparations, such as enemas.

Minimizing radiation

■ Many doctors do not realize how much radiation dosage their patients are exposed to during radiological investigations. One study found that 77% of non-radiologists

underestimated the dose of radiological examinations.
■ The risk of inducing a cancer from a single chest X-ray (CXR) is very small, around 1 in 200,000. The risk from a single CT brain scan is much higher, around 1 in 7000.
■ In terms of radiation, different procedures are ranked as indicated in Table 14.1.

Common concerns about X-rays

Patients are usually concerned about being X-rayed. Therefore, wherever possible, tell the patient:

1 What is about to happen to them

2 Why they are having this done

3 Duration of imaging

Table 14.1 Radiation doses of radiological investigations.

Investigation	Number of CXR equivalents (1 CXR = 0.02 mSv)	Equivalent background radiation dose
Abdomen X-ray	35	105 days
Chest X-ray	1	3 days
CT abdomen	500	4.1 years
CT chest	400	3.3 years
CT head	100	300 days
MRI brain/abdomen/limbs	0	0
IVU	120	1 year
Barium swallow	75	225 days
Barium enema	360	3 years
Leg arteriogram	100	300 days
Thyroid isotope scan	50	150 days
PET scan	250	2 years

Lee RKL et al. (2012) Knowledge of radiation exposure in common radiological investigations: a comparison between radiologists and non-radiologists. *Emergency Medical Journal* 29:306–308. RCR Working Party (1998) Making the Best Use of a Department of Clinical Radiology: Guidelines for Doctors, 4th ed. The Royal College of Radiologists, London.

4 Whether or not they will be sedated or have a general anaesthetic

5 If they might experience any discomfort

6 What to do if they have pain or other symptoms after the procedure

7 When they can expect to receive the result

Pregnancy

■ Referring clinicians (i.e. you) are responsible for informing the radiologist if a patient is pregnant. It is negligent not to do this. Where possible tell the radiologist and radiographer yourself.

■ If you need to X-ray a pregnant patient, ask the radiologist for advice; they may suggest an alternative.

■ Pregnant patients will be particularly concerned about the dose of radiation exposure so it is important to know the differences between investigations, alternative tests and the risks and benefits of proceeding with a test.

Plain films

Chest X-rays

CXRs use ionizing radiation in the form of X-rays to generate an image. It is able to provide views of the bones, lungs, heart, great vessels and trachea. As a result, they are one of the most commonly performed investigations when a patient is admitted to hospital (Fig. 14.1). A CXR can be used to diagnose a number of conditions including:

1 Pneumonia

2 Pulmonary oedema

3 TB

4 Pulmonary fibrosis

5 Lung cancer

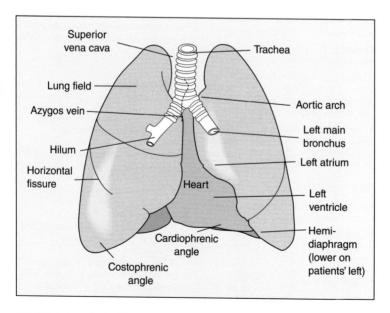

Figure 14.1 Anatomy of a chest X-ray.

6 Pleural effusions

7 Sarcoidosis

8 Pneumothorax

9 Rib fractures

10 Lung collapse

Checking the CXR: The bare bones

1 Patient's name, the date of the film and whether the film is anterior–posterior projection or posterior–anterior projection.

2 Trace the diaphragm and the lateral outline of the rib cage (look for pleural effusions, air under the diaphragm, raised hemi-diaphragm, pneumothorax).

3 Check the size and shape of the heart (look for enlarged heart, atrial shadows, calcified valve rings). Also look 'through' the heart for lesions that it partially obscures such as hiatus hernia or a cancer.

4 Check the position of trachea and heart (look for displacement or if the film is rotated).

5 Look at the mediastinum (look for air, widened mediastinum, lymphadenopathy).

6 Examine the hilar shadows (look for enlarged pulmonary arteries and veins).

7 Examine the lungs (look for opacities – consolidation, fluid or nodules). For interstitial oedema, look for straight lines (normal interstitial shadows are 'never' straight).

8 Check the bony structures (ribs, clavicles, spine) and the soft tissues (fractures, densities or lucencies, air in the tissues – surgical emphysema after trauma).

Abdominal films

An abdominal film can be used to diagnose the following conditions:

1 Obstruction

2 Constipation

3 Volvulus

4 Pneumoperitoneum

5 Renal calculi (although not the best imaging modality for this pathology)

6 Toxic megacolon

7 Ulcerative colitis flare

8 Abdominal aortic aneurysms, particularly if calcified

Checking an abdominal plain film

1 Patient's name and date of the film; whether erect, supine or lateral decubitus.

2 Gas pattern and intestinal diameter (a small bowel >2.5 cm and colon >6 cm indicate obstruction).

3 Look for ascites and soft tissue masses.

4 Identify the liver and spleen.

5 Check the borders of the kidneys, bladder and psoas muscles if possible.

6 Calculi (gall stones, renal and pancreatic calculi, aortic calcification).

7 Sub-diaphragmatic gas (or clear outline of organ) indicates perforation or recent surgery. (Note: sub-diaphragmatic gas is best seen on an erect CXR. The absence of free gas under the diaphragm does not rule out perforation.) A decubitus film is an alternative if the patient is too ill to sit up.

Ultrasound

No radiation or contraindications!
Preparation
■ Abdominal ultrasound (US): NBM 6 hours before.
■ Pelvic US: Requires full bladder.
■ The patient should start drinking a few hours before the pelvic US.
Tell the radiologist
■ For Doppler US of legs, make sure you identify which leg is the problem.
Tell the patient
■ No radiation dose or known hazards, painless unless for legs in patients with significant peripheral arterial disease, relatively quick.

Computed tomography

Preparation
- Nil; IV access needed if contrast is needed – ask the radiologist.

Tell the radiologist
- Any metalwork in situ. This can cause streak artefact on imaging.

Tell the patient
- Painless

General

- Do CTs *before* requesting barium studies. Barium hides detail on CT and takes at least 3 days to clear. Gastrografin (water soluble) can be used instead of barium if this is a problem.

CT head: Some emergency indications

Strokes: To differentiate haemorrhage from infarct. May have poor sensitivity if done too early but this is not a reason to delay. Once a haemorrhage is excluded, the patient can be given thrombolysis or given antiplatelets as required.

Subarachnoid haemorrhage: For diagnosis (but misses 10–15% of subarachnoid haemorrhages) and to exclude a contraindication to lumbar puncture (like obstructive hydrocephalus) or to assess the cause of deterioration (re-bleed, hydrocephalus, vasospasm).

In head injury: Indicated if there is skull fracture or serious scalp injury, impaired consciousness, focal neurology, epilepsy, new-onset confusion or deteriorating conscious level. The NICE guidelines clearly outline which scans need to be done and reported within 1 hour or 8 hours or not at all. Review the quick reference guide at www.nice.org.uk/CG176. It includes guidance on indications for imaging and management of suspected cervical spine injuries. Some examples of common CT head findings associated with traumatic mechanisms of injury are demonstrated in Figure 14.2.

Magnetic resonance imaging

- MRI does not emit ionizing radiation, but scans are expensive; there is a shortage of scanners and the waiting list is often long.
- Book your patient in as early as possible and discuss with radiologist.

Resource limitations mean that the magnets are often turned off overnight, meaning scanning may not be available 24 hours in all hospitals. Similarly, it is common for elective outpatient scanning lists to run on weekends, and this again limits semi-urgent inpatient scanning.

- Inform the radiologist and get his or her advice if the patient has a pacemaker, metal heart valves or other metallic implants. Many modern implants are now 'MRI safe', although you will need to check the brand and MRI compatibility with the radiologist.
- T1-weighted images give good anatomical detail. Fat is white, and flowing blood is black.
- T2-weighted images are good at showing abnormal tissue pathology but have poorer anatomical detail (though often still excellent). Fat and fluid are bright.
- There are numerous newer MRI modalities with specific clinical and research applications, for example, functional MRI and diffusion-weighted imaging.

Preparation
- Sedation may be necessary if the patient is claustrophobic (usually given by the radiologist). 1–2 mg lorazepam orally should suffice. If the patient is very agitated, the scan may need to be done under general anaesthetic with the aid of the anaesthetists. an You should only sedate patients in compliance with your local hospital's safe sedation policy. This usually requires an anaesthetist, an intensivist or an emergency physician. Never allow yourself to be pressurized into giving sedation if you have not had specific training. Patient responses to sedatives can be unpredictable and disasters do happen.

Tell the radiologist
- If the patient is pregnant.

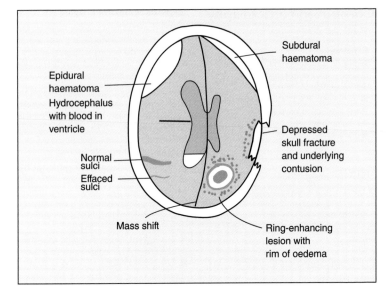

Figure 14.2 CT head pathology.

Do not allow the patient to be scanned unless you are certain that any implants are MRI-safe.

■ Even non-ferrous (i.e. non-magnetic) implants are subject to 'eddy currents' that can cause heating effects in the metalwork and have severe consequences. Often, the scan sequences need to be individualized in these patients.

■ Warn the radiographers about any tattoos the patient has. If large, these can also undergo significant heating.

Tell the patient

■ No irradiation is used.

■ The procedure is painless.

■ The patient will be in a very noisy, confined space for approximately 25–30 minutes. Often, the radiographers will give them headphones so they can listen to music, so the patient may be able to bring their own CD if they like.

Radioisotope scanning

Used to assess:

1 Bony metastases and sites of inflammation – technetium (Tm) is the radioactive isotope used for the scan:

● Radioisotope scanning delivers variable radiation doses. Ensure that the patient is not pregnant.

2 Pulmonary embolism – ventilation–perfusion (VQ) scans:

● There is no preparation for a VQ scan. These may only be available on certain days of the week, so make sure you book one well in advance. The ventilation phase of the test requires inhalation of a gaseous radionuclide (e.g. technetium) through a mask or mouthpiece. The perfusion phase involves intravenous injection of radioactive technetium. A gamma camera is used to acquire the images for both phases. Often, there is a 2–3 hour delay between the two phases of the test, so the procedure can take around half a day for the patient to complete.

• If the CXR is abnormal, it will be very difficult to interpret the VQ scan and an alternative investigation may be more appropriate.

3 Assessment of thyroid nodules, thyroid cancer and hyperthyroidism – iodine-131 or iodine-123:

• Ensure that the patient does not have an allergy to iodine.

4 Non-invasive evaluation of coronary artery disease – myocardial perfusion scans with thallium-201.

Chapter 15
APPROACH TO THE SURGICAL PATIENT

With contributions from Dr Roxanna Zakeri

Introduction

Your surgical placement is likely to be one of the most demanding periods of your Foundation training. Few other specialties will give you such a pivotal role in the team. Though this may seem daunting, it will be one of the best learning experiences you will have, from which you can take multiple transferable skills relevant to any specialty you wish to pursue.

In this chapter we will explore the main tasks you can expect to face in your surgical job, giving practical tips and advice to guide you in becoming a proficient, confident, multi-tasking junior surgeon. Essentially, you will be required to handle any medical issues the patient develops during their admission and escalate to the relevant medical teams as necessary.

Preoperative care

All patients undergoing elective surgery will be assessed preoperatively, usually in pre-assessment clinics a few weeks prior to surgery but also on the ward if admitted in advance. You may be involved at either or both of these stages; however, the points to consider when clerking are the same for both.

Clerking

- Patient details (name, DOB, hospital number)
- Procedure planned + indication
- History of presenting complaint:

○ Has the clinical picture changed significantly from when the patient was booked for surgery?
○ Note down relevant reports of scans/blood tests and other investigations

■ Fitness for surgery + anaesthesia:

- Past medical + surgical history
  ○ If possible, obtain operation reports from prior surgery. This will help in planning of surgical technique and may note previous adverse events, including anaesthetic risks. They are often filed in the patient's old notes.
  ○ Previous deep venous thrombosis (DVT)/pulmonary embolism (PE) and treatment given.
  ○ **Methicillin-resistant *Staphylococcus aureus* (MRSA)** status.
  ○ Obstructive sleep apnoea – patients may be on nightly continuous positive airway pressure (CPAP) which will be required post-operatively so planning is needed to ensure equipment is available (patients often bring their own CPAP device).
  ○ Patient's cardiac history – previous myocardial infarction (MI)/ischaemic heart disease, echo results and left ventricular ejection fraction %.
- Drug and allergy history
  ○ Allergies to dressings, latex, reactions to anaesthesia, antiseptic preparations (chlorhexidine/iodine) and antibiotics.
  ○ Anticoagulant/antiplatelet medications and when these have been stopped.

The Hands-on Guide to the Foundation Programme, Fifth Edition. Anna Donald, Michael Stein, Ciaran Scott Hill and Selina J Chavda.
© 2015 John Wiley & Sons, Ltd. Published 2015 by John Wiley & Sons, Ltd.

o Steroids (they may need extra at the time of surgery).

o Diabetic medication (they may need a sliding scale preoperatively).

o Antiepileptics – note date of last seizure as perioperative bridging with IV valproate or phenytoin may be required

o Contraception and hormone replacement therapy – increased risk of DVT/PE in major/lower limb surgery.

• Weight

o If BMI is high, special operating tables may need to be used so inform theatre staff in advance.

• Smoking history

o Consider optimizing oxygenation preoperatively, proven to improve outcomes, and ensure nicotine patch prescribed post-operatively.

• In women of childbearing age

o Date of last menstrual period.

o Contraception.

o Exclude pregnancy. Always get a urinary beta-human chorionic gonadotropin (bHCG) and document in notes. Some trusts also require serum levels of bHCG.

• It is good practice to determine the ASA (American Society of Anesthesiologists physical status classification system) grade to assess fitness for surgery.

• Examination

o Check observations carefully, especially blood pressure. This may be the first time they are having it checked.

o Perform a general physical examination, noting any cardiac murmurs, abnormal breath sounds, etc.

Address any questions or concerns the patient may have. Although the procedural details, indication, risks and benefits should have been discussed by a surgeon in clinic, the anxiety of impending surgery may result in these being forgotten. Explain the procedure and address concerns, but if unsure, reassure them that a senior colleague will come to explain further. Do not be surprised if you have patients arrive on the morning of surgery having decided they do not want to go ahead, after all of your previous efforts! Above all, ensure that they are making a fully informed decision. Usually such changes of

heart are temporary and simply require reassurance. Having said that, they are perfectly within their rights to change their minds, even if they have previously signed a consent form. In these cases, you should inform your seniors early so they can make alternative treatment arrangements and adjust the operating list as required.

Check if the patient has any current/recent symptoms of viral illness, for example, cough, sore throat, diarrhoea and vomiting. Depending on the procedure planned, patient fitness and anaesthetic risks, this may be a contraindication to proceed. Notify the consultant surgeon and anaesthetist immediately if you are concerned.

Preoperative tests

For a comprehensive guide to which tests to perform in different grades of surgery and patient ASA grade, consult the latest NICE guideline (Clinical Guideline 3 – Preoperative Tests, June 2003 – The use of routine preoperative tests for elective surgery).

You should consider requesting the following:

■ Blood tests

• Full blood count (FBC) – baseline haemoglobin (Hb) in case of bleeding and white cell count if infection is suspected

• Sickle cell screen in North African, West African, South/sub-Saharan African, Afro-Caribbean ethnic groups, Eastern Mediterranean and Middle Eastern groups. Ensure that counselling services are available in case of a positive test result

• Urea and electrolytes (U&E) – if suspected/known renal impairment; if taking steroids, diuretics and angiotensin-converting enzyme inhibitor, prior to aminoglycoside use

• Liver function test (LFT) – if known/suspected hepatic impairment, prior to antibiotic prescription

• Coagulation studies

• Random blood glucose

■ Group and save (G&S) and crossmatch (see the following table).

■ Plain chest radiograph – age >60 years, unexplained shortness of breath, cardiorespiratory disease, malignancy and thoracic/upper GI surgery. The Royal College of Radiologists advises against routine chest X-ray use in a pre-op setting for young, healthy individuals.

- Resting electrocardiogram – age >50 years, cardiovascular disease, diabetic and smoker.
- Urinalysis.
- Cardiopulmonary co-morbidities may necessitate arterial blood gas, exercise testing, echocardiography and pulmonary function tests – for ASA grades 2 and 3.

Requesting blood preoperatively

Check local hospital guidelines on transfusion requirements for specific procedures but the commonly requested amounts are presented in the following table. There is no evidence-based justification for routine G&S in all surgical cases; therefore, check with your consultant and local transfusion policy and send if needed.

Blood request	Procedure
No request	Minor day case procedures: excision of skin lesion/lipoma/incision and drainage of abscess/haemorrhoid surgery/carpal tunnel release/arthroscopy/laparoscopy
Group and save	Appendicectomy/cholecystectomy/hernia repair/mastectomy/varicose vein surgery/digital amputation/ERCP/PTC/liver biopsy
2 units, crossmatched	Laparotomy/colectomy/gastrectomy/splenectomy/TURP/Hysterectomy/hemi-arthroplasty/limb amputation/dynamic hip screw/thyroidectomy/tonsillectomy/craniectomy/burr hole, laminectomy
4 units, crossmatched	Abdominoperineal repair/resection/pancreatic/liver surgery, oesophagectomy/total joint replacement/cardiothoracic surgery, radical neck dissection
≥ 6 units, crossmatched	Vascular reconstruction (aortobifemoral, femoropopliteal bypass)/aneurysm repair/extensive liver surgery/emergency repair bleeding peptic/duodenal ulcer

Timing of G&S requests should also be considered. Bear in mind it takes a minimum of 45 minutes for a full crossmatch, often longer in practice in a busy blood bank. Some blood banks require two separate G&S samples to be sent for each patient at separate times before they will issue type-specific blood. Check with your hospital how long preoperative blood samples are saved and valid for. On average, G&S samples are saved for 14 days; however, a history of recent blood transfusion complicates matters and will require an up-to-date sample to be taken as follows (timings may vary).

Last transfusion	New sample to be taken a maximum of
Within 3–14 days	24 hours prior to surgery/transfusion
Within 15–28 days	72 hours prior to surgery/transfusion
29 days–3 months	7 days prior to surgery/transfusion

Preoperative fasting

To reduce the risk of aspiration during anaesthesia, patients are fasted preoperatively. Traditionally, a 'nil by mouth from midnight' approach was taken, but now, the general rule is no oral intake of solids for ≥6 hours prior to induction of anaesthesia. Only *clear* fluids are allowed within 2–6 hours of surgery, that is, water/black tea/coffee. Chewing gum and soluble mints/sweets are the equivalent of eating in terms of producing gastric juices; therefore, ensure they are avoided for ≥6 hours. Many cases have been cancelled because of missing the occult gum-chewing patient!

The above timings are the absolute minimum times for elective cases. In absolute emergency, rapid sequence induction can be carried out regardless of fasting time, involving complete paralysis and maintained cricoid pressure to reduce the risk of passive gastric reflux. However, aspiration risk can still be high and rigorous oropharyngeal monitoring and suction may be needed during recovery.

Factors that increase the risk of aspiration include:

- Pregnancy
- Obesity
- Elderly
- Gastric disorders: hiatus hernia and gastro-oesophageal reflux disease
- Pain + opiate use

Consent

Criteria for consent

- Consent must be given voluntarily, free from coercion. Patient autonomy must always be respected, so ensure you have informed them fully and respect their decision:
  - Relatives/friends may help or hinder the process, for example, when views are conflicting. You should always ask the patient if they would like someone to be present with them before consenting. Be wary of social/financial/family situations that may make this patient vulnerable and discuss with your senior.
- The patient must have the *capacity* to give consent:
  - Can understand, believe, retain and weigh all necessary information and relay it back to you
- You must *inform the patient fully*, explaining:
  - What the procedure entails
  - Where and when it will take place
  - Intended benefits
  - Common and serious risks/complications
  - Expected outcomes including failure
  - Possibility of any further procedure to be carried out simultaneously depending on the operative findings
  - What should happen if the patient refuses consent for the procedure

Obtaining consent is an art combining communication skills, surgical knowledge and perception. It takes practice and the best way to learn is to watch your senior colleagues in action.

Do not think of obtaining consent as an isolated process where a patient signs a piece of paper moments before being wheeled away, though this has been known to happen in practice. It is advisable to take the time to discuss the patient's overall management, not just this procedure, and ensure they are fully informed of the plan, including alternative treatments. Although this may have been explored prior to admission, unless the patient is aware and understands the plan at the time of surgery, consent would not be valid. Written consent alone is not legally adequate proof of consent. It takes time for these discussions, but you benefit by developing your relationship with the patient. Unless the patient objects, it is usually best to have a member of close family present during the consent process. This helps the family to understand the process and risk, and it also helps in building the therapeutic relationship that will be important for the remainder of their treatment.

Before embarking on consenting a patient, consider the following; firstly, are you the right person to be obtaining consent? You should only accept this responsibility if you are performing the procedure, are able to do the procedure yourself or are satisfied that you know fully the indications and potential complications. It is still the responsibility of the operator, however, to ensure that adequate consent is given. If you are not happy signing the form, that is perfectly acceptable. Do not be pressured or rushed into doing it by seniors. The deaneries take a very hard line on this and you are likely to be specifically asked at your annual review whether you were ever put in a situation where you were asked to obtain consent at a level beyond your competency.

To help with the consent process, use language that the patient can understand. The patient should have an understanding of every word that you use – do not forget that phrases such as 'anterior, supine, intubation, etc.' are all alien to the majority of even well-educated patients. My particular favourite is when anaesthetic colleagues tell patients they intend to paralyze them! Occasionally a little imagination and abstract analogies may be required but you must persist. Diagrams are invaluable. Practice drawing relevant anatomy and/or steps of the procedure that you can use when explaining them to patients. Alternatively, look in your department for patient information leaflets. Often they can be in different languages, ideal for when your patient does not speak English.

If you feel confident to obtain consent, fill in the appropriate consent form and sign with your name, grade and date. Obtain the patient's signature and then document in the notes what was discussed.

There are many different types of consent forms. In general use a yellow consent form 1 for routine informed consent. If an adult patient lacks capacity and you are performing a procedure in their best interests, use a form 4. This does not require patient signature but relatives can sign to show they were involved in a discussion about care. The different forms available are as follows.

Consent forms

Form 1	Patient agreement to investigation or treatment
Form 2	Parental investigation to investigation or treatment for a child or young person
Form 3	Patient/parental agreement to investigation or treatment which does not require general anaesthesia or sedation
Form 4	Form for adults who are unable to consent to investigation or treatment. This must be signed by two healthcare professionals involved in the patient's care. Next of kin may be consulted but legal consent falls to the medical provider

In all cases of surgery, it is important to inform patients of:

- Fatigue – length of time varies according to patient and procedure.
- Anaesthetic risk – anaesthetists will explore this area in detail.
- Bleeding – reassure patients that major bleeding is uncommon but it is a risk they should be aware of.
- Infection – antibiotics will be given prophylactically if the procedural risk of infection is high.

- Multiple drains, tubes, oxygen masks, etc. may be in place for several days post-operatively.
- Risk of conversion to open surgery for laparoscopic procedures.
- For bowel surgery, always explain the risks of colostomy/ileostomy formation and put this on the consent form.

If possible, check the actual figures for risks common to the procedure in question, both in the literature and locally.

Some of the common or serious risks of specific procedures are listed below.

Procedure	Complication
Amputation	Cramp, phantom limb pain, wound slough/dehiscence, psychological distress, need for revision
Aortic aneurysm repair	Bleeding, VTE, ureteric damage, paraplegia (anterior spinal artery damage), bowel ischaemia, adult respiratory distress syndrome, renal failure, aortoenteric fistula
Biliary surgery	Jaundice, damage to bile ducts causing strictures or bile leakage requiring further intervention (radiological/open), pancreatitis, hepatorenal syndrome
Gastrointestinal surgery	Post-op ileus/pseudo-obstruction, obstruction, fistula, anastomotic leak, ureteric damage. Stoma complications: dehiscence, prolapse, leak, bleeding, obstruction, infection, need for revision
Genitourinary surgery	Ureteric and renal damage, strictures, leaks, further intervention, infection – high-risk recurrent urinary tract infection (UTI)
Haemorrhoid surgery	Bleeding, anal stricture
Mastectomy	Seroma, haematoma, infection, damage to neurovasculature, especially lateral pectoral, long thoracic, serratus anterior, intercostobrachial nerves – may cause cutaneous numbness/paraesthesia, muscle weakness, lymphoedema if LN removed
Splenectomy	Infection (pneumococcal septicaemia), need for prophylactic antibiotics for life – will need vaccination (Hib, pneumococcus, meningococcus) ≥1 week prior to surgery
Thyroid surgery	Bleeding, hoarseness, replacement therapy (may be lifelong), damage to parathyroids, transient hypocalcaemia
Tracheostomy	Stenosis, mediastinitis, surgical emphysema
Prostatectomy	Urinary retention, urethral stricture, incontinence, bleeding, retrograde ejaculation, transurethral retrograde prostatectomy syndrome (water overload – electrolyte imbalance)

Marking

As there have been cases where the wrong side was operated on (wrong-site surgery), the UK National Patient Safety Agency and the Royal College of Surgeons have recommended the following for surgical site marking:

- **How:** Using an indelible marker, mark an arrow that extends to the incision site and remains visible after application of skin cleaning preparations and drapes.
- **Where:** Procedures involving laterality should be marked near the intended incision clearly differentiating the correct side needing operating.
- **Who:** The operating surgeon or a nominated deputy who will be in the operating theatre at the time of procedure.

- **When:** Prior to transferring to the operating theatre, prior to any anaesthesia/premedication, usually on the ward/day case unit or at time of consenting patient.
- **Verify:** Checked upon arrival to theatre and again prior to starting surgery as part of theatre checklist.

Robust marking pro formas are encouraged to ensure multiple stages of site verification. Here is an example of one you may be expected to complete (Table 15.1).

Booking theatre lists

For hospitals that still require juniors to book elective lists, prepare the list by the morning prior to operating day by the latest. Check

Table 15.1 Preoperative marking verification checklist

Patient's name:	Date:
Hospital no./DOB:	Intended procedure:
Addressograph label	

	Responsibility	Signature to confirm check completed
Check 1 • Check patient's identity • Check reliable documentation and/or images to ascertain intended surgical site • Mark intended site with an arrow using an indelible pen	The operating surgeon, or nominated deputy, who will be present in theatre at the time of the procedure	Signed: Print name
Check 2 • Prior to leaving ward/day care area, mark is inspected and confirmed against patient's supporting documentation • Relevant imaging studies accompany patient/are available in operating theatre	Ward or day care staff	Signed: Print name
Check 3 • In anaesthetic room prior to anaesthesia, mark is inspected and checked against patient's supporting documentation • Re-check imaging studies accompany patient/available in operating theatre • Availability of correct implant (if applicable)	Operating surgeon or a senior member of team	Signed: Print name
Check 4 Surgical, anaesthetic and theatre team involved in intended operative procedure prior to commencement of surgery should pause for verbal briefing to confirm: • Presence of correct patient • Marking of correct site • Procedure to be performed	Theatre staff directly involved in intended procedure	Signed: Print name

when the consultant and his/her secretary require finalized details. If you continue with surgical training this will become routine for you. Things to include are:

• Theatre number
• Date/time of list – a.m. versus p.m.
• Name of consultant doing each case
• Patient name, DOB, gender, hospital number and location

• Operation and side (written in full 'right/left')
• Special requirements – diabetic, MRSA positive, latex allergy, bariatric equipment needed, crossmatch requested and ITU bed needed post-operatively
• Order the list:
  ○ Children first
  ○ Older patients and those with co-morbidities before young and fit

- ○ Clean operations before 'dirty'
- ○ Longer procedure, more complex anaesthesia earlier

  Sign, date and bleep number

For booking emergency operations you should:

- List the patient details, location and procedure.
- Note time patient is fasted from.
- Inform on-call anaesthetist.
- Inform theatre coordinator.
- Inform ward staff and nurse in charge.
- Check patient has consented.
- Check all relevant investigation results are available.
- Check if G&S is needed and done.
- Check pregnancy test done if appropriate.
- Check patient is marked and pro forma filled correctly.

WHO checklist

Further to all the checks you have done so far, further perioperative checks are done according to the WHO Surgical Safety Checklist. There are three points of verification:

- Prior to anaesthesia
- Prior to commencing surgery
- Prior to moving the patient out of theatre to the recovery area

The simple checklist shown in Figure 15.1 has proven to reduce the incidence of the most common avoidable perioperative risks and improve outcomes. Familiarize yourself with your hospital's version. The current version can be found at http://www.who.int/patient safety/safesurgery/tools_resources.

Perioperative prescribing

When admitting a patient for elective surgery, prescribe as much as possible on the drug chart whilst clerking as it saves time and ensures the patient will not go without necessary medications for long periods. In addition to the regular medications, which may need modifying or withholding, you should also prescribe symptomatic relief

for the post-operative period (analgesia/anti-emetics/laxatives), thromboprophylaxis and any prophylactic or routine post-operative antibiotics.

Here are some suggestions of common medications to prescribe. Always consult the **BNF** to check for drug interactions and contraindications for specific cases.

Anti-emetics

- Cyclizine 50 mg TDS IV/PO.
- Ondansetron 4–8 mg TDS IV/PO.
- Metoclopramide and domperidone should generally be avoided due to their prokinetic GI effects.

Analgesia

Every patient's experience of post-operative pain varies. Aiming for adequate pain control on regular analgesia, rather than on an as-required basis, is the ideal. When prescribing, follow the WHO analgesic ladder. If control of symptoms is difficult, consult your hospital's Specialist Pain Team or the on-call anaesthetist.

Laxatives

Patients post-operatively are less mobile and do not drink as much fluids as they would at home. Their diet is altered and they can often be taking multiple analgesics with constipating side effects. Prescribing laxatives **pro re nata** (as required) (PRN) is helpful to try and prevent significant constipation.

Bowel preparation

For patients undergoing colorectal surgery or endoscopy, bowel preparation is often required. Check your consultant's preference or local guidelines. Commonly used treatments include Klean-Prep (non-absorbable iso-osmotic solutions that pass through the bowel without absorption) or Picolax (stimulates peristalsis and osmosis). Make sure you counsel patients fully on the expected effects! In elderly, immobile patients or those with

APPROACH TO THE SURGICAL PATIENT

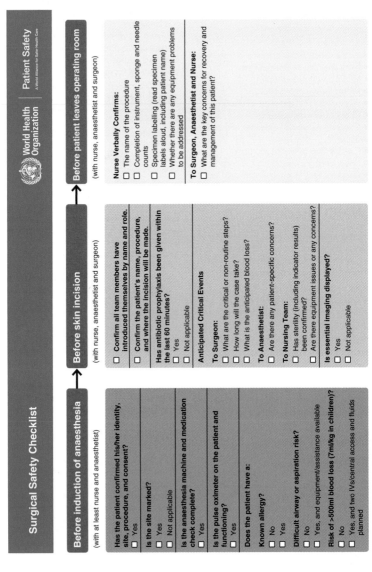

Surgical Safety Checklist

World Health Organization | Patient Safety
A World Alliance for Safer Health Care

Before induction of anaesthesia

(with at least nurse and anaesthetist)

Has the patient confirmed his/her identity, site, procedure, and consent?
☐ Yes

Is the site marked?
☐ Yes
☐ Not applicable

Is the anaesthesia machine and medication check complete?
☐ Yes

Is the pulse oximeter on the patient and functioning?
☐ Yes

Does the patient have a:

Known allergy?
☐ No
☐ Yes

Difficult airway or aspiration risk?
☐ No
☐ Yes, and equipment/assistance available

Risk of >500ml blood loss (7ml/kg in children)?
☐ No
☐ Yes, and two IVs/central access and fluids planned

Before skin incision

(with nurse, anaesthetist and surgeon)

☐ Confirm all team members have introduced themselves by name and role.

☐ Confirm the patient's name, procedure, and where the incision will be made.

Has antibiotic prophylaxis been given within the last 60 minutes?
☐ Yes
☐ Not applicable

Anticipated Critical Events

To Surgeon:
☐ What are the critical or non-routine steps?
☐ How long will the case take?
☐ What is the anticipated blood loss?

To Anaesthetist:
☐ Are there any patient-specific concerns?

To Nursing Team:
☐ Has sterility (including indicator results) been confirmed?
☐ Are there equipment issues or any concerns?

Is essential imaging displayed?
☐ Yes
☐ Not applicable

Before patient leaves operating room

(with nurse, anaesthetist and surgeon)

Nurse Verbally Confirms:
☐ The name of the procedure
☐ Completion of instrument, sponge and needle counts
☐ Specimen labelling (read specimen labels aloud, including patient name)
☐ Whether there are any equipment problems to be addressed

To Surgeon, Anaesthetist and Nurse:
☐ What are the key concerns for recovery and management of this patient?

© WHO, 2009

This checklist is not intended to be comprehensive. Additions and modifications to fit local practice are encouraged. Revised 1 / 2009

multiple co-morbidities, have a low threshold for admitting for inpatient prep or using a less aggressive preparation regime.

Thromboprophylaxis

Thromboprophylaxis is essential in the surgical setting. Patients who are immobile due to their operation and dehydrated from being NBM are prone to develop DVTs/PE. Encourage your patients to remain well hydrated by drinking plenty, and prescribe prophylactic LMWH:

■ Patients should stop taking anticoagulants at least a week before surgery unless they have a condition that requires continuous anticoagulation (e.g. patients with artificial heart valves). Patients with artificial heart valves or other conditions requiring continuous anticoagulation should be bridged with treatment-dose LMWH. These bridging plans are made in conjunction with haematologists, and so the patients may need to be seen in clinic prior to surgery. Some surgeons prefer not to operate on patients on aspirin. If aspirin needs to be stopped, it should be 7 days preoperatively, so remind the patient at any pre-admission clinic. The same is true of clopidogrel.

Oral contraception
■ The **BNF** recommends that people stop taking the oral contraceptive pill at least 4 weeks before major surgery. The pill does not

need to be stopped for minor surgery such as laparoscopic sterilization. Progestogen-only pills do not need to be stopped. In people who have stopped or have not been using contraception, exclude pregnancy with a formal pregnancy test.

Insulin
■ Diabetics may need to stop their regular anti-hypoglycaemics and be placed on an insulin sliding scale. The hospital pharmacist can advise you about this.

Insulin infusion

■ Draw up 50 units of short-acting insulin (e.g. Actrapid) in a 50 ml syringe and then fill the syringe with 50 ml of normal saline. This means that there is 1 unit of insulin per millilitre, allowing easy adjustment on the sliding scale shown in Table 15.2.
■ Label the syringe.
■ Make sure you check U&E at least once daily whilst the patient is on a sliding scale of insulin. Adjust K^+ accordingly.
■ Measure blood glucose regularly. If the capillary blood glucose is persistently >10 or constantly <4.0 mmol/l, modify the sliding scale.

Post-operative care

One of your most important roles on the wards will be management of post-operative patients. You will need a constant degree of

Table 15.2 Surgical protocols for people with diabetes.

	Minor surgery (eating same day)	Major surgery (not eating for several days)
Type II diabetes mellitus on oral agents	Omit morning hypoglycaemic drugs	Omit hypoglycaemic drugs Monitor blood glucose four times a day (QDS) Insulin sliding scale if uncontrolled glucose levels
Type I and II diabetes mellitus on insulin	Omit morning insulin Monitor blood glucose	Needs an insulin sliding scale until eating Return to usual insulin regime as soon as eating

suspicion for emerging complications, which may be directly related to surgery or indirect responses to the physiological stresses of surgery and anaesthesia (PE, hospital acquired pneumonia, MI, pain, drug reactions, atelectasis). As surgical ward rounds are typically fast paced, it is a good idea to do your own daily review of inpatients, running through the checklist below to ensure you do not miss any early signs of complications. Obtain senior help early if you detect any concerning features:

- Review the operation note:

  o What was done?
  o Any intraoperative complications?
  o Instructions for post-op care and follow-up?

- Ask about pain, nausea and vomiting, breathing difficulties, ability to eat and drink, bladder and bowel output and current mobility compared to baseline.
- Examine the wound site, chest, abdomen and legs (oedema, calf swelling).
- Look at drains, stomas, catheters, venous access lines, NG/NJ tubes and oxygen requirements:

  o Calculate input–output balance.
  o Document nature of output (e.g. drain content serous/sanguinous/purulent/bilious).

- Ask your seniors what level of drain output is sufficient for removal (e.g. <30 ml in 24 hours). All drains are a common source of sepsis, and you should aim to remove them as soon as appropriate – usually at 24 hours post-operation.

- Review the observation charts. Note tachycardia, pyrexia, BP changes and fluid balance.
- Review the drug chart:

  o Optimize analgesia and anti-emetic.
  o Prescribe IV fluids if needed.
  o Review antibiotics, response and duration of treatment.

- Check blood results:

  o Hb level – Is transfusion needed?
  o Electrolytes and renal function.
  o Inflammatory markers – look at the trend for sign of developing sepsis.
  o Procedure-specific bloods.

- Consider need for multidisciplinary input:

  o Physiotherapy for mobilization and respiratory exercises to avoid atelectasis and chest infection.
  o Occupational therapy and social services to begin discharge planning. This can often be a lengthy process so involve them early.

For the cause of post-operative pyrexia, consider the following 7 C's:

Chest (atelectasis, aspiration)
Cut (wound infection)
Catheter (UTI)
Cannula
Central line
Collection
Calves (DVT)

Wound checks

Wounds should ideally be examined daily. The risk of infection varies according to the type of procedure and contamination of the tissues involved.

Category	Description	Infection risk (%)
Clean	Incising uninfected skin without opening a viscus	<2
Clean–contaminated	Intraoperative breach of a viscus (but not colon)	8–10
Contaminated	Breach of a viscus + spillage OR breach of the colon	12–20
Dirty	Site already contaminated with pus/faeces/dirt (e.g. trauma)	25

Erythema of the wound may be a normal feature of healing but rapidly spreading erythema, induration, increased temperature and purulent discharge from the wound suggest developing infection. If cellulitis does occur, it is good practice to draw around the erythematous area and review progress daily. Ensure swabs are taken and sent for microscopy, culture, and sensitivity. Start empirical antibiotics without delay. Also be wary of the possibility of underlying serous, purulent or haemorrhagic collections that may require drainage and washout. Releasing staples or sutures in small parts of the wound is often the simplest, most reliable test you can do to check for a wound collection, but notify your seniors prior to doing this and have a low threshold for requesting an ultrasound scan for large or deep wounds.

Stoma care

• Patients with stomas usually have rigorous follow-up by Stoma Care Clinical Nurse Specialists. However, you will still be expected to assess stomas daily and monitor for features of complications. Patients can also be significantly distressed about new stomas, embarrassed about leaks, or unsure of changing regimens. Surgical nurses are usually good at helping with this, but you should familiarize yourself with the equipment used and normal post-operative behaviour of different stoma types.
• Stoma types: colostomy/ileostomy/urostomy/mucus fistula
• Common complications:

  ○ Electrolyte and fluid imbalance
  ○ Stoma ischaemia/necrosis
  ○ Obstruction
  ○ Prolapse
  ○ Parastomal hernia
  ○ Skin erosion/infection
  ○ Psychological distress, social implications for stoma care in community

• On a daily basis, you should **assess and document** the following:

  • Stoma colour + condition
  ○ Pink (healthy)
  ○ Dusky (poor venous outflow/impending ischaemia)
  ○ Black (necrotic)
  ○ Sloughy
  ○ Detached
  • Peristomal skin
  ○ Intact/broken
  ○ Erythematous
  ○ Wet/dry (if wet, is discharge serous/purulent?)
  • Functional status
  ○ No output
  ○ Flatus
  ○ Output contents: colour, viscosity, volume + over what time period
  • Hydration status

  ○ Observations
  ○ Electrolyte levels
  ○ Urine output

Enhanced recovery after surgery

Enhanced recovery has been described as a 'multi-modal, evidence-based, patient-centred method of optimising surgical outcome' (The 1000 Lives Plus ERAS mini-collaborative). It is essentially a structured perioperative programme for the rapid, accelerated recovery of patients undergoing major surgery, in whom day surgery is not appropriate. It has been shown to produce fitter patients who recover from surgery faster and report higher satisfaction rates. Thus far in the United Kingdom, ERAS programmes are established in colorectal, breast, urology, gynaecology, and orthopaedic surgery.

Important points that you should know about ERAS are outlined below, in the context of colorectal surgery:

Day of operation

• **Fasting**: 6 hours for solids and 2 hours for clear fluids.
• Review and **stop relevant medications**.
• **Preload IV fluid** 400 ml, 2–3 hours preoperatively.
• **Phosphate enema** 2 hours preoperatively (left-sided resections only).

- *Anaesthesia*: epidural/spinal/TAPP block.
- *Post-operatively*:

  o Sit out for 2 hours.
  o Oral fluids and diet as tolerated. Offer nutrient drinks if not tolerating solids.
  o Maintenance IV fluids (approximately 100 ml/hour).
  o *Thromboprophylaxis*: LMWH (e.g. clexane 20–40 mg SC), TEDS.

Post-operative day 1

- *Diet*: diet and fluids as tolerated. Offer nutrient drinks if not tolerating solids. Stop IV fluids if possible.
- *Analgesia*: epidural and oral (paracetamol 1 g QDS, ibuprofen 400 mg QDS, PRN tramadol 50–100 mg QDS).
- *Mobility*: 4 walks along length of ward.
- *Catheter*: out once mobile (except in low pelvic dissection).
- *Stoma*: start stoma care.
- *Bloods*: FBC, U&E and LFT.
- *Thromboprophylaxis.*

Post-operative day 2

- *Diet*: normal diet. Stop IV fluids if not done previously.
- *Analgesia*: epidural stopped (except in low pelvic dissection); bridge with PRN oramorph and continue oral analgesia.
- *Mobility*: 4 walks along length of ward.
- *Catheter*: out once mobile.
- *Stoma*: continue stoma care.
- *Bloods*: FBC and U&E.
- *Thromboprophylaxis.*

Post-operative day 3

- *Diet*: normal diet.
- *Analgesia*: oral only.
- *Mobility*: should be independently mobile, but continue as physiotherapist deems appropriate.
- *Catheter*: should be out.
- *Stoma*: learn and practise how to manage stoma independently.
- *Bloods*: FBC and U&E.
- *Thromboprophylaxis.*
- *Consider discharge.*

If the patient has progressed smoothly through the preceding steps, ensure the following criteria have been achieved prior to discharge:

- *Diet*: tolerating oral diet.
- *Analgesia*: pain well controlled with oral analgesia.
- *Mobility*: independently mobile.
- *Stoma*: able to manage stoma independently. Plan for outpatient review and support is in place.
- *Bloods*: acceptable results.

Theatre

Having worked tirelessly on all the above, there may still be opportunities during your surgical job to go to theatre. Even if you think you're not destined to be one of the 'cutters', there is great reward in seeing those patients you have meticulously prepared for theatre undergoing their procedure. It also allows you to put many of the ward patients into context, having seen the extent of surgery they underwent. You may also get the chance to learn some basic surgical skills, such as suturing, knot-tying and dressing application. These are guaranteed to come in use in your future posts, especially Emergency Medicine. If anything, it also affords you some valuable time with your consultant supervisors which, other than rapid sprints behind them on ward rounds and succinct e-portfolio meetings, can be very hard to come by.

Further reading

Andrews S., MRCS Core Modules: Essential Revision Notes, 2nd Edn. PasTest.

Brady M. C., Kinn S., Stuart P., Ness V. (2003), Preoperative fasting for adults to prevent perioperative complications. Cochrane Database of Systematic Reviews, Issue 4. Art. No.: CD004423. DOI: 10.1002/14651858.

Dunn D.C., Rawlinson N. (1999), Surgical Diagnosis and Management: A Guide to General Surgical Care. Blackwell Science, Oxford.

General Medical Council (2008), Consent: patients and doctors making decisions together. http://www.gmc-uk.org/guidance/

ethical_guidance/consent_guidance_index. asp (accessed on September 4, 2014).

NHS Improvement, Enhanced Recovery Partnership. http://www.improvement.nhs. uk/enhancedrecovery/ (accessed on September 4, 2014).

NICE Clinical Guideline 3 – Preoperative Tests, The use of routine preoperative tests for elective surgery (June 2003).

NPSA (2005), Patient Safety Alert 6, Pre-operative marking recommendations http://www.nrls.npsa.nhs.uk/resources/? entryid45=59799&p=15 (accessed on September 4, 2014).

The 1000 lives plus ERAS mini-collaborative. http://www.1000livesplus.wales.nhs. uk/eras (accessed on September 4, 2014).

WHO Surgical Safety Checklist, 1st Edn. (2008). http://www.who.int/patientsafety/ safesurgery/tools_resources/SSSL_ Checklist_finalJun08.pdf (accessed on September 4, 2014).

Chapter 16
GENERAL PRACTICE

General practice is a very different experience to hospital medicine. You will meet many new people and encounter all sorts of conditions. You may be exposed to a lot of uncertainty: strange skin rashes, lumps and bumps, aches and sprains, odd-sounding symptoms, to name a few. Do not be afraid to ask. The general practitioner (GP) partners know you are in training and are happy to review patients if you are unsure. Use the opportunity to learn – general practice is one of the few times where you have the privilege of being the sole trainee to several tutors, most of whom are keen to teach. Working in general practice can take some time to adjust to. There is a lot more reliance on clinical skills and picking up signs. Blood tests and imaging aren't always immediately available to you, which can be daunting at first. However, as you adapt to these challenges most people find that the job can be very rewarding.

What you can and cannot do

You can

■ Run your own surgeries and decide patient management independently.
■ Write and sign referral letters, but always write the name of the GP in charge of the patient underneath your name.
■ Perform any duty expected of a doctor that you are trained for and feel comfortable doing, for example, smear tests, minor surgery, adjusting medication.

You cannot

■ Sign legal documents, for example, prescriptions, sick notes and abortion certificates, whilst you are still 'preregistration'. Most GP rotations are now in your FY2 year, when this no longer applies.

Referral letters and note keeping

The most important thing is to write referral letters as soon as possible after seeing patients. Practice notes are much briefer than hospital notes, so they may not provide sufficient detail for referral letters weeks later. Some GP computer systems allow you to generate a referral letter from your consultation documentation. This is a really easy way to write a referral letter, as all the relevant information is available when the patient's history is still fresh in your mind.

General points

■ Stick to a simple format:

  o The first line should tell the specialty team exactly what is wrong, for example, 'Thank you for seeing this 17-year-old girl with recurrent bouts of tonsillitis'.
  o The next line/s should provide a brief summary of the history and a summary of any relevant examination findings.
  o The last paragraph should clearly state what you would like the consultant to do, for example, 'I would be grateful if you could therefore consider this woman for tonsillectomy'. Note the wording; you can ask but never tell another professional what to do. In other cases you may simply be seeking their specialist opinion 'I would be

The Hands-on Guide to the Foundation Programme, Fifth Edition. Anna Donald, Michael Stein, Ciaran Scott Hill and Selina J Chavda.
© 2015 John Wiley & Sons, Ltd. Published 2015 by John Wiley & Sons, Ltd.

grateful if you could give me your opinion about…'.
o Always send a list of their medications with the letter.

Public health and health promotion

The most common public health and health promotion matters you are likely to encounter are as follows:

■ *Contraception.* You need to be able to discuss the pros and cons of the different kinds of contraception in detail with any woman over the age of 16 and any Gillick[1] – competent female below 16 who asks for advice, especially the oral contraceptive pill (one of the most common consultations). There are multiple different kinds, each containing different hormones.

The combined oral contraceptive pill contains oestrogen and progesterone. The combined pill is usually given to younger women but can be given to women up to the age of 50. Most GPs use the combined oral contraceptive pill (COCP) in women under 35. In general, you should use a pill with the lowest concentration of both hormones that gives the patient effective contraception and regulation of menstrual cycles.

There are several issues you must address when starting a patient on the COCP.

As with all patients it is important to take a history and then perform an examination.

Make sure the following points are covered:

• Sexual health and sexually transmitted infection (STI) risks.
• Reproductive health.
• Any regular medications including herbal remedies that may affect absorption of the COCP.
• Compliance with medication and previous use of COCP or other contraception.

[1] Gillick v West Norfolk and Wisbech Area Health Authority [1985] 3 All ER 402 (HL) states parental right to determine whether or not their minor child below the age of 16 will have medical treatment is terminated if and when the child has competence to make the decision in question, that is, is able to weigh, understand and retain the information, make a decision based on this and communicate this decision to the healthcare provider.

• History of migraines.
• Smoking history.
• Venous thromboembolism (VTE) risks.
• BMI.
• BP monitoring – the COCP is contraindicated in patients with a BP persistently greater than 140/90.

The patient should then be counselled on the risks and benefits of using the COCP, so that they can make an informed decision.

Risks

• Use of COCP will prevent pregnancy but not STIs including HIV and so a second method of barrier contraception is advised, such as condoms.
• The risk of VTE increases by fivefold when on the COCP.
• There is a very small absolute increased risk of stroke but no absolute increased risk of myocardial infarction (MI).
• After 5 years of using the COCP, the risk of cervical cancer increases.
• The risk of breast cancer increases with use of the COCP but this is small.

Benefits

• Protects against pregnancy
• No evidence that use of COCP causes weight gain
• Protects from endometrial cancer
• Reduces risk of ovarian Ca and ovarian cysts
• Reduces menstrual pain and blood loss by menstruation
• Regulates menstrual cycles

If the patient gives her consent, prescribe a 4-week pack and ask for her to come back in for a check-up thereafter to review use of pill, BP, compliance and side effects. There are multiple different types of pills, so if one does not agree with the patient reassure them and prescribe a different pill.

The mini pill or POP (progesterone only pill) tends to be used in women over the age of 35 who smoke or who have hypertension or VTE risks and so cannot use the COCP. The issues with this pill are that they have to be taken at the same time every day, as missing pills or taking pills as little as 3 hours late could make the contraception ineffective. For this reason, they are much less popular than the COCP.

There are multiple other forms of contraception that you can offer to patients. A brief list is presented in the following. For more information visit the following NHS website: http://www.nhs.uk/Conditions/contraception-guide/Pages/contraception.aspx

Condoms

There are both male and female condoms available in an array of shapes, sizes, colours and flavours. Condoms are a form of barrier contraception and prevent pregnancy in 98% of cases, as well as preventing transmission of STIs such as gonorrhoea and chlamydia. Importantly, they also protect against transmission of HIV. Free condoms are available from the local GUM clinic. Condoms are usually made from latex, but latex-free versions are also available. Always advise patients that condoms can only be used once and if they slip off during intercourse should not be reused. Similarly, all condoms have a sell by date on them, and out-of-date condoms should not be used.

Intrauterine system

This is a long-term type of contraception. A coil-releasing progesterone is inserted into the uterus by a healthcare professional. The progesterone causes thickening of the cervical mucus, preventing sperm from reaching the ova, and in some women prevents ovulation. It is more than 99% effective at preventing pregnancy. Other benefits include reducing heavy menstrual bleeding (some females stop menstruating all together) and can be fitted at any time during the menstrual cycle. 'Spotting' or irregular menstrual bleeding can occur however, and it does not protect against STIs, so advise patients to also use barrier contraception. There is a small risk of ectopic pregnancy with this device if the patient does become pregnant, so always warn your patient about this.

Intrauterine device

This is also known as the copper coil and is another type of long-term contraception. They are more than 99% effective. Intrauterine devices last for 5–10 years once inserted. Unfortunately, they can make periods longer, heavier and more painful. They do not protect against STIs and there is an increased risk of ectopic pregnancy if the patient does become pregnant. They are usually not suitable in patients who have had pelvic inflammatory disease in the past.

Contraceptive injection

Contraceptive injections contain progesterone. There are two types – Depo-Provera which lasts 12 weeks or Noristerat which lasts 8 weeks. It is useful for women with poor compliance or those who forget to take the pill. It is more than 99% effective. The injection gives no protection against STIs so barrier contraception should be used. Common side effects include weight gain, breast tenderness, mood swings and irregular bleeding. Amenorrhea is also a possible side effect. Unfortunately, these side effects last as long as the injection does and some side effects can persist after as well. Patients on long-term Depo-Provera are at increased risk of osteoporosis in the long term, and patients should be counselled on this.

Contraceptive implants

This is a plastic tube about 4 cm in length that is inserted subcutaneously commonly in the upper arm. It is a form of long-term contraception and provides protection for 3 years at least. It is therefore not a good form of contraception for patients who are thinking of conceiving in the near future, as fertility can be affected for a few months after the implant is removed. The implant continuously releases progesterone to prevent ovulation and causes mucous thickening within the cervix. It does not protect against STIs and should be used in conjunction with barrier contraception.

Smoking

Actively encourage patients to stop smoking and offer them as much advice and support as you can. This may include patches, gum or just a friendly chat when willpower is fading. Be aware of smoking cessation clinics and other local services available such as text message services.

Lifestyle advice

This is important, particularly for preventing coronary heart disease. You can offer advice about diet, alcohol and exercise. Thirty minutes of exercise a day can make a big difference to a patient with cardiovascular risk factors. This can be simple things like walking briskly home rather than taking the bus or getting off a stop earlier than the patient would usually. Encourage overweight patients to lose weight and explain the potential long-term health problems. Referral to the practice dietician can also be helpful.

Notifiable diseases

Ask practice staff for a form with a list of notifiable diseases. The most common is food poisoning. The important thing to remember when filling out these forms is the person's work address, or name and address of any school or institution they are attending. This helps keep track of outbreaks.

Vaccinations

Flu jabs should be offered to all people who are 65 years old or older, as well as those with immunosuppression or chronic illness such as heart failure, asthma and COPD. Pneumococcal vaccines are currently offered for people older than 75, patients with splenectomies and those with chronic illnesses such as COPD and heart failure, but are not used routinely for people with asthma. Immunizations for children are usually performed by the practice nurse or health visitors, but you may need to give them too.

Breast screening

You are rarely involved in routine screening. You do, however, need to be confident in breast examination and be aware of the local facilities offered, such as one-stop breast clinics. Between ages 50 and 70, a mammogram screening test is offered every 3 years, and females over 70 can continue screening but need to 'opt in'. Current NICE guidance states that those with a moderate to severe family history should be tested from their 40s. The evidence for women picking up breast lumps on self-examination is poor so if indicated you should perform the examination or refer to a one-stop breast clinic where they will receive triple investigation with history, examination and ultrasound scan/mammogram. The NHS screening protocol for breast cancer is currently undergoing change with digital mammography use being extended into a wider age range (47–73). This is likely to be complete by 2016.

Cervical screening

Cervical screening is common in general practice. Women eligible are those between 25 and 64. It is your job to encourage any women who are overdue their smear to book an appointment (you will usually be prompted by the desktop computer). Cervical smears are repeated every 3 years between ages 25 and 49 then every 5 years between ages 50 and 64. Smears in the eligible age range are free. Those over the age of 65 are normally only eligible for a smear if they have had a recent abnormal result or have not been screened since age 50. The technique used now is liquid-based cytology, and this has replaced the traditional Pap smear. Early detection can prevent 75% of cervical cancers. Cervical cancer is strongly linked to human papilloma virus (HPV). Therefore the chance of developing it is very small (but not zero) if a woman has never been sexually active. Pilot screening for HPV by cervical smear is currently being undertaken in the United Kingdom.

■ All girls aged 12–13 are now being offered HPV vaccination in the United Kingdom

(Gardasil). It protects against HPV strains 16 and 18, and these account for around 70% of all cervical cancers, and it is thought that this scheme will save around 400 lives a year. This vaccine is offered in secondary schools and delivered over 12 months in a course of three injections.

Sexual health

With the numerous GUM clinics around, you may not encounter many people with sexual health issues. However, you should remember to promote safe sex and remind anyone who is considering non-barrier contraception that it will not protect them from STIs.

The hidden agenda and health beliefs

What a patient presents with may not be what is really bothering them. The most common example is depression. Depression can manifest as a variety of physical conditions. Be alert to people who keep returning with seemingly minor ailments. To give people the opportunity to reveal their real underlying concern, try the following:

■ Asking if there is anything more they would like to tell you
■ Asking why they feel they are not getting better
■ Allowing for a longer consultation (many GPs operate on a 7–10 minutes appointment slot although trainees should be allocated more time)

You will also encounter people from different social and cultural backgrounds with different health beliefs to yours. To avoid mistrust and dissatisfaction with your care, try:

■ Explaining clearly your diagnosis and why you are treating them as you are.
■ Asking what the person expects or would like.
■ Providing leaflets and information explaining their condition and what they should expect. This is more realistic, as time is not always sufficient for a verbal explanation and people rarely remember everything you tell

them. NHS Choices (www.nhs.uk) has a fairly comprehensive and well-written encyclopaedia (Health A–Z) for most conditions.

The key to dealing with both issues is being alert to people with repeat attendances or strange symptoms, and to allow people to talk. Ask open questions and let them lead the consultation. A good way to see this being done well is to sit in on a consultation with one of the senior GPs and see how they handle the issue. You can then use the skills you saw being demonstrated to you in your own consultations.

Follow-up

One of the main differences and benefits of general practice is that you get to follow-up most patients. This provides good continuity of care for patients and gives you the satisfaction of seeing your treatment working. Always tell people to come back if things do not improve. Sometimes, the only way to realize that trivial symptoms are part of a bigger illness is when those symptoms persist. There are some people, however, whom you should insist return for a follow-up appointment. These include:

■ Depressed or anxious people who are starting medication. At first, you should only give them 28 days of antidepressants and follow them up 2 weeks after starting treatment to see if their symptoms are improving. You should review them again 2 weeks after this, before issuing a repeat prescription. Further follow-ups can be monthly or less frequent if you feel they are stable on their current medications.
■ Women on the oral contraceptive pill (OCP) should have their blood pressure checked every 6 months before offering a repeat prescription. Some specialist family planning clinics may extend this to 12 months if the patient has been taking the pill without concern for several repeats. Also remember that when starting somebody on the OCP for the first time or when changing to a different brand, they should only be given 3 months supply and reviewed before a further prescription is given.

■ Hypertension. Any person with a single high BP reading should have at least two further readings before being diagnosed as hypertensive. Give lifestyle advice and arrange tests for end-organ damage. Any confirmed hypertensive patients started on medications should have their BP checked monthly at least.

■ Diabetics. Because BP, lipid and arterial risk factor checks are performed annually, you will probably not follow these patients up during a short stint in general practice. If the BP or lipid profile is abnormal you will need to bring the person back for earlier repeat testing or intervention.

Home visits

Most home visits will either be to people who are housebound, in residential/nursing homes or with chronic illnesses. They can be a bit daunting at first. Try reading the person's notes beforehand to understand their medical problems.

■ Make sure the home visit is warranted before setting out. Find out why they cannot come to the surgery. Some diagnoses might be clear cut from the phone and warrant hospital admission, such as suspicion of an MI, or some visits may simply be for prescriptions which can be done and left at the reception for a relative to pick up.

■ Don't forget your equipment. You never know what you are going to face on a home visit so be prepared with your kit, for example, thermometer, stethoscope, sats probe, BP monitor, emergency meds, otoscope.

■ Be safe. As you will be travelling alone and going into people's homes, make sure that the practice knows where you are and you have a mobile phone in case of an emergency.

■ If you have any concerns that the patient is acutely unwell, discuss with your seniors and refer the patient to the local emergency department. If you are happy, always arrange a follow-up appointment to ensure that the patient is improving with the treatments you have instigated. Providing the patient with a 'safety net' in terms of either further follow-up or a plan in case of deterioration is vital.

Chapter 17
SELF-CARE

How are doctors supposed to take care of patients if they don't take care of themselves? If you overwork yourself consistently sooner or later you will experience burnout. Most of us are not taught much about self-care in medical school. Look after yourself and become a better doctor in the process.

Accommodation

Sadly, the days of doctors being provided with free on-site accommodation are at an end. This used to be available because doctors were resident on-site for long periods of time. However, many hospitals still offer accommodation at favourable rates. Living in hospital accommodation is a good way to meet people that you could rent with at a later date. It is also likely to be within walking distance to the hospital. This may not sound important now but after a week of long shifts the 45 minute commute into work may seem far less tolerable. If a hospital offers accommodation, it must comply with national regulations governing minimum acceptable standards which are non-negotiable:

■ Your room should contain a 3-by-6 foot bed, telephone, cupboards, drawers, desk, chair, washbasin, be carpeted and have curtains. It should be heated and regularly cleaned.
■ There should be a nearby bathroom and toilet, cooking facilities, a common room and on-site laundry facilities. Common areas should be regularly cleaned.

If you have a specific problem with your quarters, contact the designated 'accommodation officer' or equivalent through switchboard.

There are often websites advertising rooms for rent or check the noticeboard as there are often adverts for rooms to rent.

When you are at registrar level then depending on your speciality you may be contractually allowed to rest/sleep during on calls. However, as a junior doctor this is unlikely to be the case and most trusts stance is that you should not be sleeping at night. So if you decide to rest in an empty on-call room, be aware that this may be against the trust policy. It is not uncommon for a junior to have gotten into hot water when found by the matron or security asleep! Similarly, be extremely careful about leaving the hospital grounds whilst on call unless specific cover has been agreed. Remember that patient care is your first priority so do not put yourself in a situation where you cannot deal with an emergency should it arise.

Alternative careers

What if you have come all this way and decide that you don't want to be a doctor? Or you like it, but not enough to dedicate your life to it? Little known to many medics, having a medical degree opens many great doors. Chekhov, JPR Williams, Graham Chapman,

The Hands-on Guide to the Foundation Programme, Fifth Edition. Anna Donald, Michael Stein,
Ciaran Scott Hill and Selina J Chavda.
© 2015 John Wiley & Sons, Ltd. Published 2015 by John Wiley & Sons, Ltd.

Harry Hill, Che Guevara and Keats were all once doctors – to name a few:

■ Medical training gives you multiple skills that you probably never even noticed. These include leadership, managerial, communicating, teamworking and observational skills; analytic, mechanical, adversarial skills; and the ability to work within a hierarchy and still get what you want. Sheer endurance and persistence (much prized in the workforce), great people skills and many other talents can be developed through medicine. Never think that these are wasted in a 'non-medical' career. Having medical training will enable you to bring something special to whatever you do.

■ However, *in general*, we would advise completing your Foundation Programme before saying goodbye to medicine. Many people find that they enjoy working more than being a student and having full registration is useful if you ever wish to work in the future.

■ Do not underestimate the breadth of careers available in medicine. Medicine is probably one of the few careers that gives you flexibility to work anywhere in the world, as the skills you have are translational. You can do helicopter mountain rescue in France, research anticancer drugs for pharmaceutical companies in Australia, enjoy office-based occupational health in Dubai, be a sports physician for Olympic athletes or work at the cutting edge of forensic pathology in New York. A good book for inspiration is the *Medic's Guide to Work and Electives Around the World* by Mark Wilson.

Bleep

■ Pick up your bleep from switchboard. They will replace the batteries and exchange it for a new one if it breaks.

■ Leave your bleep on the ward and switch it off if you are not on call, as switchboard may call you even when you are off-duty. If you live nearby or on hospital accommodation, this is especially important, as otherwise you may get a rude awakening in the middle of the night by your bleep going off!

British Medical Association

Becoming a member of the British Medical Association (BMA) not only brings you the *BMJ* with adverts for professional courses but also provides advice and support in all areas of your work, leave, contracts, tax and financial planning. It is also a negotiating body on behalf of all doctors and is definitely worth the subscription costs. The *BMJ* is an excellent journal in its own right, it is one of the easiest to browse with its almost magazine-like approach, but it also has summaries of up-to-date research that the *BMJ* has published that week. Specific benefits of membership include:

1 Personal advice on contracts and terms of service, which DO reap benefits and occasional upbanding, particularly if you are proactive about investigating your contractual terms.

2 Assistance and representation in disagreements with hospital management. This is becoming more important as trusts and management try to change contracts and reduce pay. For example, the BMA has threatened court action against trust management that has tried to cut pay, now protected under the New Deal terms. The BMA can assist with claims for overtime and additional hours. Simply the knowledge that you are a member of a strong representative organization can often support your case in disagreements.

3 Independent financial advice by salaried representatives on pensions, income protection, etc.

4 Insurance services. The personal contents policy is particularly useful.

5 The fee is tax deductible.

Car insurance

You may buy your first car during your first year. Whilst you may need to purchase it in July just prior to moving to your new job, cars are most expensive around July–August. Most people know where they will be working from January to February, so if you have the funds and the time, consider buying a car around January/February, when you are much more likely to pick up a bargain.

Car insurance varies a lot. The BMA offers insurance for doctors, but it may be more expensive than you need, particularly if you have bought an old car. Probably the best thing to do is to ring local brokers who deal with many different insurance firms and who can get you the best deal for the cover you need. Alternatively, a thorough Internet search is a good way forwards. Many firms give a discount for female drivers. Be aware that you can purchase third-party insurance, fire and theft, if your car is not valuable although this may not build your 'no-claims' discount, an important factor in reducing the eventual costs of insurance.

Clothes (laundry/stains)

■ Smart clothes are often touted as helping maintain professional demeanour; this is particularly so since white coats and suits are no longer in line with current infection control guidelines. If your trust has a policy on their professional dress code, be careful not to fall foul of it; these things are rarely worth getting into hot water about. Generally, don't show too much skin, have comfortable shoes, and don't wear too much flashy jewellery.

Contacting medical colleagues

After graduation, all doctors are entered into the UK *Medical Directory*. This is a reasonably reliable way of tracking down friends from medical school and beyond. The *Directory* is available in hospital libraries and also from the General Medical Council (GMC) nearest you. You can search the register at the GMC website, www.gmc-uk.org. There are now Internet services dedicated to doctors which can supply doctors with contact details of colleagues who have also subscribed. Alternatively, there are lots of professional websites such as Linked In that are popular with doctors to keep in contact. Beware of breaking patient confidentiality on these websites – keep things strictly about yourself and your career.

Contract and conditions of service

Doctors' working conditions are negotiated by the Junior Doctors' Committee. More recently, the Junior Doctors' agreement has altered the rates at which overtime is paid and stipulated the maximum hours for which you can be contracted to work. All hospitals, including trusts, have to abide by these nationally agreed guidelines.

What you need to know about your contract

Your contract is a binding agreement, regulating your hours and conditions of service, pay, holiday and notice. It cannot be altered unilaterally by either you or your employer. In particular, pay protection means that your pay cannot be cut from the time of accepting the job, even if the banding of the job changes. Having a contract is essential to ensure you are on the right pay grade.

Rotas
Virtually all junior doctors now work a full-shift rota with additional duty periods every few days (e.g. 1 in 5), meaning that they work a 40 hour working week and are also on duty every fifth night and/or every fifth weekend. Contracts stipulate the maximum number of hours you work, the amount and type of rest breaks you are entitled to during your working day and the amount of time you must have off, depending on your pay banding.

■ It is important not to get confused by colloquial use of the term 'on call' for full-shift duty periods. This is erroneous as it implies you are entitled to sleep during the duty periods.
■ Prospective cover means that when colleagues are away on holiday, the remaining junior doctors cover the duty periods the missing colleague would have done. This works out equitably if everyone takes the same amount of holiday. Virtually all contracts stipulate that you cover your colleagues if they are sick. This provision does not give authorities the power to force you to cover

foreseen and notified absences such as annual leave. Similarly, you cannot be forced into doing extra night shifts to cover those that call in sick. It is not a problem if the trust offers you locum rates or pays you at the usual rate, but ensure that you do get the money back. Alternatively, if you cannot work the extra hours, the trust is required to get a locum to cover. Do not cave to pressure from rota coordinators or bullying if you are unable to work. See Table 17.1 for information of the New Deal for Doctors regarding shift patterns.

Working time monitoring

This is a mandatory obligation of your contract. At least twice a year, your medical personnel department will run a diary card monitoring exercise over a period of 2 weeks, where the junior doctors on the same rota will be required to document what they do in hourly time slots. You need to write down on the diary card the time that you started work and the time that you left. You will be asked to write down the number of breaks you had and the duration. This is to ascertain whether the post meets European Working Time Directive requirements and also to determine the amount of pay you get. That alone should be an incentive to take part! The diary card monitoring exercise can be online or a paper exercise. The European Working Time Directive has stipulated a maximum of 56 working hours per week that was cut down to 48 in 2008 (see Table 17.2):

Table 17.1 New Deal hours.

Rotation pattern	Maximum period of continuous work (hours)	Minimum period off duty between work periods (hours)	Minimum continuous period of duty
Full shift	14	8	48 hours + 62 hours in 28 days
Partial shift	16	8	48 hours + 62 hours in 28 days
On-call rota	32 (56 hours at weekend)	12	48 hours + 62 hours in 21 days

Table 17.2 European Working Time Directive.

Maximum working time per week of 56 hours

- Working time is defined as any period during which doctors are working, at their employers' disposal and carrying out their activity or duties, and any period during which they are receiving relevant training. This includes time when resident in hospital on call (even if asleep)

The rest requirements which came into effect in August 2004 are as follows:

- A minimum daily consecutive period of 11 hours

- A minimum rest break of 20 minutes when the working day exceeds 6 hours

- A minimum rest period of 24 hours in each 7-day period (this can be averaged to be a 48 hour rest period in 14 days)

- For occasions when working time is in excess, compensatory rest must be taken immediately following the period of work which it is supposed to counteract (i.e. before commencing the next period of work)

A minimum of 4 weeks' paid annual leave

■ Monitoring exercises should not be viewed as 'checking up' on you. They are your chance to demonstrate the commitments of your job and get the remuneration you deserve. Never allow yourself to be pressurized into lying on them; you must stand up for what you deserve. It is a good way to get the trust to realize the real hours you work, especially if you are regularly staying late on the ward.

■ There is no need to document exactly what you are doing in each time slot period, just simply whether you are working, resting, eating or studying. Answering a bleep is considered work or simple administrative task. Anything requiring you to be in the hospital should be considered work and must be documented accordingly.

■ It is not your individual working time in a particular week that needs to be in line with the European Working Time Directive. It is the average weekly working time for all the junior doctors on the same rota and in order for changes to be made, at least 75% of junior doctors need to complete the exercise for it to be valid. It is therefore worth completing even if you are working 'normal' hours to help initiate change for your colleagues.

■ Monitoring exercises need not be initiated by the medical personnel department. This is significant if there is a dispute over working time arrangements or the running of the exercise. All you need to do is print diary sheets and distribute one to every doctor on the same rota and get them to fill it in. You can request monitoring at any time. It is best to do it when there are enough juniors on the ward to make the exercise valid.

Pay

National Health Service (NHS) doctors' rates of pay are agreed nationally by the Doctors and Dentists' Review Body, which negotiates the annual pay increase each April. Your pay is calculated on the basis of a banding system. The banding system takes into consideration the type of rota worked, the duration and intensity of out-of-hours work. Your band dictates the supplement received for out-of-hours work as a multiple of your basic salary. Junior doctors in general practice who have an out-of-hours commitment receive an additional 22.5% over and above basic salary regardless of the duration or frequency of that commitment. The BMA website (bma.org.uk) features a band calculator, allowing you to check that your employer is complying with national requirements (see Table 17.3). Alternatively, if you have concerns over your rota and feel the banding does not comply with your rota, you can send the BMA a copy of your rota and ask them to check to see if it is compliant with the EWTD and corresponds to your banding:

■ Your band is specified in your contract. The band allocation is based on the previous working time monitoring exercise, which should be done twice yearly.

Table 17.3 Banding.

Banding	Pay multiple	Description
'Unbanded'	0	<48 hours per week, sociable hours
1A	1.5	<48 hours per week, high proportion of antisocial hours
1B	1.4	<48 hours per week, low proportion of antisocial hours
1C	1.2	<48 hours per week, non-resident on calls
2A	1.8	48–56 hours per week, high proportion of antisocial hours
2B	1.5	48–56 hours per week, low proportion of antisocial hours
3	2.0	>56 hours per week, insufficient rest (few of these jobs now remain)

Note: Pay protection does not protect Band 3 pay, but it only protects up to Band 2A.

■ Whilst the odd hour here or there probably does not warrant special overtime claims, if you are systematically working extra hours (e.g. by starting at 8 a.m. instead of 9 and finishing at 7 p.m. instead of 5), then do not feel ashamed to ask for pay for honest work that you have done. This is best achieved through a working time monitoring exercise rather than an individual claim.

■ Your salary is protected such that even if your banding changes during the time you are working, your monthly salary cannot drop below the banding when you signed your contract. The only exception is Band 3, which is only protected up to Band 2A should the job be down-banded by a monitoring exercise.

Holiday

Junior doctors are entitled to 9 days of annual leave per 4-month rotation, excluding bank holidays:

■ Do not carry leave forwards, unless exceptional circumstances arise. You are likely to lose the annual leave days and won't be paid for the extra days you have worked! If you do have extenuating circumstances, contact personnel both at your current hospital and your future place of work to try to ensure you are granted the extra leave.

■ Leave can be supplemented by 'in lieu' days. Over the year you are likely to work several bank holidays and statutory hospital holidays. You can take a day off 'in lieu' of each holiday worked.

■ Find out the procedure for booking leave early. It may involve simply informing your consultant and his or her secretary, or there may be specific forms to be filled in and signed by your consultant (more likely). Liaise with the rota coordinator early to ensure you get the time off and swaps you want.

Notice

Junior doctors only need to give 2 weeks' notice of their intention to leave their post. However, to be eligible for full GMC registration you need to have completed 12 months as an FY1 doctor. Although rare, it is not unheard of for trainees to be given notice if the employing hospital is cutting back staff. In

this unfortunate circumstance, you will need to discuss the situation with your educational supervisor, the deanery and your representative union, for example, the BMA.

Leave

Compassionate leave

In the event of family or personal bereavement, up to 72 hours paid leave will usually be given. Tell your consultant as soon as possible and the rota coordinator. If there is any difficulty, talk to your clinical tutor and personnel and if necessary escalate the situation to your educational supervisor or the medical director.

Maternity (and paternity) leave

Regulations and rates of parental leave are complex, depending on how long you have worked and whether you intend to return to work. New female doctors are unlikely to have worked for more than 1 year and, therefore, are allowed only 18 weeks' unpaid leave. By comparison, doctors who have worked for longer than 1 year are entitled to 8 weeks' full pay, 10 weeks' half pay and up to 34 weeks of additional leave, to a total absence of 52 weeks. Doctors who have not declared intention to return to work receive fewer benefits.

■ If you or your partner is pregnant or considering it, discuss the options for leave fully with your personnel department or the BMA beforehand.

■ The United Kingdom now has up to 2 weeks paid paternity leave as an entitlement for employees. However, if you are an expectant father and need more time off, it is worth discussing with your employer and the BMA. They may be able to add on your annual leave or lieu days that can be worked at a later date.

Study leave

Preregistration (F1) doctors are not usually allocated study leave other than time during the working day to attend clinical and pathology meetings. Post-registration doctors are entitled to 30 days of study leave per year. Note that in many trusts this is not the actual time you can take off though. For example, 10 days may be automatically allocated to 'generic teaching' during bleep-free time on a given afternoon. A further 10 days may be allocated as 'taster weeks' that can be spent gaining experience in specialties you are interested in. The final 10 days are in theory for you to use as you wish (courses, conferences, etc.) – however, many foundation schools will not have allocated study leave for activities that fall outside of the rather narrow range of appointed 'foundation competencies'. Instead, it is likely to be divided into 5 days for 'external' study leave for courses and conferences and 5 days for internal study leave to attend clinics or teaching.

Study leave can be somewhat of a battle to get, so get your requests in as early as possible. Study leave tends to be easier to get for exams so be specific when you apply.

Sick leave

Physical illness: It is still the case in most hospitals that if you are sick, your colleagues must cover for you in addition to doing their own jobs. Because of this very few doctors will tell you to go home or not to come in. If you are struggling to keep up with your tasks, *just go home* rather than make a mistake potentially and cause harm to patients because you are unwell. You are doing nobody any favours by lurking around shedding your virus and if you are caring for neutropenic or immunosuppressed patients you may make them very unwell. That said, sick leave for hangovers is always unacceptable and unfair to your colleagues.

Mental illness: If you are struggling with mental burnout (depression, serious anxiety, grief or the emotional weight of your job) it is very important that you get help and rest. Mental fatigue and illness is common amongst doctors yet so little spoken about. It is also a cause of long-term absence and loss of self-esteem which can be avoided.

Prolonged illness: Even if you fall ill on the first day of work and cannot work again, you are still entitled to sick pay equal to your full salary for 1 month. After this, you will receive the usual state benefits. After completing 4-month full-time work, a junior doctor is entitled to 1 month of full pay and 2 months of half pay. If you fall ill towards the end of the

contract and the illness continues after the time when you would have finished, you are entitled to continued sick pay as long as the illness lasts or until you have had all the sick pay you are entitled to.

If you have trouble with illness of any kind, consider doing the following:

■ Tell someone who loves you that you are sick/in trouble. They can help you summon up the courage to take time off and get help.

■ See the hospital occupational health team or your general practitioner (GP). They can help you medically and psychologically. They will give you any documentation you need (e.g. sick notes) and may be able to speak with your seniors if necessary. You are obliged to tell your consultant that you are sick (after 3 days of absence). Unlike more junior colleagues, your consultant won't suffer directly if you take time off and will probably be sympathetic. If needed, they can also help organize cover for your absence.

■ Learn to care for yourself now and it will serve you throughout your life. This is preferable to a heart attack or depression or worst of all leaving the NHS because you cannot cope anymore.

■ Occupational health requirements

■ Hospitals recommend that you register with a local GP or give them details of your own GP if within the same city.

■ On arrival at the hospital, the Occupational Health Department will ask about your immunization record. Try and keep a copy of this in a memorable place; you will change jobs a lot and life will be simpler. Alternatively, ask occupational health for a copy of all your screening tests and use this when you change trusts.

■ Ask Occupational Health to check your hepatitis B immunity, which may have dramatically declined since immunization as a student. It should be around '100%' although a portion of the population will always be 'non-responders'. If you do become infected with active hepatitis B, you cannot be a surgeon or a specialist who does invasive work.

■ Contact the Occupational Health Department if you are ill for longer than 3 days. They will clear you for sick leave and may well give you help in the meantime.

Doctors' mess

The doctors' mess may be a scruffy room strewn with old newspapers and coffee cups or a comfortable lounge with a coffee machine, satellite TV and a PlayStation. Some hospitals do not even have a mess any longer! Most messes run with a Mess President, Secretary and Treasurer and a variable number of committee members. It is great to get to know colleagues and makes work so much more enjoyable!

Making money for the mess

■ Hold a party that requires payment for entry or tickets. Have free drinks before 8.30 p.m. to make sure everyone arrives early, or no one will come until the pubs close.
- Alternatively, hold a ball (Christmas, spring, summer, Halloween) and use this to raise money.

■ Ask doctors to make a regular deduction from their salary and arrange this with personnel. Many now have an automatic contribution taken from doctors' wage slip although people may opt out.

Insurance (room contents)

Probably the best room contents' insurance against theft and damage is BMA-arranged insurance, because it is designed specifically for junior doctors. Other policies may not have plans appropriate for your unusual living situation and generally cost much more. If you have time you can shop around online.

Jobs

■ Network. Tell your consultant what you're hoping to do next. If you are set on a particular job or hospital, ask the consultant if he or she knows anyone there. Do not underestimate the importance of getting your face known and having a good reputation. Such

brownie-points are also valuable for future career options.

■ Choose your referees carefully. One is usually the consultant you are currently working for. Well-known professors and consultants add a little weight to your list – provided you actually know them well enough for them to write something personal about you. Do not be afraid to ask to see your reference before it is sent. This is not easy but is very important. Always ask more consultants to be your referees than needed, then if one lets you down or writes a poor reference for you, you will always have a backup.

■ Application form. Make sure you get the basics right. If it asks to be typed or printed in a specific format, do it. Include whatever is requested. Don't jeopardize your chances at this early stage. Consider using recorded or registered delivery. Many application forms are now done online. Make sure you submit at least several days in advance as the portal often freezes or stops working the day before the deadline due to sheer volume of submissions.

■ I cannot overemphasize the importance of planning ahead when you decide on your specialty. See the form at least 6 months before you apply and ensure you tick those boxes.

Curriculum vitae

It is probably easiest to type out your curriculum vitae (CV) yourself, so you can make small changes as necessary. Use high-quality paper. Keep your CV up to date. It is much easier to add a course on an ad hoc basis rather than having to add large numbers of conferences, courses and presentations in one go.

Make sure you meticulously spellcheck and proofread your CV. Misspellings are unlikely to be forgiven. Never write anything on your CV that is not true. Beware of bending the truth, as the consequences might well be disastrous:

■ Make the most of your experience, listing skills you have acquired and responsibilities you have taken. Don't forget skills such as computing and languages. Make sure you include honours or prizes; depending on your stage and CV this may include those from school:

- Try to be concrete in demonstrating what you have done. For example, instead of saying 'Running', you might specify your running activities: 'Participation in Anglia regional running events, club secretary'. Your skill or interest can be something simple such as volunteering. You don't have to have climbed Mount Everest!

■ When applying for a post-registration job, it also helps to sell yourself and your clinical experience. The demonstration of experience is now largely displayed by logbooks and DOPS (direct observation of procedural skills) but there is still a place for this on most CVs.

■ Show your CV to your family or a close friend to make sure that you haven't left anything important out. Consider showing it to your present colleagues, registrars or consultant who have probably seen many CVs and can give you good advice on both content and style. The reviewer need not be medical.

A CV should include:

1 *Personal*: name, address and phone number/ email, date of birth, relevant memberships, brief general education, and employment history (if any)

2 *Medical*: undergraduate education including medical school, date of entry and graduation, qualifications, honours or prizes, previous and present appointments, career plans, publications and presentations, leadership and teaching experience, society memberships, referee names and contact details (you do not always need to provide these but resist the temptation to state *'References available on request'*; this is frighteningly obvious)

The interview

■ Try to visit the hospital before the interview, see the department and meet the consultants. If you have already met some of the interview panel you may be more relaxed. DO not underestimate how important this is. It is increasingly expected as you progress up the career ladder. This is particularly helpful for academic interviews where you may need to meet the person you will be doing your project with.

■ Follow the basics: clean suit, hair and shoes, be punctual and courteous.

■ Find out from the person coordinating the interview what you can expect inside the interview room, such as how many interviewers you will face and the expected length of the interview.

■ Early questions are likely to focus on why you want the job, your CV and experience. Be prepared to discuss and expand on anything you have mentioned. At this level you may be asked general clinical questions but these will be basic ones regarding safe general care. Be prepared for questions about your career plans. Try to say something concrete, even if you are unsure about your future career. At all costs avoid looking unsure. The interviewers want someone who really wants the job. *Be Enthusiastic*! Ethical issues may be discussed. Issues such as quality control, audit and clinical governance are also very likely to arise. These should be revised for, as they are not topics often covered at medical school.

■ Listen attentively to the interviewers' questions and take care to answer them directly. Don't ramble. Short punchy answers work best. Try to practise the obvious questions beforehand so you know what to say.

■ Write thank-you letters to your referees for their help and support. You may need them again in the future!

Consultant career prospects

The medical and dental staffing prospects are published annually in the journal *Health Trends*, published by the Department of Health. The prospects include the current number of SpRs, consultants, likely consultant vacancies and future consultant numbers, by specialty.

Locums

Locums pay well if you can bear working through your holidays and weekends. Get registered with one or more locum agencies. These may be much better than the basic

'NHS locum' rate you will get if unregistered and doing a locum shift in your current hospital. Note that different agencies pay very different rates. You can register with more than one. Try to negotiate travel expenses with the agency. If you secure a locum at a hospital you don't know, the following is a checklist of things to do when you arrive:

1 Sign in at the switchboard. Sign-in registers what time you arrive at the hospital – the locum agency may check when working out your pay.

2 From switchboard and reception, pick up bleep, keys, map of the hospital, identification (if necessary) and essential telephone numbers.

3 Find out (on the hospital map) where these are:

- Blood gas machines
- Canteen
- Doctors' residence
- Drinks machine
- Intensive therapy unit
- Radiology department
- Wards

4 Bleep your senior and arrange to meet.

5 Dump your overnight bag in the doctors' residence.

6 Go to the wards and introduce yourself.

7 On the wards, stuff a folder (see Chapter 2, Personal folder and the lists) with relevant forms.

8 Locate IV equipment, catheters, drug cupboard and resuscitation equipment.

9 Find out if there is a phlebotomist in the morning and where to leave requests.

10 If possible, speak to the person who usually carries your bleep about any useful information he or she may know about patients, staff and the hospital.

11 If you are required to attend a ward round when you should have finished the locum, you are entitled to extra hours' pay; contact the locum agency as soon as possible about this. If you have to leave on the dot, let your senior know this from the outset.

12 Hospitals that are desperate to fill locums will often negotiate terms with you, such as allowing you to arrive late or leave early if necessary.

13 Locums have a poor reputation but if you work hard, you will build a good reputation that will not only get you more work but will also put you in favour with consultants and colleagues who you may work with in the future. Strive to maintain your professionalism at all times.

Meals

■ Try not to miss meals; this is easy to say and hard to do! Twenty minutes for a hot evening meal makes little difference to patient care, but it will keep *you* going. The same applies to lunch. Sitting down for 10 minutes off the ward and eating a meal will do wonders for your energy levels.

■ Don't forget to drink as much liquid as possible. It's easy to get dehydrated and even more tired when you're too busy to stop for tea breaks. *Always* keep a water bottle in your bag and refill it regularly.

■ Find out about local takeaways. Some may discount hospital staff. There are almost always people on the shift who will share a meal with you and cut down the delivery cost. A pizza late in the evening is a great morale booster and good for team building.

Medical defence

Historically, it was compulsory to belong to a defence organization for representation and insurance against medico-legal complaints arising out of the care of patients. This changed in 1990 when Crown Indemnity came into force, so that the Crown, or rather the NHS employer, will pay the costs of investigation and damages for cases arising during your employment with them. Most importantly, Crown Indemnity may not support you if you have a conflict with your employer. The advantage of joining a medical defence organization is expert, round-the-clock advice with *your* interests at heart. Investigate the benefits offered by various organizations (e.g. MDU, MPS) and join whichever one suits your needs. It may be a little pricey, but they are invaluable in times of a crisis for advice in ethical scenarios and will be willing to act in your best interest.

Money

For the first time, your bank account will be filling up with up to £2000 or so each month. Be a bit careful. You should be prepared to find that for the first year or two your lifestyle may not be much better than as a student. Try and save some of your pay every month; take out an individual savings account (ISA) or a savings account where a proportion of your pay cheque is directly sent to every month. Plan your finances carefully to avoid running into debt.

Income protection if long-term sick or disabled

Various organizations offer income protection (also known as PHI or permanent health insurance). On payment of a monthly premium, you are covered for prolonged absence, even if you never work again. If you have a mortgage and family, sickness cover becomes more important. Research the various policy options carefully – some have limited payment durations. Others pay more from year to year in line with your expected career progression. Perhaps most important is to check if you will be paid if you cannot work *as a doctor* or only if you cannot do *any type of work* (the company is likely to find that this will very rarely be the case).

Student debt

Many experienced financial advisers have compiled good data to show that the best way to save money is to pay off all existing debt, as virtually all debt has an interest rate higher than the national savings rate. As medical students have 5–6 years to acquire a sizable debt, particularly with the introduction of increasingly expensive tuition fees, it is advisable to start chipping away at this as early as you can. Your governmental student loan will

automatically be repaid with deductions from your pay cheque 6 months after starting work. This has a low interest rate (but NOT zero unless there are exceptional circumstances with a very low national base rate). Because of this, it is usually best not to try and pay this off early but to just let it get chipped away at from month to month (just try and forget about it). Credit cards and personal loans are a different matter and these need to be paid off as soon as you can. Avoid *negative equity*; this is just the financial term for more going out of your bank account each month than goes in! Setting up direct debits is a good way of making sure you are strict about repayments; they can be set up for credit cards also and will help you get a good credit rating for the future.

Mortgages

Some banks and building societies provide special mortgages for professionals such as doctors and solicitors, to account for the structured career path and salary increases. These often are willing to lend larger amounts of money (e.g. 4× annual salary rather than 2.5×), but be aware that you should only borrow what you can afford to pay back on a monthly basis. As a rough guide try and avoid deductions of more than £200 a month when you start work.

Payslip deductions

National Insurance is a compulsory contribution which will pay for your future state pension, maternity pay and sick leave.

Superannuation is not compulsory but is essential for your pension. The national state pension is meagre. The NHS superannuation scheme is your employer's scheme to allow you to make additional pension contributions that the government will supplement:

■ You have to sign a form at the start of your job stating your intention to stay with or opt out of the superannuation scheme. The only people who might not want to contribute towards their own superannuation are those who are pretty sure that they will not be working for long in the NHS, such as foreign graduates.

■ You can reclaim superannuation contributions if you have worked for the NHS for *fewer than 2 years*. Otherwise your contributions will stay locked in the scheme.

■ Think long and hard before leaving the superannuation scheme to join a private pension plan. It is highly unlikely that you could ever match the security and returns of the NHS scheme despite the recent changes to the pensions scheme. It is no barrier to joining an *additional* private scheme.

Pensions

There have been many changes made to the pensions scheme that will take effect from 2015. When you retire, your pension will be based on the average of your lifetime earnings as a doctor. This is different to the previous scheme that was based on your last 3 years of earning (i.e. when you are a consultant):

■ It is possible to make additional contributions to your future pension. The most cost-effective way is to make additional voluntary contributions (AVCs) into the NHS Group Scheme. This is a well-kept secret, with low commission and charges. You should contact your local BMA office. It is also possible to buy 'added years', as if you had worked for longer than you really have.

■ You will doubtless meet financial salesmen who will offer to sell you Free Standing AVCs, that is, a way of investing your contributions in their company's policies (and earning them a bonus). Be aware that your whole first year's contribution may disappear in the salesperson's commission.

Tax

Earning a regular salary means paying serious tax. You will save time, trouble and money if you make an effort to keep basic records. Each month you should get a payslip giving details of your pay, national insurance and any other deductions you have authorized such as telephone bills or car parking charges. Check this to see you have not been overcharged – sadly, this is not uncommon.

A P60 is sent to you at the end of the tax year (April 5). It is your record of how much income you have received and tax you have paid. A P45 is given to you when you leave the job, to take to the finance department at your next job to show how much tax you have been paying. If you lose it you will probably be taxed the wrong amount (usually overtaxed) until the tax office sorts it out – which may take months. Always check your tax code as inevitably in the first few months of changing jobs this will be incorrect.

Understanding your tax

Doctors have tax deducted automatically from their pay before they receive it (known as PAYE – pay as you earn). The Inland Revenue works out how much tax you are likely to owe throughout the year and this is deducted monthly from your salary.

Junior doctors start work in August, part way through the tax year which runs from April 6 to April 5. This means that your first ever pay cheque will be larger than any of the subsequent months. The tax year ends on April 5. After this your tax office will send you a note stating how much tax you paid in the last year and how much tax you ought to pay in the next year (P60). However, it is quite likely that you have been overtaxed and could claim money back on tax-deductible items. You also have a duty to declare untaxed income so that it can be taxed (this includes money paid for completion of cremation forms or certain psychiatric documentation relating to sections of the Mental Health Act). At the simplest, you could just write a letter declaring your tax-deductible items and untaxed income; alternatively, contact your tax office for a full tax return form. Your personnel department will be able to give you full details of your tax office, which is usually determined by where you work.

Tax-deductible items (on which you can reclaim money you have paid in tax) include:

1 GMC fee (but only the renewal fee, not the initial joining-up fee)

2 Medical defence subscription

3 BMA membership

In later years, membership to the Royal Colleges and JRCPTB enrolment fees for those who go on to do a CMT job or ISCP fees for surgical trainees are also tax deductible.

Untaxed income that must be declared

The main item here is cremation fees, worth approximately £78, which you receive for completing part 1 of the cremation form. In recent years, the Inland Revenue has tightened up on this potential evasion. It is not unknown for them to investigate funeral directors' records and compare them with doctors' tax returns. Non-declaration constitutes tax evasion and is penalized accordingly. You should declare full cremation fees even if there is a deduction, for example, for mess expenses. There has been recent public criticism of doctors being paid to complete these forms, as such some people choose to give this money to charity. Whatever you choose, make sure you declare it.

Tax allowances

Everyone has a personal allowance, that is, an amount of income they can earn before being taxed. In 2013–2014, you may earn £9440 before paying tax. The rest of your earnings (above your personal allowance) up to £32,010 is taxed at 20%. The high bracket rate of 40% is paid on any income above this. Since 2013, the tax bracket for those earning over £150,000 has been reduced to 45%. See www.hmrc.gov.uk for more information.

Tax-free savings

Each person is allowed to save up to £11,520 each tax year in a tax-free savings account called an ISA. These accounts give high rates of tax-free interest and are offered by most banks. There are various types of ISA on offer. Some (called 'cash' ISAs) guarantee growth of your savings (in effect a straightforward tax-free savings account). Alternatively, you may choose an ISA where the bank will invest in named stocks and shares on your behalf. These 'equity' ISAs are more risky, especially if you may need to withdraw the money in the short term, but may have much greater yield in the longer term. ISA's rarely have instant access to savings, so don't use them instead of a current account. However, they are a good way of putting away savings for the future. Seek financial advice to help you choose between the ISA packages on offer.

Telephone and online banking

Consider switching to telephone or online banking, which allow 24 hour access to your account, in addition to all the other services provided by a high street account (including use of cash machines). *Which?* Magazine regularly reviews banking services; so look out for the next *Which?* Report. These accounts can offer a high rate of interest, although many exclusively online banks will offer these rates only as a promotion, with interest rates quickly falling back to more moderate (although often competitive) levels. Don't worry about this as you can always open another account and move your money when the interest rates fall. Also be aware that exclusively online banks may not be covered by the banking ombudsman (the government watchdog for banks).

Needlestick injuries

You should familiarize yourself with your occupational health or department's policy for needlesticks before you come across one. If you do encounter a needlestick, follow their advice, seek help from A + E/virology, or do the following:

1 Go to a sink. Run the wound under fast running, lukewarm water and clean with soap. There is no evidence for 'bleeding' the wound.

2 See your occupational health consultant immediately if within working hours (and inform your own consultant). If out of hours, go to A and E to be assessed. You may need to take post-exposure anti-HIV prophylaxis (at present this consists of triple therapy) or have a hepatitis B booster vaccine depending on your status. Always make a trip to occupational health in normal working hours after as they will perform any further steps necessary and ensure the donor samples are taken. They

will also keep a 'serum save' of your blood and the donor's blood.

3 Don't panic. Virtually all doctors needlestick themselves from time to time and very few have contracted anything undesirable, even from patients infected with HIV and hepatitis. Even if the patient is known HIV positive, the chance of a full needlestick transmitting the virus to you is only around 1 in 250.

4 If the patient consents to it and are counselled about the implications of having an HIV test done, get a colleague to take one purple tube of blood from the patient (check with your trust which bottle they prefer). This needs to be analysed immediately for HIV and hepatitis B and C.

5 Alert your senior and/or the public health unit in the hospital. They will instruct you further.

If the patient is known to be HIV positive

Don't panic. Thousands of HIV needlestick injuries have resulted in only a handful of cases of HIV worldwide. The chances of your getting HIV are very small. On the other hand, don't give yourself a hard time if you do panic. Almost everyone does. Seek help from a counsellor or GP if you are suffering from excessive anxiety about it:

1 Have one clotted tube of blood taken from yourself. Give it to the public health unit/GP for storage. This is to ascertain your hepatitis/ HIV status at the time of injury. It will only be analysed in the unlikely event that you are later found to be positive.

2 You will need to take antiretroviral triple therapy for post-exposure prophylaxis. There is always a box of PEP available in A and E so if in doubt go there to get it. Be warned, the side effects of the drugs can be impressive, with diarrhoea being the worst symptom.

3 After 3 months (at least) have an HIV test check. Over 95% of people who are going to seroconvert do so within 3 months. If this is negative, repeat it at 6 months and 1–2 years. The second test will give you peace of mind.

4 Use condoms at least until the 3-month check.

5 Having HIV tests does not usually pose a problem for getting life insurance (as it once did), if you explain that you are a health professional having a routine HIV check. However, if you are concerned, you can usually have your blood checked confidentially by your virology lab or the hospital's sexually transmitted infection clinic. The latter is preferable, as you will get proper counselling for the test.

If the patient is known to be hepatitis positive

1 Follow your doctor's instructions. Give the lab a clotted sample of your blood as soon as possible after injury to ascertain your hepatitis antibody status at the time of injury.

2 Find out what kind of hepatitis the patient has. If they have hepatitis B, you may need instant immunoglobulin (the booster vaccine); if they have hepatitis C you may need interferon treatment. There is no vaccine currently for hepatitis C.

3 You may need to be re tested for hepatitis antigen after 6 months. In the meantime, it is advisable to practise safe sex.

Not coping

Coping is not about 'just getting a grip'. You may hear this from some colleagues, but most likely they have felt the way you do at some point. You are not alone. *Everyone* has disastrous days, weeks or entire job rotations. Almost everyone thinks about giving up medicine, sometimes frequently! If you feel like giving up, this does not mean that you are less motivated or committed than your peers. In fact the chances are that if you are feeling like that, so is everyone else, except that they have not admitted it. Studies show that a substantial proportion of junior doctors become clinically depressed; most suffer depression and anxiety at least a few times during their career:

■ Confidential counselling services have been established which provide support for doctors who are not coping. The BMA can advise you where such services are and how to contact them.

■ A bullying consultant or charge nurse will make anyone's life difficult, not just yours. Consider talking to your colleagues – or even to your local representative – about such problems.

■ Remember that feeling low or anxious may just be manifestations of adjusting to a completely new way of life and will pass within a few months, however painful they seem at present. This may well reoccur with job changes but hopefully should become less frequent as you get used to the routine of changing jobs.

■ Simple fatigue can greatly exacerbate mental distress; in difficult times don't be afraid to acknowledge this to yourself. Don't underestimate the importance of regularly getting a good night's sleep, eating properly and spending time outside of the workplace having fun and socializing. These small creature comforts can make a massive difference to your mental state in the long run.

Part-time work (flexible training)

■ It is now possible to be a part-time junior doctor. At present, part-time jobs are individually negotiated and created by postgraduate tutors. Part-time usually means half-time, doing half the number of on-call nights. Unfortunately, the corollary of doing half-time is that you end up taking more time to complete your training and get paid proportionally.

■ It is possible to continue flexible part-time training as a senior house officer (SHO) up to and including consultant level. At the registrar level and above, national recognition and approval for part-time training is required. At SHO level, simple agreement with the Postgraduate Dean suffices.

■ Job shares are also now available as part of flexible training. The same applies to these jobs as working as a part-time doctor but can be very useful if you have a family and are struggling to juggle a busy life as a junior

doctor and as a parent. Speak to your training deanery if you are considering job-sharing, as there may be someone in the deanery they can pair you with.

Representation of junior doctors

You can get a great deal done if you and your colleagues work together on agreed goals. You can act as a body in several ways:

1 *Doctors mess, mess president and committee.* This may meet regularly or on an ad hoc basis. It usually has several roles: organization of social events, representation of junior doctors' interests to management and administration of mess funds. Mess presidency is a good way to begin to develop leadership and management skills for your CV.

2 *Junior doctors' division.* This is usually a hospital committee which meets every few months to discuss issues relevant to junior doctors. The main frustration for junior doctor representatives is that you rarely work at the hospital long enough to see changes implemented.

3 *New Deal committee.* Hospitals should have convened this committee or something similar to consider and implement the issues arising from the Junior Doctors' New Deal, that is, reducing doctors' hours and delegating inappropriate duties.

4 *BMA.* Junior doctors may stand as representatives for local, regional and national committees like the *BMA*. You should be allowed a reasonable amount of time off to attend to these activities. In practice, it is usually doctors beyond the initial foundation year who have the career stability to embark upon medical politics.

Sleep and on-call rooms

Thankfully, the days of 48 hour on calls are largely a thing of the past. However, long days on call with 12–13 hour shifts are still a regular occurrence and can be very draining.

You can get very run-down if you don't take care of yourself:

■ If you've had little or no sleep the night before, a shower and a filling breakfast go a long way to holding off fatigue.

■ Try to do simple admin-related tasks that do not require too much brainpower. Some people also find caffeine regularly throughout the day is beneficial! Avoid this on a regular basis if you can as caffeine withdrawal is not pleasant.

■ After long shifts, go to bed after eating something. Try not to do anything else such as checking emails. Avoid alcohol as this can disrupt your sleep pattern. You will be grateful the next morning when you wake up refreshed and ready to attack the new day.

■ Another trick is to sleep in a doctor's room or hospital accommodation whilst doing your blocks of on call. This radically cuts down time getting up and travelling long distances to work. In the morning, you only have to get up minutes before the ward round. Avoid sleeping whilst on the job if you can such as during your shifts as in some trusts it is now a disciplinary matter to sleep whilst on duty.

When things go wrong

The F1 year is one of the most challenging years you will ever experience due to the steep learning curve. Usually your problems are focused on matters like needing more sleep and not feeling experienced enough. A feeling of being unsupported is a worryingly common concern and on the rare occasion, you may encounter more difficult complex problems.

Bullying and psychological stress

It is important to stress that this rarely ever happens, but when it does it can really ruin your working life. This can be even more difficult when the person doing the bullying is senior to you or even your boss:

■ Talk to someone. There are many avenues of support available: your postgraduate tutor, your previous tutors in medical school, BMA support lines, your medical defence agency, and even your non-medical friends. If you do not feel like divulging names, you don't have to, but it helps greatly to look at the problem outside the perspective of the victim.

■ Find a witness to any bullying. This may be a nurse or colleague. Whilst patients under your care may be witness to bullying, it is considered unprofessional to enlist their help against a colleague.

■ Confrontation is one strategy for dealing with bullying but it may not be suited for a hierarchical structure like medicine. If you are being bullied by your direct senior, you should voice your concerns to the person senior to him or her (or at the least a sympathetic fellow consultant) as they may not be aware what is going on. Your educational or clinical supervisor is also a great ally.

■ If intending to confront someone, have a witness present. Ensure you are in a private place such as a seminar room. Avoid being overheard. Be as formal as possible and try to stay professional. Start with an explanation of your feelings of being threatened and how you want to avoid the situation again. Do not launch into accusations.

■ Document incidents with date, time, details of conversation and those present. If you are able to, keep a written log as evidence.

It is unacceptable for anyone to be bullied in the workplace. Do not accept this kind of behaviour.

Whistle-blowing

This has become a major issue in light of the number of high-profile medical scandals in the past decade. It is important to stress that these incidents are not scandals because they are medical disasters; they are scandalous because safeguards which should have been in place were not working. There are existing channels for voicing problems, and these should be used when available. The term whistle-blowing still holds some stigma but in essence is a professional obligation to ensure high-quality care. It should be undertaken in accordance with trust and GMC policy. It is definitely NOT the same as going to the press, something we would strongly counsel against doing!

■ Speak to your medical defence agency before taking any action.

■ Document everything (letters, memos, emails, conversations in the corridor) on paper with date, times, those present and details.

■ Before whistle-blowing, you should ensure that the person who is responsible for the problem is aware of the problem. It is unfair to whistle-blow on a problem which could easily be fixed with a phone call.

■ Whom to whistle-blow to is just as important as what to whistle-blow about. Depending on the scale of the problem, you should pick the appropriate agency to talk to. There is no point complaining to the GMC about minor problems. For hospital-scale problems or problems with doctors, the order of preference is the hospital management, the training deanery and then the GMC.

Check the GMC website that has guidance on whistle-blowing: www.gmc-uk.org/guidance/ethical_guidance/raising_concerns.asp.

Appendix I
SCORING SYSTEMS

A few of the most commonly used scoring systems, grouped by specialty, are listed in the following. Please note that scoring systems go in and out of fashion, and it is always important to concomitantly examine the patient.

Cardiovascular

CHA2DS2 VASc

This is used to assess risk of stroke in patients with atrial fibrillation. A score of 2 or more indicates high risk and consideration of warfarinisation.

Age?	<65 years old	0
	65–74 years old	1
	>75 years old	2
Congestive heart failure history?	Y	1
Hypertension history?	Y	1
Stroke/TIA/ thromboembolism?	Y	2
Vascular disease? (MI/IHD, PVD)	Y	1
Diabetes mellitus?	Y	1
Female?	Y	1

HASBLED score

This is used to calculate risk of major bleeding for patients on anticoagulation to help determine risk benefit ratio in patients with AF.

Hypertension? (uncontrolled or systolic >160 mmHg)	Y	1
Renal disease? (dialysis or serum creatinine >200 µmol/l)	Y	1
Liver disease? (cirrhosis, bilirubin >2× normal or ALT/ALP >3× normal	Y	1
Stroke history?	Y	1
Previous major bleed or predisposition to bleeding?	Y	1
Labile INR?	Y	1
Age ≥65 years?	Y	1
Medication usage predisposing to bleeding?	Y	1
Alcohol usage history?	Y	1

GRACE score

The GRACE score is used in ACS patients to assess the risk of death or death/MI in hospital and at 6 months. You will need to calculate the GRACE score when referring the patient for an urgent inpatient angiogram. The new online calculator requires the following information:

Age (years)
Heart rate (bpm)
Systolic BP (mmHg)
Congestive heart failure according to Killip Class (0 – no CHF, I – crackles and raised JVP, II – pulmonary oedema, III – cardiogenic shock)

The Hands-on Guide to the Foundation Programme, Fifth Edition. Anna Donald, Michael Stein, Ciaran Scott Hill and Selina J Chavda.
© 2015 John Wiley & Sons, Ltd. Published 2015 by John Wiley & Sons, Ltd.

Serum creatinine
ST segment changes
Cardiac arrest at admission
Elevated troponin

The best way to calculate this is online using the web version of the calculator using the address

http://www.gracescore.org/WebSite/WebVersion.aspx

You will get a result for risk of death in hospital, at 6 months, 1 year and a risk of death/MI at 1 year. Generally cardiologists quote the risk of death/MI figure to help risk stratify patients to decide when to perform a coronary angiogram.

TIMI Risk Index

The TIMI score is used to prognosticate the risk of ACS in patients using simply their heart rate, age and systolic blood pressure in a simple formula

$$\text{TIMI Risk Index} = \text{heart rate} \times (\text{age}/10)^2/\text{systolic BP}$$

There are also more detailed TIMI scoring systems to estimate mortality risk in STEMI and NSTEMI patients involving Killip's Class and time to treatment. These have largely been taken over by GRACE scoring systems.

NYHA scoring system (New York Heart Failure Association Scoring System)

This grades the severity of the patient's heart failure.

NHYA I Cardiac disease, but asymptomatic and no limitation in ordinary physical activity, for example, shortness of breath on exertion or climbing stairs

NHYA II Mild symptoms (mild shortness of breath and/or angina) and slight limitation during ordinary activity

NYHA III Marked limitation in activity due to symptoms, even during less-than-ordinary activity, for example, walking short distances (20–100 m). Comfortable only at rest

NYHA IV Severe limitations. Symptomatic *at rest*. Mostly bedbound/housebound

Neurology

MRC grading of muscle power

MRC stands for the Medical Research Council and they have a robust method of grading muscle power that is used internationally.

0 No muscle contraction visible.
1 Muscle contraction is visible but there is no movement of the joint.
2 Active joint movement is possible with gravity eliminated.
3 Movement can overcome gravity but not resistance from the examiner.
4 The muscle group can overcome gravity and move against some resistance from the examiner.
5 Full and normal power against resistance.

TIA-ABCD2 scoring

This is used to calculate risk of stroke after TIA.

A (Age):	<60 – 0
	≥60 – 1
B (Blood pressure):	<140/90 – 0
	≥140/90 – 1
C (Clinical):	No speech disturbance and no unilateral weakness – 0
	Speech disturbance but no unilateral weakness – 1
	Unilateral weakness – 2
D (Duration):	<10 minutes – 0
	10–59 minutes – 1
	60 minutes – 2
D (Diabetes):	No – 0
	Yes – 1

Low risk = 1–3
Moderate risk = 4–5
High risk = 6–7

Score of ≥4 indicates high risk of an early stroke; patient should be seen and assessed by a stroke specialist within 24 hours

Score of ≤3 and no other episodes in the last week, to be seen by a specialist within 7 days.

AMTS (abbreviated mental test score)

This is used to assess confusion levels in patients. A score of ≤8 reflects confusional state, and will require further investigation with MMSE and exclusion of other pathology.

Age	1
Date of birth	1
Time to nearest hour	1
Year	1
Name of hospital	1
Recognizes two people	1
Date of WW2	1
Name of prime minister/ monarch	1
Count back from 20 to 1	1
Can repeat address	1

AVPU score

The AVPU scale is a basic way to assess a patient's GCS (see text below). It is often used by paramedics in an emergency setting. A score of P is suggestive of a GCS of 8 or less and may indicate that the patient needs a more secure airway.

A – Alert
V – Responsive to voice
P – Responsive to pain
U – Unresponsive

(GCS) Glasgow Coma score

This scoring system is used to assess patient's state of consciousness. It is only validated in head injury. GCS <8 suggests risk of airway compromise, and so will require a more definitive airway/airway adjunct.

Eyes	None	1
	Open to pain	2
	Open to speech	3
	Spontaneous	4
Verbal	None	1
	Incomprehensible sounds	2
	Inappropriate words	3
	Confused/disoriented	4
	Oriented	5
Motor response	None	1
	Extension to pain	2
	Abnormal flexion to pain	3
	Withdraws from pain	4
	Localizes pain	5
	Obeys commands	6

Anaesthetics

ASA classification
This is used to risk stratify patients according to surgery prognosis and survival.

I	Normal healthy patient
II	Patient with mild systemic disease
III	Patient with severe systemic disease
IV	Patient with severe systemic disease that is a constant threat to life
V	A moribund patient who is not expected to survive without operation
VI	A declared brain dead patient whose organs are being removed for organ donor purposes

Mallampatti classification for intubation

This classification determines risk of intubation. Those with a higher score are likely to have more difficulty being intubated.

1 Full visibility of pillars, uvula and soft palate

2 Soft, hard palate and base of uvula present

3 Soft and hard palate visible

4 Only hard palate visible

BMI

BMI is a calculation to assess a persons' body fat based on height and weight.

$$BMI = (weight\ in\ kg)/(height\ in\ m)^2$$

- Underweight = <18.5
- Normal weight = 18.5–24.9
- Overweight = 25–29.9
- Obesity = BMI of 30 or greater

Calculating anion gap

Calculating the anion gap is useful in patients with a metabolic acidosis, to help determine whether the gap is high or normal, as there are different causes for each subgroup

Anion gap = $([Na^+] + [K^+]) - ([Cl^-] + [HCO_3^-])$

Normal anion gap <11

Causes of raised anion gap metabolic acidosis are as follows:

Raised lactic acid – shock, infection, ischaemia

Raised urate levels – renal failure

Ketones (DM, ETOH)

Drugs – salicylate, biguanides

Toxins – methanol, ethanol, ethylene glycol

Causes of normal anion gap metabolic acidosis are as follows:

Renal tubular acidosis

Addison's

Diarrhoea

Drugs – ammonium chloride ingestion, acetazolamide

Calculating serum osmolality

Serum osmolality is a measure of the electrolytes in the body. Calculating the serum osmolality is useful if you think the patient has an 'osmolar gap'. This means that the difference between the serum osmolality calculated by the lab and the manual calculation has a difference of more than 10. If this is the case, think of additional solutes in the blood, such as methanol, ethanol, ethylene glycol or diabetes.

Serum osmolality = 2(Na + K) + urea + glucose

Normal serum osmolality = 285–295 mmol/l

Respiratory

DVT and PE – Wells scoring system

This system is used to assess risk of DVT/PE and aids decision on management

Active cancer (treatment within the last 6 months or palliative)	Y	1
Paralysis, paresis or recent plaster immobilization of leg	Y	1
Major surgery or recently bedridden for >3 days in the last 4 weeks	Y	1
Local tenderness along distribution of deep vein system	Y	1
Entire leg swollen	Y	1
Calf swelling >3 cm compared to asymptomatic leg (10 cm below tibial tuberosity)	Y	1
Pitting oedema greater in the symptomatic leg	Y	1
Collateral superficial veins (non-varicose)	Y	1
Alternative diagnosis as or more likely than that of DVT	If Y then	−2

Score ≥3: high pretest probability – treat as suspected DVT and perform Doppler USS.

Score 1–2: intermediate pretest probability – treat as suspected DVT and perform Doppler USS.

Score ≤0: low pretest probability – perform D dimer. If negative, DVT is reliably excluded, if positive treat as suspected DVT and perform Doppler USS.

PERC (pulmonary embolus rule out criteria) score

This is another scoring system used to exclude PE. This system can be used to exclude PE in low risk patients. If all of the criteria are negative, no further investigations are required. The system has a sensitivity of 97.4% and a false negative rate of only 1%.

No hypoxia – $SaO_2 > 94\%$ RA

No unilateral leg swelling or signs suggestive of DVT

No haemoptysis

No prior DVT or PE

No recent surgery or trauma

Age <50

No hormone use

No tachycardia – HR <100 bpm

CURB score for pneumonia

This helps to assess risk of mortality in patients with a community acquired pneumonia, and decide on need for admission, and in some trusts antibiotic management

Confusion (new onset, with an AMTS <8)	1
Urea >7 mmol/l	1
Respiratory rate >30 breaths per minute	1
BP (systolic < 90, diastolic < 60)	1
65 (age 65 or older)	1

Score	mortality risk at 30 days
0	0.7%
1	3.2%
2	13.0%
3	17.0%
4	41.5%
5	57.0%

If score is 0–1: treat as an outpatient

2–3: short inpatient admission or close monitoring as an outpatient

4–5: requires hospitalization with consideration as to whether patient needs transfer to ITU

SIRS (systemic inflammatory response syndrome) criteria for sepsis

The SIRS criteria have been made famous by World Sepsis day and the research done into the pathogenesis of sepsis. SIRS is thought to be central to causing the sepsis response, by allowing release of free radicals, cytokines and vasodilators. It is an excellent way to stratify septic patients and can help predict those who are likely to need ITU hospitalization.

A score of 2 or more is suggestive of SIRS

Temperature >38 °C or <36 °C	Y	1
Heart rate >90	Y	1
Respiratory rate >20 or $PaCO_2 < 4.3$ kPa	Y	1
WBC >12,000/mm³, or WCC <4000/mm³, or >10% bands	Y	1

Sepsis is defined as SIRS in the presence of infection.

Severe sepsis is defined as sepsis with organ hypoperfusion, hypotension, oliguria or lactic acidosis.

Septic shock is defined as sepsis with hypotension despite adequate fluid resuscitation.

MRC dyspnoea scale

This scale is used to classify severity of breathlessness in patients with COPD

0   No dyspnoea except with strenuous exercise

1   Dyspnoea when walking up an incline or hurrying on the level

2   Walks slower than most on the level, or stops after 15 minutes of walking on the level

3   Stops after a few minutes of walking on the level

4   Dyspnoea with minimal activity such as getting dressed, too dyspnoeic to leave the house

Gastroenterology

Rockall score

This score is used to assess the risk of mortality in patients who have had an upper GI bleed. Scores can be calculated as an initial pre-OGD score and a post-OGD score to incorporate the findings at OGD.

Variable	Score 0 points	Score 1 point	Score 2 points	Score 3 points
Age (years)	<60	60–79	>80	
Shocked	SBP >100 HR <100	SBP >100 HR >100	SBP <100	
Comorbidities	Nil major	CHF/IHD/major comorbidity	Renal failure, liver failure	Metastatic cancer
Diagnosis	Mallory Weiss, no lesion or sign or recent bleeding	All other diagnoses	GI malignancy	
Evidence of bleeding	None or dark red spot		Blood in GIT, adherent clot, spurting vessel	

An initial score of 6 or more is said to be an indication for surgery. A score of 8 or more carries a 41.1% risk of mortality.

Glasgow-Blatchford bleeding score

This score calculates the likelihood that a patient having an UGIB will need an intervention such as blood transfusion or endoscopy.

The scoring system is useful as those with a score of 0 do not need to be admitted to hospital.

Child Pugh classification

The Child Pugh score is used to assess prognosis in patients with cirrhotic chronic liver disease.

Glasgow-Blatchford score

Admission risk marker	Score component value
Blood urea	
≥6.5–<8.0	2
≥8.0–<10.0	3
≥10.0–<25.0	4
≥25	6
Haemoglobin (g/dL) for men	
≥12.0–<13.0	1
≥10.0–<12.0	3
<10.0	6
Haemoglobin (g/dL) for women	
≥10.0–<12.0	1
<10.0	6
Systolic blood pressure (mmHg)	
100–109	1
90–99	2
<90	3
Other markers	
Pulse ≥100 (per minute)	1
Presentation with melaena	1
Presentation with syncope	2
Hepatic disease	2
Cardiac failure	2

	1 point	2 points	3 points
Total bilirubin, μmol/l (mg/dl)	<34	34–50	>50
Serum albumin, g/l	>35	28–35	<28
PT INR	<1.7	1.71–2.30	>2.30
Ascites	None	Mild	Moderate to severe
Hepatic encephalopathy	None	Grades I–II (or suppressed with medication)	Grades III–IV (or refractory)

Scores are calculated and patients divided into the following groups:

Score	Class	One-year survival
5–6	A	100%
7–9	B	81%
10–15	C	45%

Modified Glasgow criteria for predicting severity in pancreatitis

This scoring system helps to risk stratify patients in terms of severity. A score of ≥3 within 48 hours of onset suggests severe pancreatitis necessitating HDU/ITU transfer.

PaO_2 <8 kPa RA

Age >55

Neutrophilia (WCC >15 × 10^9 l)

Calcium <2 mmol/l

Renal function (urea >16 mmol/l)

Elevated liver enzymes AST >200 IU/l, LDH >600 IU/l

Albumin <32 g/l

Sugar (blood glucose >10 mmol/l)

True-Love and Witt's criteria

This is used to assess severity of acute UC flare.

Activity	Mild	Moderate	Severe
Number of bloody stools per day (*n*)	<4	4–6	>6
Temperature (°C)	Afebrile	37.1–37.8	>37.8
Heart rate (beats per minute)	<70	70–90	>90
Haemoglobin (g/dl)	>11	10.5–11	<10.5
Erythrocyte sedimentation rate (mm/hour)	<20	20–30	>30

Renal

AKIN criteria

The Acute Kidney Injury Network has released a new set of guidelines to help doctors diagnose acute kidney injury.

1 Rapid time course (less than 48 hours)

2 Reduction of kidney function

- Rise in serum creatinine, defined by either

  - Absolute increase in serum creatinine of ≥0.3 mg/dl (≥26.4 µmol/l)

  - Percentage increase in serum creatinine of ≥50%

- Reduction in urine output, defined as <0.5 ml/kg/hour for more than 6 hours

RIFLE criteria

This criteria has been developed by the Acute Dialysis Quality Initiative to help stage patients with AKI:

- *R*isk: GFR decrease >25%, serum creatinine increased 1.5 times or urine production of <0.5 ml/kg/hour for 6 hours

- *I*njury: GFR decrease >50%, doubling of creatinine or urine production <0.5 ml/kg/hour for 12 hours

- *F*ailure: GFR decrease >75%, tripling of creatinine or creatinine >355 µmol/l (with a rise of >44) (>4 mg/dl) OR urine output below 0.3ml/kg/hour for 24 hours

- *L*oss: persistent AKI or complete loss of kidney function for more than 4 weeks

- *E*nd-stage renal disease: need for renal replacement therapy (RRT) for more than 3 months

Trauma

Nexus

This is a system that looks for clinical signs that may be suspicious of cervical spine injury. Presence of any of the criteria suggests there may be a C-spine injury and imaging is required.

Focal neurologic deficit present?

Midline spinal tenderness present?

Altered level of consciousness present?

Intoxication present?
Distracting injury present?
Nursing scoring systems

Barthel score

The Barthel score helps you to assess quickly whether someone can manage at home. It is particularly useful at social rounds. A total score of 15 or more is 'good'.

Bathing

0 dependent

1 independent (bath and shower, in and out)

Bladder

0 incontinent or catheterized and unable to cope alone

1 occasional incontinence (1/day)

2 fully continent

Bowels

0 incontinent

1 occasional incontinence (1/week)

2 fully continent

Dressing

0 dependent

1 needs some help (e.g. with buttons, laces)

2 independent

Feeding

0 dependent

1 needs some help (e.g. with cutting)

2 independent (food within reach)

Grooming

0 dependent (hair, teeth, shaving)

1 independent

Mobility

0 immobile without help

1 independent with wheelchair (includes turning)

2 walks with one person assisting

3 independent

Stairs

0 dependent

1 needs assistance (physical, verbal, mechanical)

2 independent (up and down)

Toilet

0 dependent

1 needs some help

2 independent (transfer, wiping, dressing)

Transfer

0 unable (cannot balance to sit)

1 needs major assistance (two people) but can sit

2 needs minor assistance (physical or verbal)

3 independent

Appendix II
USEFUL TESTS, NUMBERS AND OTHER INFORMATION

Addresses

■ Diabetes UK (formerly The British Diabetic Association), 10 Queen Ann Street, London W1M 0BD (web: www.diabetes.org.uk; tel: 0207323 1531)

■ British Medical Association (and BMJ), BMA House, Tavistock Square, London WC1H 9JP (web: www.bma.org.uk; tel: 0207387 4499)

■ Central Public Health Lab, 61 Colindale Avenue, London NW9 5HT (web: http://www.phls.co.uk; tel: 020-8200 4400)

■ Communicable Disease Surveillance Centre (for notifying diseases), 61 Colindale Avenue, London NW9 5DF (web: http://www.phls.co.uk; tel: 020-8200 6868)

■ Disabled Living Foundation (for advice on equipment), 380–384 Harrow Road, London W9 2HU (web: http://www.dlf.org.uk; tel: 020-7289 6111)

■ Driving and Vehicle Licensing Authority (www.dvla.gov.uk)

■ General Medical Council, 178 Portland Street, London W1N 6JE (web: www.gmcuk.org; tel: 020-7580 7642)

■ Medical Defence Union, 230 Black-friars Rd, London SE1 8PJ (web: http://www.themdu.com; tel: 020-7202 1500)

■ Medical and Dental Defence Union of Scotland, Mackintosh House, 120 Blythwood Street, Glasgow G2 4EH (web: http://www.mddus.com; tel: 0141-221 5858)

■ Medical Protection Society, 33 Cavendish Square, London W1G 0PS (http://www.mps.org.uk; tel: 020-7399 1300)

■ Medical Sickness Society, Colmore Circus, Birmingham B4 6AR (web: http://www.medical-sickness.co.uk; tel: 0808-100 1884)

■ Multiple Sclerosis Society, 372 Edgeware Rd, London NW2 6ND (web: http://www.mssociety.org.uk; tel: 0208438 0700)

■ NHS Direct, www.nhsdirect.nhs.uk (tel: 0845 4647)

Poisons information	
Belfast	028 9024 0503
Birmingham	0121 507 5588
	0121 507 5589
Cardiff	029 2070 9901
Dublin	+353 1 837 9964
	+353 1 837 9966
Edinburgh	0131 536 2300
London	020 7635 9191

Mental Health Act

1 Always get senior advice before using the Mental Health Act.

2 Section 4 states that for an emergency admission, the nearest relative *or* an approved senior nurse *or* a social worker *or* a doctor *as well as* the medical recommendation of one doctor who must have seen the patient within the previous 24 hours can apply for 72 hours of compulsory admission on the grounds of

• Urgent necessity
• Mental disorder requiring hospital admission
• Danger to him/herself or others

The Hands-on Guide to the Foundation Programme, Fifth Edition. Anna Donald, Michael Stein, Ciaran Scott Hill and Selina J Chavda.
© 2015 John Wiley & Sons, Ltd. Published 2015 by John Wiley & Sons, Ltd.

3 Section 5(2) states that a patient already in hospital as a voluntary patient can be detained for 72 hours under the same conditions as Section 4, except that it only requires a single medical recommendation by the doctor in charge of the patient's care or another doctor on the staff of the hospital who is nominated by the doctor in charge.

4 Sectioning a patient does not permit you to treat a concurrent physical condition unless it is life-threatening.

Notifiable diseases

Doctors are legally required to report notifiable diseases to their local medical officer for environmental health. The microbiology department know who this is, as do people at the town hall. Alternatively you can contact the Communicable Disease Surveillance Centre: 61 Colindale Avenue, London NW9 5EQ (tel: 020-8200-6868).

The following are the recognized notifiable diseases:

Acute encephalitis
Acute poliomyelitis
Anthrax
Cholera
Diphtheria
Dysentery
Food poisoning
Leptospirosis
Malaria
Measles
Meningitis
    Meningococcal
    Pneumococcal
    Haemophilus influenzae
    Viral
    Other specified
    Unspecified
Meningococcal septicaemia (without meningitis)
Mumps
Ophthalmia neonatorum
Paratyphoid fever
Plague
Rabies
Relapsing fever
Rubella
Scarlet fever
Smallpox
Tetanus
Tuberculosis
Typhoid fever
Typhus fever
Viral haemorrhagic fever
Viral hepatitis
    Hepatitis A
    Hepatitis B
    Hepatitis C
    Other
Whooping cough
Yellow fever

Results

The following are normal ranges for results of tests. However, every lab is different; make sure that you use their values, particularly for unusual tests, which require local calibration of lab equipment.

Consider copying the normal ranges that are important for your job onto a single sheet, which you can stick at the back of a folder or Filofax for easy reference.

Haematology

APTT (factors VIII, IX, XI, XII)	35–45 seconds
Eosinophils	0.04–0.44 (1–6%) × 10^9/l
ESR (female)	(Age + 10)/2
ESR (male)	Age/2
FDP	Lab-dependent
Hb (male)	13.5–18 g/dl
Hb (female)	11.5–16 g/dl
INR (factors I, II, VII, X)	(expressed as ratio versus control) Normal INR is 1.0
Lymphocytes	1.3–3.5 (20–45%) × 10^9/l
MCV	76–96 fl
Monocytes	0.2–0.8 (2–10%) × 10^9/l
Neutrophils	2–7.5 (40–75%) × 10^9/l
Platelets	150–400 × 10^9/l
Prothrombin	10–14 seconds
RCC (female)	3.9–5.6 × 10^{12}/l
RCC (male)	4.5–6.5 × 10^{12}/l
Reticulocytes	0.8–2% (25–100 × 10^9/l)
WCC	4–11 × 10^9/l

Biochemistry

Acid phosphatase (prostate)	0–1 IU/l
Acid phosphatase (total)	1–5 IU/l
ACTH	3.3–15.4 pmol/l
ADH	0.9–4.6 pmol/l
Albumin	35–50 g/l
Aldosterone	100–500 pmol/l
Alkaline phosphate	30–300 IU/l
Alpha fetoprotein	<10 IU/l
ALT	5–35 IU/l
Amylase	0–18 0U
Angiotensin II	5–35 units
AST	5–35 IU/l
Bicarbonate	24–30 mmol/l
Bilirubin	3–17 mmol/l
Ca (ionized)	1–1.25 mmol/l
Ca (total)	2.12–2.65 mmol/l
Chloride	95–105 mmol/l
Cholesterol	3.9–7.8 (>5 is high) mmol/l
Cortisol (am)	280–700 nmol/l
Cortisol (pm)	140–280 nmol/l
Creatine kinase (males)	25–195 IU/l
Creatine kinase (females)	25–170 IU/l
Creatinine	70–120 mmol/l
CSF glucose	>2/3 of plasma glucose
Ferritin	20–300 mmol/l
Folate	5–6.3 nmol/l
FSH	2–8 U/l
GGT (males)	11–51 IU
GGT (females)	7–33 IU
Glucose (fasting)	4–6 mmol/l
Glycosylated Hb	6–8.5%
Haptoglobin	20–125 mmol/l
Iron (male)	14–31 mmol/l
Iron (female)	11–30 mmol/l
LDH	240–545 IU/l
Magnesium	0.75–0.15 mmol/l
Osmolality	278–305 mOsm/kg
PTH	<0.1–0.7 mg/l
Phosphate	0.8–1.45 mmol/l
Potassium	3.5–5.0 mmol/l
Prolactin (males)	<450 units
Prolactin (females, non-pregnant)	<600 units
Protein (total)	60–80 g/l

Red cell folate	0.36–1.44 mmol/l
Sodium	135–145 mmol/l
Troponin	Lab-dependent
TSH	0.5–5.7 U/l
T_4	70–140 nmol/l
Thyroxine (free)	9–22 pmol/l
TIBC	54–75 mmol/l
Triglyceride	0.55–1.9 mmol/l
T_3	1.2–3.0 nmol/l
Urea	2.5–6.7 mmol/l
Uric acid (males)	210–480 mmol/l
Uric acid (females)	150–390 mmol/l
Vitamin B_{12}	0.13–0.68 nmol/l or >150 ng/l

Arterial blood gases

pH	7.35–7.45
PaO_2	>10.6 kPa
$PaCO_2$	4.7–6.0 kPa
Base excess	±2 mmol/l
Bicarbonate	22–26 mmol/l
Type 1 respiratory failure	$Pao_2 < 8$ $Paco_2 < 6$
Type 2 respiratory failure	$Pao_2 < 8$ $Paco_2 > 6$

Useful biochemical formulae

- The anion gap is made up of ions such as phosphate, sulphate, lactate.
- It is high in any condition with reduced clearance or excess production of any unmeasured anions (e.g. DKA, lactic acidosis).
- It is low in hyperalbuminaemia, liver disease and paraproteinaemias.

Corrected calcium = reported total Ca + 0.2 × (40 − the actual albumin)

Creatinine clearance (males)

$$= \frac{1.23 \times (140 - \text{age}) \times \text{weight(kg)}}{\text{creatinine}}$$

Creatinine clearance (females)

$$= \frac{1.04 \times (40 - \text{age}) \times \text{weight(kg)}}{\text{creatinine}}$$

Fitness to drive

Condition	Normal licence	Notification of DVLA	Vocational licence
Anaesthetic	Avoid for 48 hours post general anaesthetic	No	
Angina, chronic and stable		No	Many restrictions; refer to DVLA
Angioplasty	1 month	No	Check with DVLA
Aortic aneurysm	No restrictions	Yes	Permanent ban
Arrhythmias	Avoid driving if symptomatic whilst driving. Driving may continue once symptoms are controlled	Yes	
Occasional ventricular premature beats	No restrictions	No	
Frequent or polymorphic premature beats	Stop driving, pending CVS investigation	Yes	Check with DVLA
Ventricular tachycardia	Stop driving, pending CVS investigation. Driving may continue once symptoms are controlled with annual review	Yes	
Implanted defibrillator	Avoid driving forever	Yes	
CNS disorders	Where definite diagnosis of progressive disability; refer to DVLC for specific advice with consent of patient	Yes	Check with DVLA
Complete heart block	Driving forbidden until 1 month after pacing	Yes	Forbidden
Conduction abnormalities	If symptomatic, avoid driving pending CVS investigation. Can drive when symptoms are controlled	Yes	Check with DVLA
Congenital heart anomalies	No restrictions unless arrhythmia, angina or syncope	No	Check with DVLA
Post-surgery	1 month	No	
Congenital heart block (usually bradycardia)	3-year licence after CVS investigation, including stress test and 24-hour ECG, repeated annually	Yes	Usually forbidden

Diabetes mellitus	Can hold licence for 1, 2 or 3 years depending on type and complications. Insulin-requiring patients need to demonstrate ■ Understanding of disease ■ Reasonable control ■ No frequent or unexplained hypoglycaemic attacks. Always carry sugar in car	Yes	Need to notify DVLC if becomes IDDM, with individual review Established type I diabetes will not be granted new vocational licences
Drugs (if impairs consciousness or motor response)	Avoid driving whilst taking drug. Warn patient that alcohol potentiates side effects of many drugs	No	
Epilepsy	Can hold (renewable) licence for up to 3 years if ■ Free of fits for 2 years ■ Fits only whilst asleep for 3 years ■ Avoid for 6 months during treatment changes	Yes Yes Yes	Allowed if fit-free since 5 years of age or fit-free for 10 years and off medication and annual review to confirm fit-free
Single fit	■ Cannot drive until investigated ■ Possible 1-year ban	Yes	Fit-free for 10 years and off medication and annual review to confirm fit-free
Hypertension (uncomplicated)	No restriction	No	
Impaired locomotor system	Avoid driving. If permanent disability, refer to DVLA	Yes	Refer to DVLA
MI	Avoid driving for 1 month	No	Many restrictions; refer to DVLA
Pacemakers	Can hold licence for up to 3 years 1 month post-implantation if ■ Followed up annually ■ Asymptomatic	Yes	Refer to DVLA
PVD	No restriction		
Syncope, TIA, LOC	Avoid driving until problem solved; 3-month ban	Yes	Permanent ban
Valvular heart disease	No restrictions if no arrhythmia, angina or syncope	No	Check with DVLA

From Raffel A. (ed.) (1985) Medical Aspects of Fitness to Drive: A Guide for Medical Practitioners. Medical Commission on Accident Prevention, London.

Index

The Hands-on Guide to the Foundation Programme, Fifth Edition. Anna Donald, Michael Stein,
Ciaran Scott Hill and Selina J Chavda.
© 2015 John Wiley & Sons, Ltd. Published 2015 by John Wiley & Sons, Ltd.